clinical course or to require management that is complicated by HIV infection. Examples of conditions in clinical Category B include but are not limited to:

- Bacillary angiomatosis
- Candidiasis, oropharyngeal (thrush)
- Candidiasis, vulvovaginal; persistent, frequent, or poorly responsive to therapy
- Cervical dysplasia (moderate or severe)/cervical carcinoma in situ
- Constitutional symptoms, such as fever (38.5 C) or diarrhea lasting >1 month
- Hairy leukoplakia, oral
- Herpes zoster (shingles), involving at least two distinct episodes or more than one dermatome
- Idiopathic thrombocytopenic purpura
- Listeriosis
- Pelvic inflammatory disease, particularly if complicated by tubo-ovarian abscess
- Peripheral neuropathy

For classification purposes, Category B conditions take precedence over those in Category A. For example, someone previously treated for oral or persistent vaginal candidiasis (and who has not developed a Category C disease) but who is now asymptomatic should be classified in clinical Category B.

Category C

Category C includes the clinical conditions listed in the AIDS surveillance case definition. For classification purposes, once a Category C condition has occurred, the person will remain in Category C.

Conditions included in the 1993 AIDS surveillance case definition

- Candidiasis of bronchi, trachea, or lungs
- Candidiasis, esophageal
- Cervical cancer, invasive*
- Coccidioidomycosis, disseminated or extrapulmonary
- Cryptococcosis, extrapulmonary
- Cryptosporidiosis, chronic intestinal (>1 month's duration)
- Cytomegalovirus disease (other than liver, spleen, or nodes)
- Cytomegalovirus retinitis (with loss of vision)
- Encephalopathy, HIV-related
- Herpes simplex: chronic ulcer(s) (>1 month's duration); or bronchitis, pneumonitis, or esophagitis
- Histoplasmosis, disseminated or extrapulmonary
- Isosporiasis, chronic intestinal (>1 month's duration)
- Kaposi's sarcoma
- Lymphoma, Burkitt's (or equivalent term)
- Lymphoma, immunoblastic (or equivalent term)
- Lymphoma, primary, of brain
- *Mycobacterium avium* complex or *M. kansasii,* disseminated or extrapulmonary
- *Mycobacterium tuberculosis,* any site (pulmonary* or extrapulmonary)
- *Mycobacterium,* other species or unidentified species, disseminated or extrapulmonary
- *Pneumocystis carinii* pneumonia
- Pneumonia, recurrent*
- Progressive multifocal leukoencephalopathy
- *Salmonella* septicemia, recurrent
- Toxoplasmosis of brain
- Wasting syndrome due to HIV

*Added in the 1993 expansion of the AIDS surveillance case definition.

AIDS AND HIV INFECTION

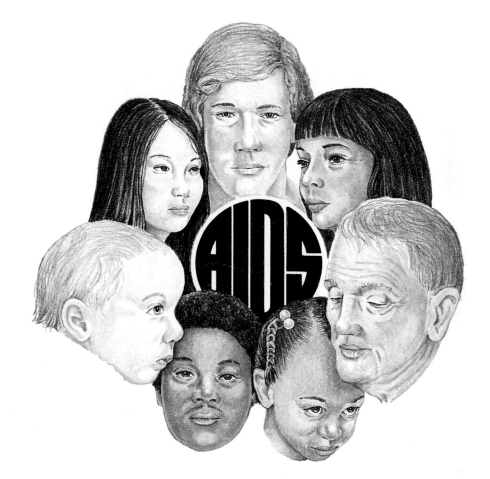

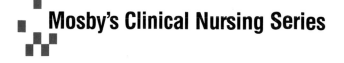
Mosby's Clinical Nursing Series

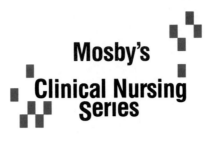

Mosby's Clinical Nursing Series

Cardiovascular Disorders

by Mary Canobbio

Respiratory Disorders

by Susan Wilson and June Thompson

Infectious Diseases

by Deanna Grimes

Orthopedic Disorders

by Leona Mourad

Renal Disorders

by Dorothy Brundage

Neurologic Disorders

by Esther Chipps, Norma Clanin, and Victor Campbell

Cancer Nursing

by Anne Belcher

Genitourinary Disorders

by Mikel Gray

Immunologic Disorders

by Christine Mudge-Grout

Gastrointestinal Disorders

by Dorothy Doughty and Debra Broadwell Jackson

Blood Disorders

by Anne Belcher

Ear, Nose, and Throat Disorders

by Barbara Sigler and Linda Schuring

Women's Health Care

by Valerie Edge and Mindi Miller

AIDS and HIV Infection

by Deanna Grimes and Richard Grimes

Skin Disorders

by Marcia Hill

AIDS AND HIV INFECTION

DEANNA E. GRIMES, R.N., Dr.P.H.

Associate Professor,
School of Nursing,
University of Texas Health Science Center,
Houston, Texas

RICHARD M. GRIMES, Ph.D.

Associate Professor,
The School of Public Health,
Director, AIDS Education and Training Center,
University of Texas Health Science Center,
Houston, Texas

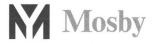 Mosby

St. Louis Baltimore Boston Chicago London Madrid Philadelphia Sydney Toronto

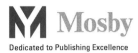
Dedicated to Publishing Excellence

Publisher: Alison Miller
Editor: Sally Schrefer
Developmental Editor: Penny Rudolph
Project Manager: Mark Spann
Production Editor: Stephen C. Hetager
Manuscript Editor: Christine O'Neil
Layout: Doris Hallas
Design: David Zielinski
Manufacturing Supervisor: Betty Richmond

Composition by The Clarinda Company
Printed by Von Hoffmann Press
Printed in the United States of America

Mosby–Year Book, Inc.
11830 Westline Industrial Drive
St. Louis, Missouri 63146

ISBN 0-8016-8012-3

94 95 96 97 98 / 9 8 7 6 5 4 3 2 1

CONTRIBUTORS

Chapter 10, HIV-related malignancies, contributed by
James Halloran, R.N., M.S.N., O.C.N., A.N.P.
HIV Clinical Specialist,
AIDS Regional Education and Training Center,
School of Public Health,
University of Texas Health Science Center,
Houston, Texas

Chapter 12, Issues affecting women and injection drug users, contributed by
Deborah L. Brimlow, Ph.D.
Assistant Professor,
School of Public Health,
AIDS Regional Education and Training Center,
University of Texas Health Science Center,
Houston, Texas

Chapter 13, Law, AIDS, and nurses, contributed by
Carl S. Hacker, Ph.D., J.D.
Associate Professor,
School of Public Health,
University of Texas Health Science Center,
Houston, Texas

Julie R. Watson, B.S., J.D., R.D.H.
Attorney at Law,
Houston, Texas

Chapter 15, Therapeutic procedures, contributed by
Kristin K. Ownby, R.N., C.S., M.P.H., M.S.N., O.C.N.
Medical Oncology Nurse Specialist,
Houston, Texas

CONSULTANTS

Philip C. Johnson, M.D.
Chief, General Internal Medicine
Medical School,
University of Texas Health Science Center
Houston, Texas

Gene C. Stevenson, D.D.S.
Assistant Professor,
Dental Branch,
University of Texas Health Science Center
Houston, Texas

Original illustrations by
George J. Wassilchenko
Tulsa, Oklahoma
and
Donald P. O'Connor
St. Peters, Missouri

Original photography by
Patrick Watson
St. Louis, Missouri

PREFACE

The choice of content for this book was, in part, based on research conducted by Deanna Grimes and James Halloran, the author of Chapter 10. Dr. Grimes and Mr. Halloran conducted nine separate focus groups with nurses experienced in HIV/AIDS care. The nurses who participated in the focus groups practiced in hospitals, outpatient HIV clinics, nursing homes, public health agencies, and home health care. During the group sessions, the nurses focused on the question "What are the critical knowledge and skills that nurses need to deliver safe, adequate nursing care to persons with HIV disease?" The authors are extremely grateful to these busy nurses who shared their time, knowledge, and insights.

These experienced HIV nurses expressed a need for a ready reference to conditions that should alert them to the potential for HIV infection in patients. We have tried to respond to this need by providing color plates of most of the visible conditions that are associated with HIV infection. Many of these conditions, such as Kaposi's sarcoma, were quite rare prior to the HIV epidemic and, often, have never been seen by health care providers who are not involved in HIV care. The color plates can be a ready reference for nurses new to HIV care.

Almost all of the focus groups expressed a desire to better understand the function of the immune system. So much new knowledge about immunology is constantly becoming available that it is difficult to stay current in the area. Fortunately, the National Cancer Institute and the National Institute of Allergy and Infectious Disease have co-authored a booklet called "Understanding the Immune System," which has been updated frequently to reflect expanding knowledge of this complex system. The Institutes have given permission to reproduce their booklet, and it appears, with slight modifications, as Chapter 1 of this book.

Nurses practice in a variety of specialized settings (e.g., inpatient, outpatient, and home care), providing care to patients at varying stages of disease. During the focus groups nurses expressed a need to understand all phases of infection, even though they may only be caring for patients at one phase, such as acute care or end-stage disease. Therefore, Chapters 2, 3, and 4 were developed. Chapter 2 provides an overview of HIV infection, its progressive phases, pathophysiology, modes of transmission, epidemiology, and management. Chapter 3 describes the opportunistic diseases

and conditions associated with impairment of the immune system, which eventually result in the acquired immunodeficiency syndrome (AIDS). This chapter also presents the common psychological responses that accompany progression to AIDS. Chapter 4 provides a brief overview of the bacterial, mycobacterial, protozoan, fungal, and viral infections that occur during HIV infection. Together, these four chapters provide the scientific base for the remainder of the book.

Chapter 5 focuses on patient assessment and general diagnostic procedures that may be applied at any time during the course of infection. Specific instructions are given about procedures for collecting and handling of specimens of body tissue, fluids, and exudates.

In the pre-antibiotic era, there was a common saying that, if a physician knew syphilis, he or she knew all of internal medicine. This was true because syphilis could manifest dermatologically, neurologically, cardiovascularly, etc. In the postretroviral era of HIV, one can say that, if a nurse knows HIV/AIDS care, he or she knows all of nursing. This disease calls upon all of one's nursing knowledge and skills because the effects of this infection can manifest in almost every body system and at any stage of life. Chapters 6, 7, 8, and 9 cover the major systems (dermatologic, gastrointestinal, neurologic, and respiratory systems, respectively) and the HIV-related conditions associated with each system. Each of these chapters presents an overview table describing the conditions, a brief discussion of each condition, summary tables of the diagnostic studies, and the medical management for the conditions.

While HIV-related malignancies affect more than one body system, they have many characteristics in common. These are presented in Chapter 10, together with diagnostic tests and medical and nursing management of persons with HIV-related malignancies.

Nursing HIV-infected persons involves caring for individuals who, during the long course of the infection, will experience pathology in almost every body system. Consequently, their nursing caregivers may diagnose and intervene in a wide range of patient problems, many of which coincide in time. For this reason, nursing management was consolidated into one chapter. Chapter 11 presents a complete nursing care plan for the extensive nursing diagnoses that many occur sometime during HIV infection.

Much of the early information about HIV disease was developed from experience of caring for HIV-infected homosexual men. Recently, however, the epidemic in the United States has been affecting more and more injecting drug users and women. Chapter 12 discusses the issues associated with providing care to these two groups, with emphasis on epidemiologic, diagnostic, and social considerations for these populations.

Chapter 13 presents the legal issues associated with HIV/AIDS, from the standpoints of the health care worker, the employer, and the HIV-infected person. Legal issues of concern to HIV-infected persons include power of attorney and living wills.

Chapter 14 focuses on infection control to safeguard health care workers and patients. It contains recommendations from the Centers for Disease Control on universal precautions, category-specific isolation procedures, and controlling transmission of tuberculosis in the health care setting.

Chapter 15 highlights some of the technical therapeutic procedures (aerosolized pentamidine, chemotherapy, total parenteral nutrition, and vascular access devices) most frequently used by nurses in caring for HIV-infected patients. Each procedure is described, together with its indications and contraindications, administration techniques, safety issues, and implications for patient teaching.

Because of the variety of opportunistic organisms and infections associated with HIV, an arsenal of antiinfective drugs is utilized. Chapter 16 describes the major antiinfective drugs that are presently approved for use in the United States. Drugs are grouped by category of action (e.g., antiviral, antifungal) into tables for quick reference. Tables delineate chemical and brand names as well as routes of administration. The chapter provides further details on each drug or drug category's indications and contraindications, precautions, side effects, adverse reactions, pharmacokinetics, and interactions, and the nursing considerations for administering the drug.

Chapter 17 contains 18 patient teaching guides, which can be copied and distributed to patients. These cover a wide range of topics that may be encountered at different phases of HIV infection, such as male and female condoms, HIV testing, food safety, taking antiretroviral drugs, and caring for an implanted port.

We began this preface with a discussion of the valuable assistance provided to the authors by a large number of experienced HIV nurses. These nurses identified the critical knowledge base for HIV nursing in the hospital, nursing home, clinic, and home. But these nurses have provided the authors with more than just information. They and their nursing colleagues, who have been involved in this epidemic, have inspired us. We stand in awe of all nurses providing HIV/AIDS care. We admire your professional dedication, caring, and concern. We dedicate this book to you in recognition of your living out the best traditions of nursing.

Deanna E. Grimes
Richard M. Grimes

CONTENTS

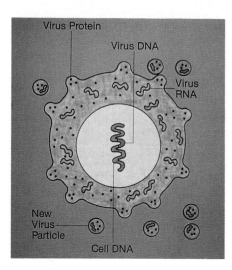

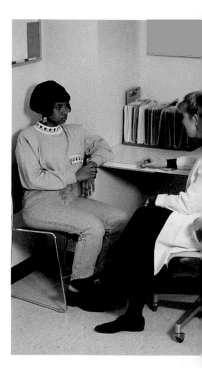

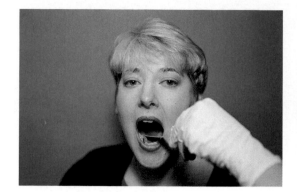

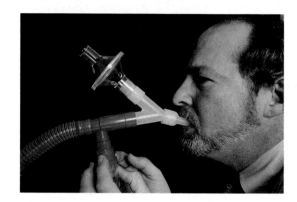

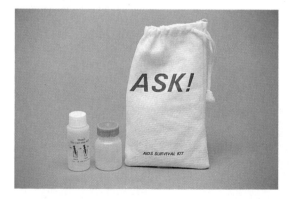

14 Infection Control, 196

15 Therapeutic Procedures, 210

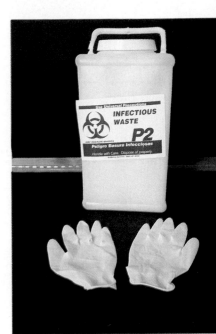

16 Pharmacology, 226

17 Patient Teaching Guides, 245

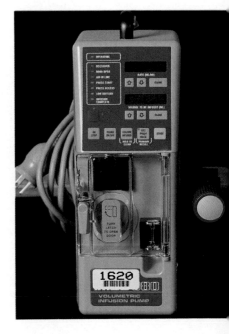

COLOR PLATES

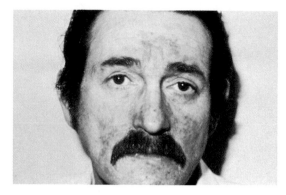

PLATE 1 Drug reaction on face.

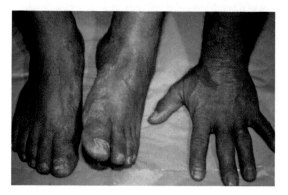

PLATE 2 Drug reaction on hands and feet.

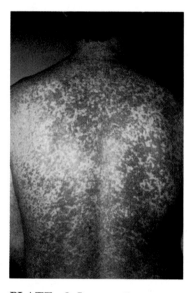

PLATE 3 Drug reaction on back.

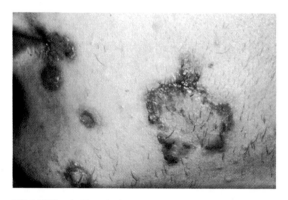

PLATE 4 *Staphylococcus aureus* "impetigo" on face.

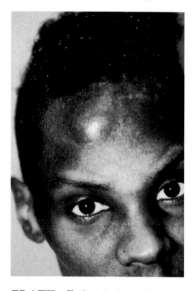

PLATE 5 *Staphylococcus aureus* "boil" on forehead.

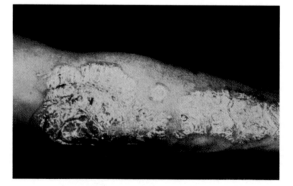

PLATE 6 Severe psoriasis on arm.

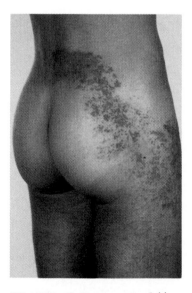

PLATE 7 Herpes zoster "shingles" on hip.

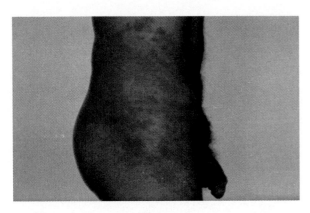

PLATE 8 Severe herpes zoster "shingles" in male.

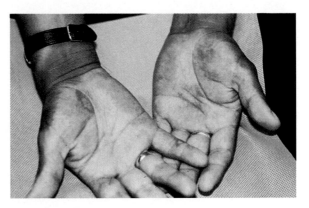

PLATE 9 Erythema multiforme on hands.

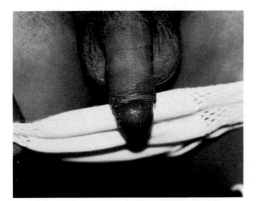

PLATE 10 Erythema multiforme on penis of male with herpes.

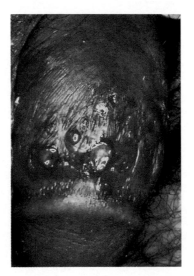

PLATE 11 Herpes corona.

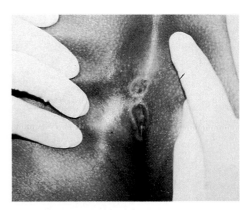

PLATE 12 Anal herpes.

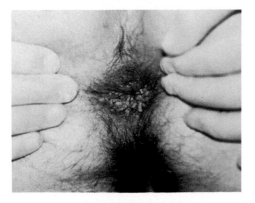

PLATE 13 Anal condylomata "warts."

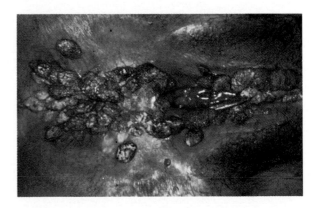

PLATE 14 Genital condylomata "warts" in female.

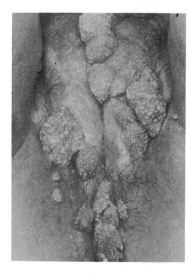

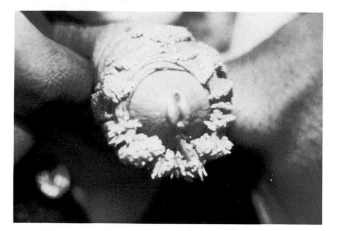

PLATE 16 Genital warts in male.

PLATE 15 Genital warts in female.

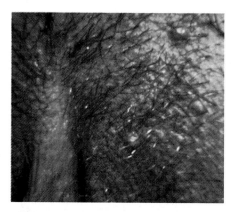

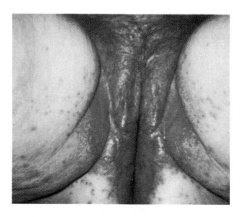

PLATE 17 Molluscum in male.

PLATE 18 *Candida* vulvitis.

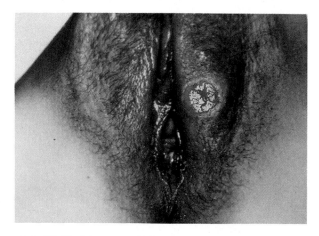

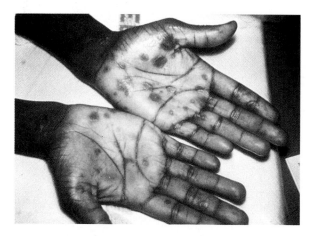

PLATE 19 Primary syphilis—chancre on labia.

PLATE 20 Secondary syphilis—rash on hands.

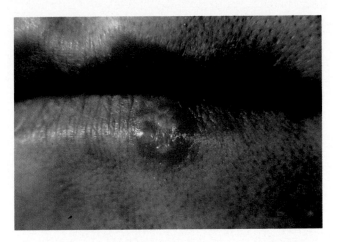

PLATE 21 Herpes simplex lesion of lower lip—second day after onset.

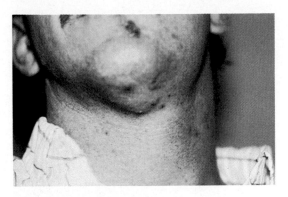

PLATE 22 Herpes on chin.

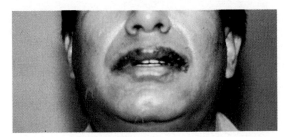

PLATE 24 Herpes on lips; person being treated with acyclovir.

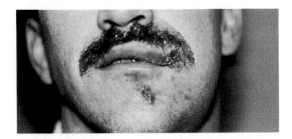

PLATE 23 Herpes with crusting on face and lips.

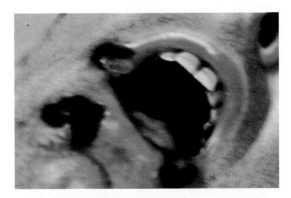

PLATE 26 Severe oral/facial herpes on day that patient died.

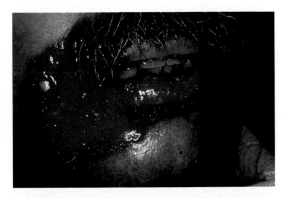

PLATE 25 Severe oral/facial herpes resistant to acyclovir.

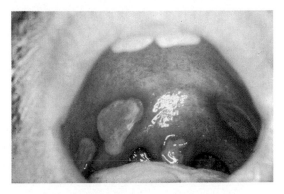

PLATE 27 Recurrent aphthous ulcers.

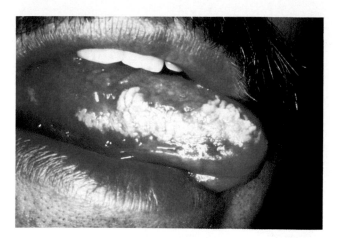

PLATE 28 Hairy leukoplakia on tongue.

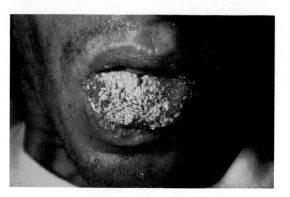

PLATE 29 Severe pseudomembranous candidiasis of tongue.

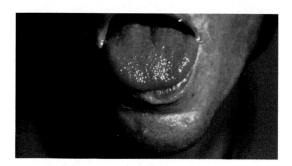

PLATE 30 Candidiasis of tongue in patient in Plate 29 after 48 hours of treatment with fluconazole.

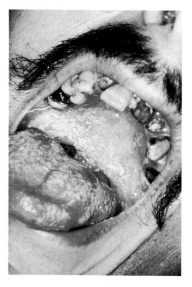

PLATE 31 Fluconazole-resistant candidiasis.

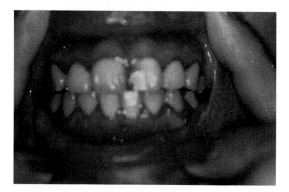

PLATE 32 Gingivitis.

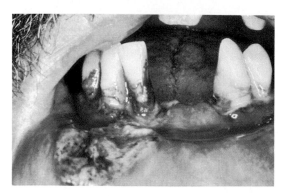

PLATE 33 Periodontitis.

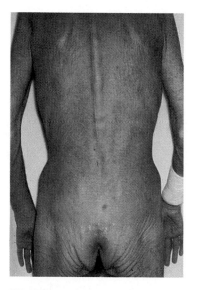

PLATE 34 Severe wasting.

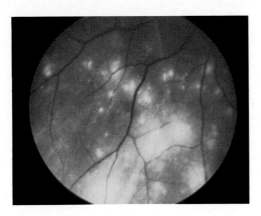

PLATE 35 CMV retinitis.

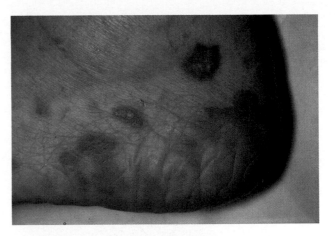

PLATE 36 Kaposi's sarcoma of heel and lateral foot.

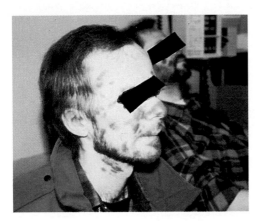

PLATE 37 Kaposi's sarcoma on face.

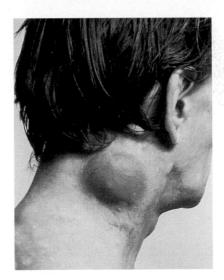

PLATE 38 Lymphoma on neck.

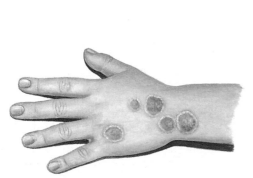

PLATE 39 Annular formation (annular granuloma).

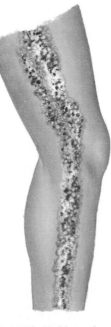

PLATE 40 Linear formation (psoriasis linearis).

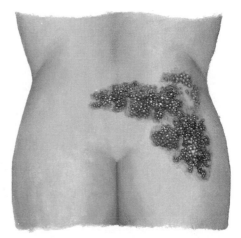

PLATE 41 Clustering of lesions (herpes zoster).

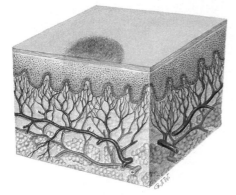

PLATE 42 Macule.

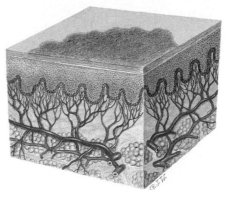

PLATE 43 Patch.

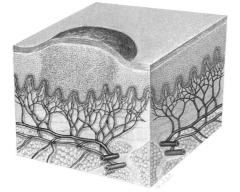

PLATE 44 Papule.

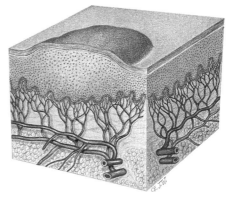

PLATE 45 Wheal.

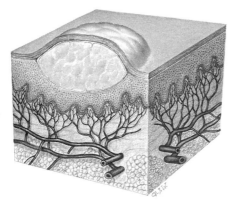

PLATE 46 Tumor.

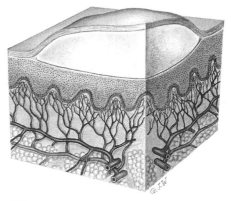

PLATE 47 Bulla.

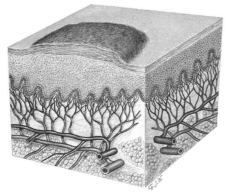

PLATE 48 Plaque.

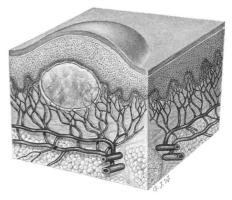

PLATE 49 Nodule.

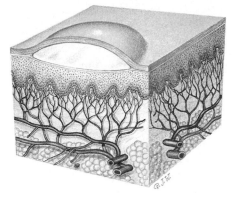

PLATE 50 Vesicle.

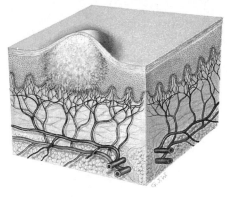

PLATE 51 Pustule.

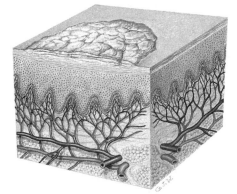

PLATE 52 Scale.

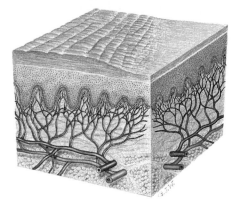

PLATE 53 Lichenification.

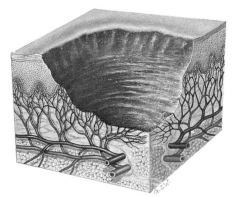

PLATE 54 Ulcer.

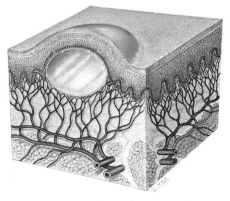

PLATE 55 Cyst.

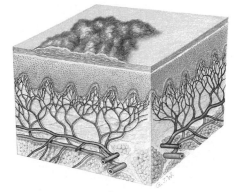

PLATE 56 Crust.

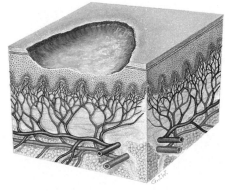

PLATE 57 Erosion.

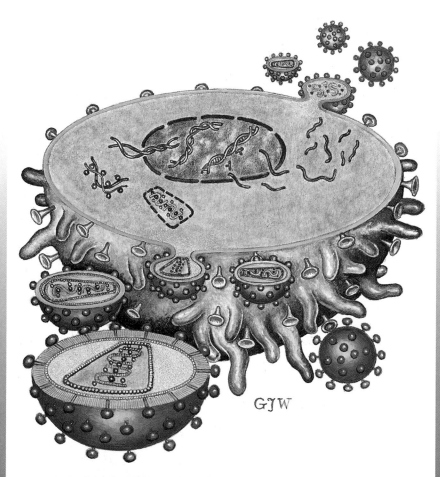

AIDS VIRUS LATCHING ONTO A CD4+ CELL AND REPLICATION CYCLE

Understanding the Immune System

The immune system is a complex network of specialized cells and organs that has evolved to defend the body against attacks by "foreign" invaders. When functioning properly it fights off infections by agents such as bacteria, viruses, fungi, and parasites. When it malfunctions, however, it can unleash a torrent of diseases, from allergy to arthritis to cancer to AIDS.

The immune system evolved because we live in a sea of microbes. Like man, these organisms are programmed to perpetuate themselves. The human body provides an ideal habitat for many of them and they try to break in; because the presence of these organisms is often harmful, the body's immune system will attempt to bar their entry or, failing that, to seek out and destroy them.

The immune system, which equals in complexity the intricacies of the brain and nervous system, displays several remarkable characteristics. It can distinguish between "self" and "nonself." It is able to remember previous experiences and react accordingly: once you have had chicken pox, your immune system will prevent you from getting it again. The immune system displays both enormous diversity and extraordinary specificity: not only is it able to recognize many millions of distinctive nonself molecules, it can produce molecules and cells to match up with and counteract each one of them. And it has at its command a sophisticated array of weapons.

The success of this system in defending the body relies on an incredibly elaborate and dynamic regulatory-communications network. Millions and millions of cells, organized into sets and subsets, pass information back and forth like clouds of bees swarming around a hive. The result is a sensitive system of checks and balances that produces an immune response that is prompt, appropriate, effective, and self-limiting.

This chapter contains material from *Understanding the Immune System*, as revised in October, 1991, by the US Department of Health and Human Services, National Institute of Allergy and Infectious Diseases, and the National Cancer Institutes.

SELF AND NONSELF

At the heart of the immune system is the ability to distinguish between self and nonself. Virtually every body cell carries distinctive molecules that identify it as self.

The body's immune defenses do not normally attack tissues that carry a self marker. Rather, immune cells and other body cells coexist peaceably in a state known as self-tolerance. But when immune defenders encounter cells or organisms carrying molecules that say "foreign," the immune troops move quickly to eliminate the intruders.

Any substance capable of triggering an immune response is called an *antigen*. An antigen can be a virus, a bacterium, a fungus, or a parasite, or even a portion or product of one of these organisms. Tissues or cells from another individual, except an identical twin whose cells carry identical self-markers, also act as antigens; because the immune system recognizes transplanted tissues as foreign, it rejects them. The body will even reject nourishing proteins unless they are first broken down by the digestive system into their primary, nonantigenic building blocks.

An antigen announces its foreignness by means of intricate and characteristic shapes called epitopes, which protrude from its surface. Most antigens, even the simplest microbes, carry several different kinds of epitopes on their surface; some may carry several hundred. However, some epitopes will be more effective than others at stimulating an immune response (Figure 1-1).

In abnormal situations, the immune system can wrongly identify self as nonself and execute a misdirected immune attack. The result can be a so-called autoimmune disease such as rheumatoid arthritis or systemic lupus erythematosus.

In some people, an apparently harmless substance such as ragweed pollen or cat hair can provoke the immune system to set off the inappropriate and harmful response known as allergy; in these cases the antigens are known as allergens.

THE ANATOMY OF THE IMMUNE SYSTEM

The organs of the immune system are stationed throughout the body (Figure 1-2). They are generally referred to as lymphoid organs because they are concerned with the growth, development, and deployment of lymphocytes, the white cells that are the key operatives of the immune system. Lymphoid organs include the bone marrow and the thymus, as well as lymph nodes, spleen, tonsils and adenoids, the appen-

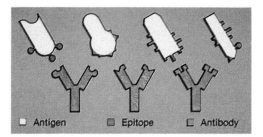

FIGURE 1-1
Antigens and antibodies.

GENES AND THE MARKERS OF SELF

Molecules that mark a cell as self are encoded by a group of genes that is contained in a section of a specific chromosome known as the major histocompatibility complex (MHC). The prefix "histo" means tissue; the MHC was discovered in the course of tissue transplantation experiments. Because MHC genes and the molecules they encode vary widely in the details of their structure from one individual to another (a diversity known as polymorphism), transplants are very likely to be identified as foreign by the immune system and rejected.

Scientists eventually discovered a more natural role for the MHC. It is essential to the immune defenses. MHC markers determine which antigens an individual can respond to, and how strongly. Moreover, MHC markers allow immune cells such as B cells, T cells, and macrophages to recognize and communicate with one another.

One group of proteins encoded by the genes of the MHC are the markers of self that appear on almost all body cells. Known as class I MHC antigens, these molecules alert killer T cells to the presence of body cells that have been changed for the worse—infected with a virus or transformed by cancer—and that need to be eliminated.

A second group of MHC proteins, class II antigens, are found on B cells, macrophages, and other cells responsible for presenting foreign antigen to helper T cells. Class II products combine with particles of foreign antigen in a way that showcases the antigen and captures the attention of the helper T cell.

This focusing of T cell antigen recognition through class I and class II molecules is known as MHC (or histocompatibility) restriction.

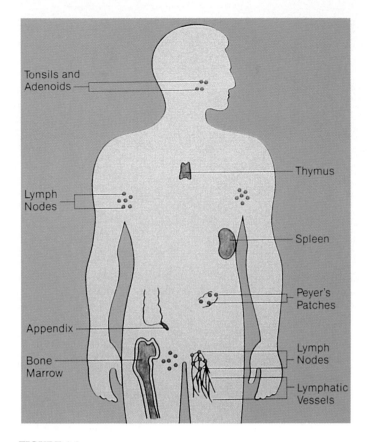

FIGURE 1-2
Organs of the immune system.

dix, and clumps of lymphoid tissue in the small intestine known as Peyer's patches. The blood and lymphatic vessels that carry lymphocytes to and from the other structures can also be considered lymphoid organs.

Cells destined to become immune cells, like all other blood cells, are produced in the *bone marrow*, the soft tissue in the hollow shafts of long bones. The descendants of some so-called stem cells become lymphocytes, while others develop into a second major group of immune cells typified by the large, cell- and particle-devouring white cells known as phagocytes.

The two major classes of lymphocytes are B cells and T cells. B cells complete their maturation in the bone marrow. T cells, on the other hand, migrate to the *thymus,* a multilobed organ that lies high behind the breastbone. There they multiply and mature into cells capable of producing an immune response—that is, they become immunocompetent. In a process referred to as T cell "education," T cells in the thymus learn to distinguish self cells from nonself cells; T cells that would react against self antigens are eliminated.

Upon exiting the bone marrow and thymus, some lymphocytes congregate in immune organs or lymph nodes. Others—both B and T cells—travel widely and continuously throughout the body. They use the blood circulation as well as a bodywide network of *lymphatic vessels* similar to blood vessels.

Laced along the lymphatic routes—with clusters in the neck, armpits, abdomen, and groin—are small, bean-shaped *lymph nodes.* Each lymph node contains specialized compartments that house platoons of B lymphocytes, T lymphocytes, and other cells capable of enmeshing antigen and presenting it to T cells. Thus, the lymph node brings together the several components needed to spark an immune response.

The *spleen,* too, provides a meeting ground for immune defenses. A fist-sized organ at the upper left of the abdomen, the spleen contains two main types of tissue—the red pulp, where worn-out blood cells are disposed of, and the white pulp, which contains lymphoid tissue. Like the lymph nodes, the spleen's lymphoid tissue is subdivided into compartments that specialize in different kinds of immune cells. Microorganisms carried by the blood into the red pulp become trapped by the immune cells known as macrophages. (Although people can live without a spleen, persons whose spleens have been damaged by trauma or by

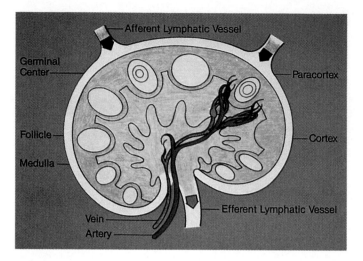

FIGURE 1-3
Lymph node. T cells concentrate in the paracortex, B cells in and around the germinal centers, and plasma cells in the medulla.

disease such as sickle cell anemia are highly susceptible to infection; surgical removal of the spleen is especially dangerous for young children and the immunosuppressed.)

Nonencapsulated clusters of lymphoid tissue are found in many parts of the body. They are common around the mucous membranes lining the respiratory and digestive tracts—areas that serve as gateways to the body. They include the tonsils and adenoids, the appendix, and Peyer's patches.

The lymphatic vessels carry *lymph*, a clear fluid that bathes the body's tissues. Lymph, along with the many cells and particles it carries—notably lymphocytes, macrophages, and foreign antigens, drains out of tissues and seeps across the thin walls of tiny lymphatic vessels. The vessels transport the mix to lymph nodes (Figure 1-3), where antigens can be filtered out and presented to immune cells.

Additional lymphocytes reach the lymph nodes (and other immune tissues) through the bloodstream. Each node is supplied by an artery and a vein; lymphocytes enter the node by traversing the walls of very small specialized veins.

All lymphocytes exit lymph nodes in lymph via outgoing lymphatic vessels. Much as small creeks and streams empty into larger rivers, the lymphatics feed into larger and larger channels. At the base of the neck large lymphatic vessels merge into the *thoracic duct*, which empties its contents into the bloodstream.

Once in the bloodstream, the lymphocytes and other assorted immune cells are transported to tissues throughout the body. They patrol everywhere for foreign antigens, then gradually drift back into the lymphatic vessels, to begin the cycle all over again.

THE CELLS AND SECRETIONS OF THE IMMUNE SYSTEM

The immune system stockpiles a tremendous arsenal of cells (Figure 1-4). Some staff the general defenses, while others are trained on highly specific targets. To work effectively, however, most immune cells require the active cooperation of their fellows. Sometimes they communicate through direct physical contact, sometimes by releasing versatile chemical messengers.

In order to have room for enough cells to match millions of possible foreign invaders, the immune system stores just a few of each specificity. When an antigen appears, those few specifically matched cells are stimulated to multiply into a full-scale army. Later, to prevent this army from overexpanding wildly, like a cancer, powerful suppressor mechanisms come into play.

LYMPHOCYTES

Lymphocytes are small white blood cells that bear the major responsibility for carrying out the activities of the immune system; they number about one trillion. The two major classes of lymphocytes are B cells, which grow to maturity independent of the thymus, and T cells, which are processed in the thymus. Both B cells and T cells recognize specific antigen targets.

B cells work chiefly by secreting soluble substances called antibodies into the body's fluids, or humors. (This is known as humoral immunity.) Antibodies typically interact with circulating antigens such as bacteria and toxic molecules, but are unable to penetrate living cells. T cells, in contrast, interact directly with their targets, attacking body cells that have been comman-

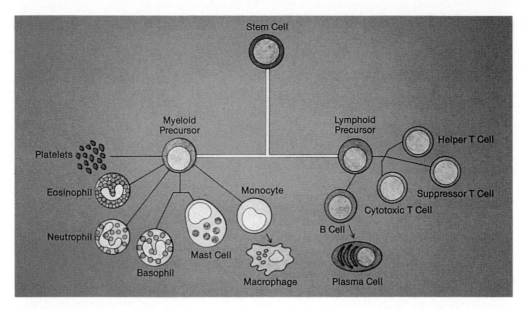

FIGURE 1-4
Cells of the immune system.

deered by viruses or warped by malignancy. (This is cellular immunity.)

Although small lymphocytes look identical, even under the microscope, they can be told apart by means of distinctive molecules they carry on their cell surface. Not only do such markers distinguish between B cells and T cells, they distinguish among various subsets of cells that behave differently. Every mature T cell, for instance, carries a marker known as T3 (or CD3); in addition, most helper T cells carry a T4 (CD4) marker, a molecule that recognizes class II MHC antigens. A molecule known as T8 (CD8), which recognizes class I MHC antigens, is found on many suppressor/cytotoxic T cells. In addition, different T cells have different kinds of antigen receptors—either alpha/beta or gamma/delta.

B Cells and Antibodies

Each *B cell* is programmed to make one specific antibody. For example, one B cell will make an antibody that blocks a virus that causes the common cold, while another produces antibody that zeroes in on a bacterium that causes pneumonia.

When a B cell encounters its triggering antigen (along with collaborating T cells and accessory cells), it gives rise to many large *plasma cells*. Every plasma cell is essentially a factory for producing antibody. Each of the plasma cells descended from a given B cell (which are all members of the same family, or clone) manufactures millions of identical antibody molecules and pours them into the bloodstream (see the box on p. 10).

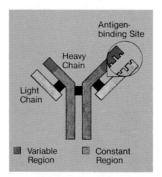

FIGURE 1-5
Antibody.

A given *antibody* matches an antigen much as a key matches a lock. The fit varies: sometimes it is very precise, while at other times it is little better than that of a skeleton key. To some degree, however, the antibody interlocks with the antigen and thereby marks it for destruction.

Antibodies belong to a family of large molecules known as immunoglobulins. Immunoglobulins are proteins, made up of chains of polypeptides, strings of the basic units known as amino acids. Each antibody has two identical heavy polypeptide chains and two identical light chains, shaped to form a Y. The sections that make up the tips of the Y's arms vary greatly from one antibody to another, creating a pocket uniquely shaped to enfold a specific antigen (Figure 1-5). This is called the variable (V) region. The stem of the Y serves to link the antibody to other participants in the immune

Table 1-1

IMMUNOGLOBULIN CLASSES

Immunoglobulin	Characteristics	Functions
IgG	Four distinct types account for about 80% to 85% of antibodies in normal serum; most abundant in blood but also found in lymph, cerebrospinal, synovial, and peritoneal fluids, and breast milk; the only immunoglobulin that crosses placenta and provides temporary immunity in neonate	Develops slowly during primary response, appearing about 1 wk or more after IgM, then reaches a peak in 1-3 wk or longer after IgM peaks; may persist for years; highest concentration during secondary immune response; activates complement system, involved in opsonization; attacks antigens directly
IgM	Accounts for about 5% of antibodies in normal serum	First antibody to form during viral or bacterial infection; usually peaks 1-2 wk after clinical symptoms appear; highest concentration during primary response; is increased in chronic infections; binds with viral and bacterial antigens in the circulation, which activates the complement cascade
IgA	Two types account for about 15% of antibodies in normal serum; found in blood and secretions (tears, saliva, colostrum, respiratory tract, and stomach and accessory organs)	Secretory antibody; increased in chronic infections and chronic inflammation
IgE	Accounts for <1% of antibodies in normal serum; found also in tissues	Sensitizing antibody; triggers release of histamine; involved with certain allergic disorders, especially atopic diseases; increased in parasitic diseases
IgD	Accounts for <1% of antibodies in normal serum	Function unclear, but increases in chronic infection

From Grimes.[82]

defenses. This area is identical in all antibodies of the same class, and is called the constant (C) region.

Scientists have identified nine chemically distinct classes of human immunoglobulins (Ig) (Table 1-1)—four kinds of IgG and two kinds of IgA, plus IgM, IgE, and IgD. Each type plays a different role in the immune defense strategy. IgG, the major immunoglobulin in the blood, is also able to enter tissue spaces; it works efficiently to coat microorganisms, speeding their uptake by other cells in the immune system. IgM, which usually combines in star-shaped clusters, tends to remain in the bloodstream, where it is very effective in killing bacteria. IgA concentrates in body fluids—tears, saliva, the secretions of the respiratory and gastrointestinal tracts—guarding the entrances to the body. IgE, which under normal circumstances occurs only in trace amounts, probably evolved as a defense against parasites, but it is more familiar as the villain in allergic reactions (see Allergy). IgD is almost exclusively found inserted into the membranes of B cells, where it somehow regulates the cell's activation.

Antibodies can work in several ways, depending on the nature of the antigen. Antibodies that interlock with toxins produced by certain bacteria can disable them directly (and are known as antitoxins). Other antibodies, by coating (or opsonizing) bacteria, make the microbes highly palatable to scavenger cells equipped to engulf and destroy them. More often, an antigen-antibody combination unleashes a group of lethal serum enzymes known as complement (see Complement). Yet other antibodies block viruses from entering into cells (a quality that is exploited in making vaccines). And, in a phenomenon known as antibody-dependent cell-mediated cytotoxicity (ADCC), cells coated with antibody become vulnerable to attack by several types of white blood cells.

T Cells and Lymphokines

T cells contribute to the immune defenses in two major ways (see the box on T cell subsets). Regulatory T cells are vital to orchestrating the elaborate system. (B cells, for instance, cannot make antibody against most substances without T cell help.) Cytotoxic T cells, on the other hand, directly attack body cells that are infected or malignant.

T CELL SUBSETS

Effector cells

- Cytotoxic T cells (also known as killer T cells) are attracted to antigens, including microorganisms, cells that contain viruses, cancer cells, and transplanted cells. Cytotoxic T cells bind to the surface of an antigen, disrupt its cell membrane, and kill it directly with lymphokines. In addition, the release of lymphokines promotes phagocytosis.
- Delayed hypersensitivity T cells stimulate allergic reactions, anaphylaxis, and autoimmune reactions.

Regulator cells

- Helper T cells "turn on" the immune system by enhancing the response of B cells and cytotoxic T cells to antigens, stimulating the activity of all other T cells, and activating the macrophage system.
- Suppressor T cells "turn off" the action of helper and cytotoxic T cells, preventing them from causing excessive, potentially harmful immune reactions.

From Grimes.[82]

Chief among the regulatory T cells are "helper/inducer" cells. Typically identifiable by the T4 cell marker, helper T cells are essential for activating B cells and other T cells as well as natural killer cells and macrophages. Another subset of T cells acts to turn off or "suppress" these cells.

Cytotoxic T cells, which usually carry the T8 marker, are killer cells. In addition to ridding the body of cells that have been infected by viruses or transformed by cancer, they are responsible for the rejection of tissue and organ grafts. (Although suppressor/cytotoxic T cells are often called T8 cells, in reality the two are not always synonymous. The T8 molecule, like the T4 molecule, determines which MHC molecule—class I or class II—the T cell will recognize, but not how the T cell will behave.)

T cells work primarily by secreting substances known as cytokines or, more specifically, *lymphokines*. Lymphokines (which are also secreted by B cells) and their relatives, the *monokines* produced by monocytes and macrophages, are diverse and potent chemical messengers. Binding to specific receptors on target cells, lymphokines call into play many other cells and substances, including the elements of the inflammatory response. They encourage cell growth, promote cell activation, direct cellular traffic, destroy target cells, and incite macrophages. A single cytokine may have many functions; conversely, several different cytokines may be able to produce the same effect.

One of the first cytokines to be discovered was interferon. Produced by T cells and macrophages (as well as by cells outside the immune system), interferons are a family of proteins with antiviral properties. Interferon from immune cells, known as immune interferon or gamma interferon, activates macrophages. Two other cytokines, closely related to one another, are lymphotoxin (from lymphocytes) and tumor necrosis factor (from macrophages). Both kill tumor cells; tumor necrosis factor (TNF) also inhibits parasites and viruses.

Many cytokines are initially given descriptive names but, as their basic structure is identified, they are renamed as "interleukins"—messengers between leukocytes, or white cells. Interleukin-1, or IL-1, is a product of macrophages (and many other cells) that helps to activate B cells and T cells. IL-2, originally known as T cell growth factor, or TCGF, is produced by antigen-activated T cells and promotes the rapid growth or differentiation of mature T cells and B cells. IL-3 is a T-cell derived member of the family of protein mediators known as colony-stimulating factors (CSF); one of its many functions is to nurture the development of immature precursor cells into a variety of mature blood cells. IL-4, IL-5, and IL-6 help B cells grow and differentiate; IL-4 also affects T cells, macrophages, mast cells, and granulocytes.

A number of cytokines, obtained in quantity through recombinant DNA technology (see Genetic Engineering), are now being used—alone, in combination, linked to toxins—in clinical trials for patients with cancers, blood disorders, and immunodeficiency diseases (including AIDS), as well as people receiving bone marrow transplants. Their versatility, however, makes it difficult to predict the full range of their effects.

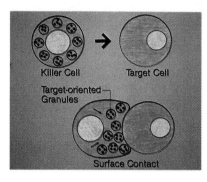

FIGURE 1-6
Killer cell makes contact with target cell, orients its weapon toward the target, and delivers a burst of lethal chemicals.

Natural Killer Cells

Natural killer (NK) cells (Figure 1-6) are yet another type of lethal lymphocyte. Like cytotoxic T cells, they contain granules filled with potent chemicals. They are called "natural" killers because they, unlike cytotoxic T cells, do not need to recognize a specific antigen before swinging into action. They target tumor cells and protect against a wide variety of infectious microbes. In several immunodeficiency diseases, including AIDS, natural killer cell function is abnormal. Natural killer cells may also contribute to immunoregulation by secreting high levels of influential lymphokines.

Both cytotoxic T cells and natural killer cells kill on contact. The killer binds to its target, aims its weapons, and then delivers a lethal burst of chemicals that produces holes in the target cell's membrane. Fluids seep in and leak out, and the cell bursts.

PHAGOCYTES, GRANULOCYTES, AND THEIR RELATIVES

Phagocytes (literally, "cell eaters") (Figure 1-7) are large white cells that can engulf and digest marauding microorganisms and other antigenic particles. Some phagocytes also have the ability to present antigen to lymphocytes.

Important phagocytes are *monocytes* and *macrophages*. Monocytes circulate in the blood, then migrate into tissues where they develop into macrophages ("big eaters"). Macrophages are seeded throughout body tissues in a variety of guises. Specialized macrophages include alveolar macrophages in the lungs, mesangial phagocytes in the kidneys, microglial cells in the brain, and Kupffer cells in the liver.

Macrophages are versatile cells that play many roles. As scavengers, they rid the body of worn-out cells and other debris. Foremost among the cells that "present" antigen to T cells, having first digested and processed it, macrophages play a crucial role in initiat-

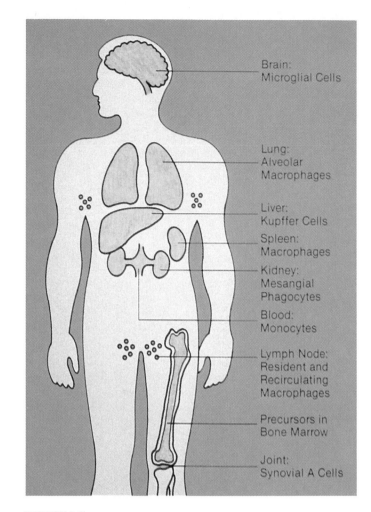

FIGURE 1-7
Phagocytes in the body.

ing the immune response. As secretory cells, monocytes and macrophages are vital to the regulation of immune responses and the development of inflammation: they churn out an amazing array of powerful chemical substances (monokines), including enzymes, complement proteins, and regulatory factors such as interleukin-1. At the same time, they carry receptors for lymphokines that allow them to be "activated" into single-minded pursuit of microbes and tumor cells.

Macrophages are not the only cells to present antigen to lymphocytes. Other antigen-presenting cells include B cells, as noted above, and dendritic cells, irregularly shaped white blood cells found in the spleen and other lymphoid organs. Dendritic cells typically have long threadlike tentacles that enmesh lymphocytes and antigens. Langerhans cells are dendritic cells that travel about in the skin, picking up antigen and transporting it to nearby lymph nodes. Many other types of body cells, properly stimulated, can also be recruited to present antigens to lymphocytes.

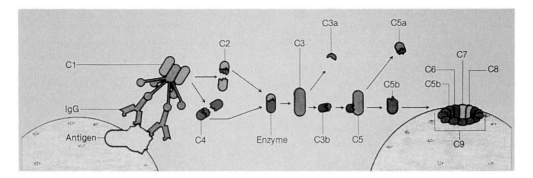

FIGURE 1-8
The complement cascade. The classical complement pathway becomes activated when the first complement molecule, C1, recognizes an antigen-antibody complex. Each of the remaining complement proteins, in turn, performs its specialized job, cleaving or binding the complement molecules next in line. The end product is the cylindrical membrane attack complex.

Another critical phagocyte is the *neutrophil*. Neutrophils are not only phagocytes but also granulocytes: they contain granules filled with potent chemicals. These chemicals, in addition to destroying microorganisms, play a key role in acute inflammatory reactions.

Also known as polymorphonuclear leukocytes or polymorphs (because their nuclei come in "many shapes"), granulocytes include *eosinophils* and *basophils* as well as neutrophils. (The cells are named for the way they stain in the laboratory: eosinophils, for instance, have an affinity for acidic dyes such as eosin.) The phagocytic neutrophil uses its prepackaged chemicals to degrade the microbes it ingests; eosinophils and basophils typically "degranulate," releasing their chemicals to work on cells or microbes in their surroundings.

The *mast cell* is a noncirculating counterpart of the basophil. Located in the lungs, skin, tongue, and linings of the nose and intestinal tract, the mast cell is responsible for the symptoms of allergy (see Allergy).

Another related structure is the blood *platelet*. Platelets, too, contain granules. In addition to promoting blood clotting and wound repair, platelets release substances that activate components of the immune system.

COMPLEMENT

The complement system is made up of a series of about 25 proteins that work to "complement" the activity of antibodies in destroying bacteria, either by facilitating phagocytosis or by puncturing the bacterial cell membrane. Complement also helps to rid the body of antigen-antibody complexes. In carrying out these tasks, it induces an inflammatory response.

Complement proteins circulate in the blood in an inactive form. When the first of the complement substances is triggered—usually by antibody interlocked with an antigen—it sets in motion a ripple effect. As each component is activated in turn, it acts upon the next in a precise sequence of carefully regulated steps known as the "complement cascade" (Figure 1-8).

In the so-called "classical" pathway of complement activation, a series of proteins gives rise to a complex enzyme capable of cleaving a key protein, C3. In the "alternative" pathway—which can be triggered by suitable targets in the absence of antibody—C3 interacts with a different set of factors and enzymes. But both pathways end in the creation of a unit known as the membrane attack complex. Inserted in the wall of the target cell, the membrane attack complex constitutes a channel that allows fluids and molecules to flow in and out. The target cell rapidly swells and bursts.

Meantime, various fragments flung off during the course of the cascade can produce other consequences. One byproduct causes mast cells and basophils to release their contents, producing the redness, warmth, and swelling of the inflammatory response. Another stimulates and attracts neutrophils. Yet another, C3b, opsonizes or coats target cells so as to make them more palatable to phagocytes, which carry a special receptor for C3b.

The C3b fragment also appears to play a major role in the body's control of immune complexes. By opsonizing antigen-antibody complexes, C3b helps prevent the formation of large and insoluble (and thus potentially damaging) immune aggregates. Moreover, receptors for C3b are also present on red blood cells, which appear to use the receptors to pick up complement-coated immune complexes and deliver them to the Kupffer cells in the liver.

A BILLION ANTIBODIES

Scientists were long puzzled by the opulence of the immune system's resources. The body apparently could recognize and mount unique responses to an endless variety of antigens—but how in the world could all that information be crammed into a limited number of genes?

The answer came as a surprise. A typical gene consists of a fixed segment of DNA, which directs the manufacture of a given protein molecule such as insulin. Antibody genes (Figure 1-9), in contrast, are assembled from bits and pieces of DNA scattered widely throughout the genetic material. As the B cell matures, it rearranges or shuffles these gene components, picking and choosing among hundreds of DNA segments—some for each of the antibody's variable (V), diversity (D), joining (J), and constant (C) regions. Intervening segments of DNA are cut out; the selected pieces are spliced together.

The new gene—and the antibody it encodes—are virtually unique. When the B cell containing this uniquely rearranged set of gene segments proliferates, all its descendants will make this unique antibody. Then, as the cells continue to multiply, numerous mutants arise; these allow for the natural selection of antibodies that provide better and better "fits" for the target antigen. The result of this entire process is that a limited number of genetically distinct B cells can respond to a seemingly unlimited range of antigens.

A similar mechanism was found to control a comparable structure on the T cell, the T cell's antigen receptor. The variable regions of T cell antigen receptors, like those of antibodies, are encoded by V, D, and J segments originally far apart, but which are brought together and fused into a single gene. With numerous candidates for each segment, the number of possible combinations becomes astronomical. However, in contrast to antibody genes, T cell receptor genes do not mutate as the T cells proliferate. This ensures that the self-tolerance imposed in the thymus will not be overthrown by the inadvertent generation of mutant T cell receptors that are anti-self.

A WEB OF IDIOTYPES

The unique and characteristic pocket on an antibody that recognizes a specific antigen—its variable region—can itself act as an antigen. More precisely, the variable region contains a number of antigen-like segments, and these are known collectively as an idiotype (Figure 1-10). Like any other antigen, an idiotype can trigger complementary antibody. This second-round antibody is known as an antiidiotype. An antiidiotype, in turn, can trigger an antiantiidiotype. Like a series of mirrored reflections, the process can go on and on.

Interactions between idiotypes and antiidiotypes, it has been proposed, constitute a mechanism whereby the immune system regulates itself. According to the "network theory," not only antibodies but B cells and T cells carry—in their unique antigen-receptors—idiotypes. The B cells and T cells that proliferate in response to a certain antigen carry a complementary idiotype. Antiidiotype B cells secrete antiidiotype antibodies, which may neutralize the original idiotypes (antibodies), or bind to idiotypes on regulatory T cells. Alternatively, antiidiotypes may trigger antiantiidiotypes, creating a spiraling response within the network—turning on, amplifying, and shutting down immune responses.

The concept of the idiotype is being put to practical use today in the development of experimental antigen-free vaccines (see Vaccines through Biotechnology).

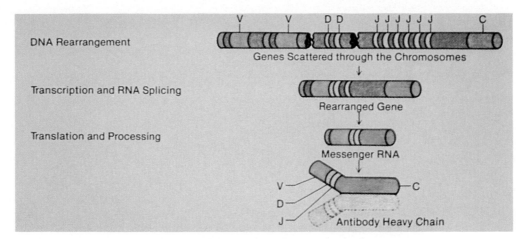

FIGURE 1-9
An antibody gene is pieced together from widely scattered bits of DNA. A typical IgM heavy chain gene consists of variable *(V)*, diversity *(D)*, joining *(J)*, and constant *(C)* segments.

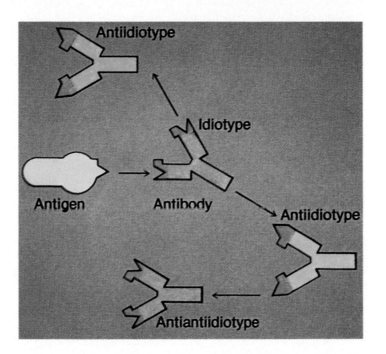

FIGURE 1-10
Idiotypes. Every antibody's unique structures can themselves act as an antigen. Known as idiotypes, these structures can trigger a complementary antibody, or antiidiotype. The antiidiotype can sometimes be substituted for the original antigen.

MOUNTING AN IMMUNE RESPONSE

Infections remain the most common cause of human disease. Produced by bacteria, viruses, parasites, and fungi, infections may range from relatively mild respiratory illnesses such as the common cold, to debilitating conditions like chronic hepatitis, to life-threatening diseases such as AIDS and meningitis.

To fend off the threatening horde, the body has devised astonishingly intricate defenses. Microbes attempting to enter the body must first find a chink in the body's external protection. The skin and the mucous membranes that line the body's portals not only pose a physical barrier, they are also rich in scavenger cells and IgA antibodies.

Next, invaders must elude a series of *nonspecific* defenses—those cells and substances equipped to tackle infectious agents without regard for their antigenic peculiarities. Many potential infections are cut short when microbes are intercepted by patrolling scavenger cells or disabled by complement or other

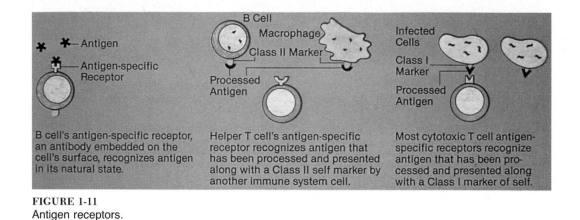

FIGURE 1-11
Antigen receptors.

RECEPTORS FOR RECOGNIZING ANTIGEN

In order to recognize and respond to the antigens that are their specific targets, both B cells and T cells carry special receptor molecules on their surface (Figure 1-11). For the B cell this receptor is a prototype of the antibody the B cell is prepared to manufacture, anchored in its surface. When a B cell encounters a matching antigen in the blood or other body fluid, this antibody-like receptor allows the B cell to interact with it very efficiently.

The T cell receptor is more complex. Structurally it is somewhat similar to an antibody, made of a pair of chemically linked chains with variable and constant regions. (But to work it needs the help of an associated set of signaling and anchoring cell surface molecules called T3.) Unlike a B cell, however, a T cell cannot recognize antigen in its natural state; the antigen must first be broken down, and the fragments bound to an MHC molecule, by an antigen-presenting cell.

Helper T cells (T4 cells) look for antigen bound to a class II MHC molecule—a combination displayed by macrophages and B cells. Most cytotoxic T cells (T8 cells), on the other hand, respond to antigen bound to MHC class I molecules, which are found on almost all body cells.

The T cell receptor molecule thus forms a three-way complex with its specific foreign antigen and an MHC protein. This complicated arrangement assures that T cells—which affect other cells through either direct contact or bursts of secretions—act only on precise targets and at close range.

The major antigen receptor, named alpha/beta for its two chains, is found on most T4 and T8 cells. A second, more recently discovered antigen receptor also has two chains and is known as gamma/delta; it is found on a distinct subset of mature T cells. Like the alpha/beta receptor, the more primitive gamma/delta receptor works in conjunction with T3. The function of T cells that carry gamma/delta receptors is not known.

enzymes or chemicals. Virus-infected cells, for instance, secrete interferon, a chemical that rouses natural killer cells.

Microbes that breach the nonspecific barriers are confronted by *specific* weapons tailored to fit each one. These may be cellular responses directed both by cells, primarily T lymphocytes and their secretions (lymphokines), and against cells that have been infected. Or they may be humoral responses, the work of antibodies secreted by B lymphocytes into the body's fluids or humors.

Most antigens are recognized by a limited number of specific immune cells (and their offspring). A few antigens, however, are capable of rousing large classes of T cells, setting off an immune response so massive that it is harmful. Dubbed "superantigens," these substances include bacterial toxins such as those responsible for the toxic shock syndrome.

Although immunologists traditionally distinguished between cellular and humoral immunity, it has become increasingly clear that the two arms of the immune response are closely intertwined. Almost all antigens evoke both a humoral response and a cellular response—and most B cell responses require T cell help. In practice, however, one arm is usually more effective than the other, and regulatory mechanisms end up skewing the response toward either the cellular or the humoral side.

The *cell-mediated* response is initiated by a macrophage or other antigen-presenting cell (Figure 1-12). The macrophage takes in the antigen, digests it, and then displays antigen fragments on its own surface. Bound to the antigen fragment is an MHC molecule. It takes both of these structures, together, to capture the T cell's attention.

A T cell whose receptor fits this antigen-MHC complex binds to it. The binding can stimulate the macrophage to secrete interleukin-1, which is required for the activation of certain T cells.

Once activated, T cells go to work. Some subsets of T cells synthesize and secrete lymphokines.

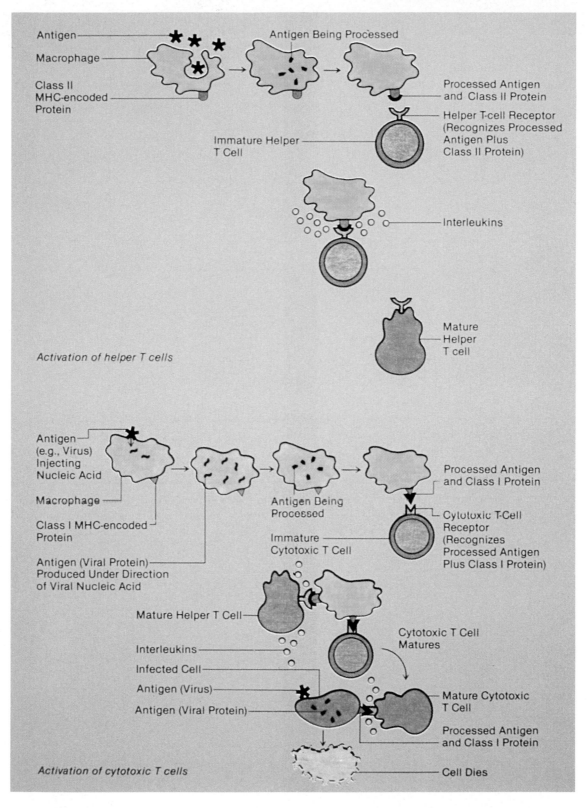

FIGURE 1-12
Activation of cytotoxic T cells. After macrophage internalizes and processes antigen, it presents antigen fragments on its surface. Antigen, combined with class II protein, attracts helper T cell; interleukins help T cell mature. Antigen plus class I protein binds to cytotoxic T cell; aided by helper T cell, cytotoxic T cell matures.

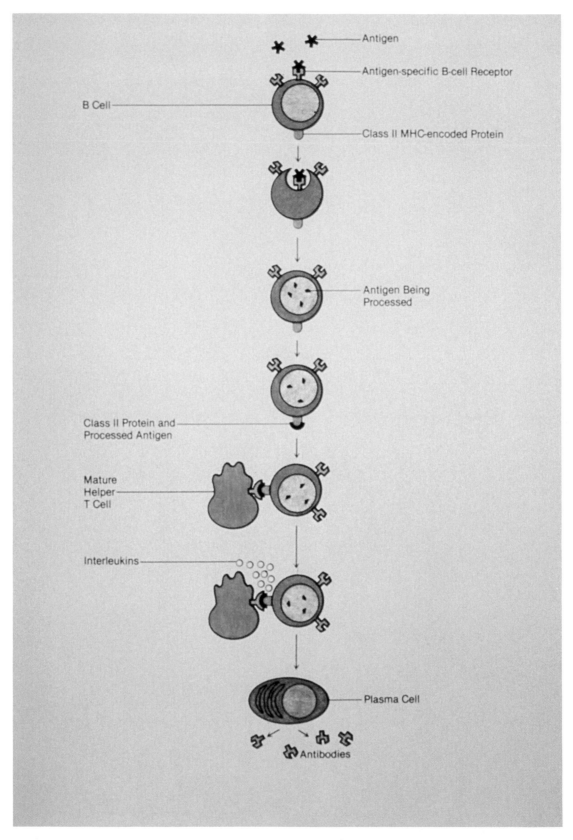

FIGURE 1-13
Activation of B cells to make antibody. B cell uses receptor to bind matching antigen, which it engulfs and processes. B cell then presents a piece of antigen, bound to class II protein, on its surface. Complex binds to mature helper T cell, which releases interleukins that transform B cell into antibody-secreting plasma cell.

Interleukin-2, for instance, spurs additional T cell growth. Other lymphokines attract other immune cells—fresh macrophages, granulocytes, and other lymphocytes—to the site of the infection, while yet others direct the cells' activities once they arrive on the scene. Some subsets of T cells become killer (or cytotoxic) cells, and set out to track down body cells infected by viruses. And when the infection has been brought under control, suppressor T cells draw the immune response to a close.

Humoral immunity chiefly involves B cells, although the cooperation of helper T cells is almost always necessary. B cells, like macrophages, take in and process circulating antigen. Unlike macrophages, however, a B cell can bind only that antigen that specifically fits its antibody-like receptor.

To enlist the help of a T cell, the B cell exhibits antigen fragments bound to its class II MHC molecules (Figure 1-13). This display attracts mature helper T cells (which may have been already activated by macrophages presenting the same antigen). The B cell and T cell interact, and the helper T cell secretes several lymphokines. These lymphokines set the B cell to multiplying, and soon there is a clone of identical B cells. The B cells differentiate into plasma cells and begin producing vast quantities of identical antigen-specific antibodies.

Released into the bloodstream, the antibodies lock onto matching antigens. The antigen-antibody complexes trigger the complement cascade or are removed from the circulation by clearing mechanisms in the liver and the spleen. The infection is overcome and, in response to suppressor influences wielded by yet other subsets of T cells, antibody production wanes.

Clinically, infections manifest themselves through the five classic symptoms of the *inflammatory response*—redness, warmth, swelling, pain, and loss of function. Redness and warmth develop when, under the influence of lymphokines and complement components, small blood vessels in the vicinity of the infection become dilated and carry more blood. Swelling results when the vessels, made leaky by yet other immune secretions, allow fluid and soluble immune substances to seep into the surrounding tissue, and immune cells to converge on the site.

IMMUNITY

As long ago as the fifth century B.C., Greek physicians noted that people who had recovered from the plague would never get it again—they had acquired immunity. (Table 1-2 summarizes types of acquired immunity.) This is because, whenever T cells and B cells are activated, some of the cells become "memory" cells. Then, the next time that an individual encounters that same antigen, the immune system is primed to destroy it quickly.

The degree and duration of immunity depend on the kind of antigen, its amount, and how it enters the body. An immune response is also dictated by heredity; some individuals respond strongly to a given antigen, others weakly, and some not at all.

Infants are born with relatively weak immune responses. They have, however, a natural "passive" immunity; they are protected during the first months of life by means of antibodies they receive from their mothers. The antibody IgG, which travels across the placenta, makes them immune to the same microbes to which their mothers are immune. Children who are

Table 1-2 ◥◥◥

TYPES OF ACQUIRED IMMUNITY

Type of immunity	How acquired	Length of resistance
Natural		
Active	Natural contact and infection with the antigen	May be temporary or permanent
Passive	Natural contact with antibody transplacentally or through colostrum and breast milk	Temporary
Artificial		
Active	Inoculation of antigen	May be temporary or permanent
Passive	Inoculation of antibody or antitoxin	Temporary

From Grimes.[82]

VACCINES THROUGH BIOTECHNOLOGY

Through genetic engineering, scientists can isolate specific genes and insert them into DNA of certain microbes or mammalian cells; the microbes or cells become living factories, mass producing the desired antigen. Then, using another product of biotechnology, a monoclonal antibody that recognizes the antigen, the scientists can separate the antigen from all the other material produced by the microbe or cell. This technique has been used to produce immunogenic but safe segments of the hepatitis B virus and the malaria parasite.

In another approach, scientists have inserted genes for desired antigens into the DNA of the vaccinia virus, the large cowpox virus familiar for its role in smallpox immunization. When the reengineered vaccinia virus is inoculated, it stimulates an immune reaction to both the vaccinia and the products of its passenger genes. These have included, in animal experiments, genes from the viruses that cause hepatitis B, influenza, rabies, and AIDS.

Instead of adding a gene, some scientists have snipped a key gene out of an infectious organism. Thus crippled, the microbe can produce immunity but not disease. This technique has been tried with a bacterium that causes the severe diarrheal disease cholera; such a vaccine is commercially available against a virus disease of pigs.

A totally different approach to vaccine development lies in chemical synthesis. Once scientists have isolated the gene that encodes an antigen, they are able to determine the precise sequence of amino acids that make up the antigen. They then pinpoint small key areas on the large protein molecule, and assemble it chemical by chemical. Wholly synthetic vaccines are being explored for malaria and for the major diarrheal diseases that are so devastating in developing countries.

Another pioneering vaccine strategy exploits antiidiotype antibodies (see A Web of Idiotypes, on page 10). The original antibody (or idiotype) provokes an antiantibody (or antiidiotype) that resembles the original antigen on the disease-causing organism. The antiidiotype will not itself cause disease, but it can serve as a mock antigen, inducing the formation of antibodies that recognize and block the original antigen. To make such a vaccine, scientists inject animals with a monoclonal antibody (idiotype) against a disease-causing microorganism, then harvest the antiidiotypes produced in response.

nursed also receive IgA from breast milk; it protects the digestive tract.

Passive immunity can also be conveyed by antibody-containing serum obtained from individuals who are immune to a specific infectious agent. Immune serum globulin or "gamma globulin" is sometimes given to protect travelers to countries where hepatitis is widespread. Passive immunity typically lasts only a few weeks.

"Active" immunity—mounting an immune response—can be triggered by both infection and vaccination. *Vaccines* contain microorganisms or parts of microorganisms that have been altered so they will produce an immune response but will not be able to induce full-blown disease. Some vaccines are made from microbes that have been killed. Others use microbes that have been changed slightly so they can no longer produce infection. They may, for instance, be unable to multiply. Some vaccines are made from a live virus that has been weakened, or attenuated, by growing it for many cycles in animals or cell cultures.

Recent research, benefiting from the biotechnology revolution, has focused on developing vaccines that use only part of the infectious agent (see the box). Such subunit vaccines, which are now available for meningitis, pneumonia, and hepatitis B, produce the desired immunity without stirring up separate and potentially harmful immune reactions to the many antigens carried, for instance, on a single bacterium.

DISORDERS OF THE IMMUNE SYSTEM

ALLERGY

The most common types of allergic reactions—hay fever, some kinds of asthma, and hives—are produced when the immune system responds to a false alarm. In a susceptible person, a normally harmless substance—grass pollen or house dust, for example—is perceived as a threat and is attacked.

Such allergic reactions are related to the antibody known as immunoglobulin E (Figure 1-14). Like other antibodies, each IgE antibody is specific; one reacts against oak pollen, another against ragweed. The role of IgE in the natural order is not known, although some scientists suspect that it developed as a defense against infection by parasitic worms.

The first time an allergy-prone person is exposed to an allergen, he or she makes large amounts of the corresponding IgE antibody. These IgE molecules attach to the surfaces of mast cells (in tissue) or basophils (in the circulation). Mast cells are plentiful in the lungs, skin, tongue, and linings of the nose and intestinal tract.

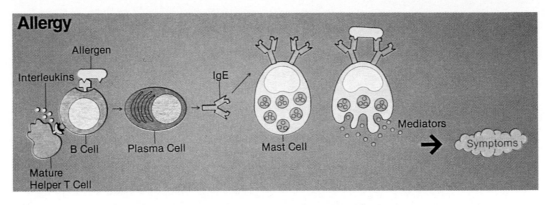

FIGURE 1-14
Allergic reactions. Allergen triggers B cell to make IgE antibody, which attaches to mast cell. When that allergen reappears, it binds to the IgE and triggers the mast cell to release its chemicals.

When an IgE antibody sitting on a mast cell or basophil encounters its specific allergen, the IgE antibody signals the mast cell or basophil to release the powerful chemicals stored within its granules. These chemicals include histamine, heparin, and substances that activate blood platelets and attract secondary cells such as eosinophils and neutrophils. The activated mast cell or basophil also synthesizes new mediators, including prostaglandins and leukotrienes, on the spot.

It is such chemical mediators that cause the symptoms of allergy, including wheezing, sneezing, runny eyes, and itching. They can also produce anaphylactic shock, a life-threatening allergic reaction characterized by swelling of body tissues, including the throat, and a sudden fall in blood pressure.

AUTOIMMUNE DISEASES

Sometimes the immune system's recognition apparatus breaks down, and the body begins to manufacture antibodies and T cells directed against the body's own constitutents—cells, cell components, or specific organs. Such antibodies are known as autoantibodies, and the diseases they produce are called autoimmune diseases. (Not all autoantibodies are harmful; some types appear to be integral to the immune system's regulatory scheme.)

Autoimmune reactions contribute to many enigmatic diseases. For instance, autoantibodies to red blood cells can cause anemia, autoantibodies to pancreas cells contribute to juvenile diabetes, and autoantibodies to nerve and muscle cells are found in patients with the chronic muscle weakness known as myasthenia gravis. Autoantibody known as rheumatoid factor is common in persons with rheumatoid arthritis.

Persons with systemic lupus erythematosus (SLE), whose symptoms encompass many systems, have antibodies to many types of cells and cellular components. These include antibodies directed against substances found in the cell's nucleus—DNA, RNA, or proteins—which are known as antinuclear antibodies, or ANAs. These antibodies can cause serious damage when they link up with self antigens to form circulating immune complexes, which become lodged in body tissues and set off inflammatory reactions (see Immune Complex Diseases).

Autoimmune diseases affect the immune system at several levels. In patients with SLE, for instance, B cells are hyperactive while suppressor cells are underactive; it is not clear which defect comes first. Moreover, production of IL-2 is low, while levels of gamma interferon are high. Patients with rheumatoid arthritis, who have a defective suppressor T cell system, continue to make antibodies to a common virus, whereas the response normally shuts down after about a dozen days.

No one knows just what causes an autoimmune disease, but several factors are likely to be involved. These may include viruses and environmental factors such as exposure to sunlight, certain chemicals, and some drugs, all of which may damage or alter body cells so that they are no longer recognizable as self. Sex hormones may be important, too, since most autoimmune diseases are far more common in women than in men.

Heredity also appears to play a role. Autoimmune reactions, like many other immune responses, are influenced by the genes of the MHC. A high proportion of human patients with autoimmune disease have particular histocompatibility types. For example, many persons with rheumatoid arthritis display the self marker known as HLA-DR4.

Many types of therapies are being used to combat autoimmune diseases. These include corticosteroids, immunosuppressive drugs developed as anticancer agents, radiation of the lymph nodes, and plasmapheresis, a sort of "blood washing" that removes diseased cells and harmful molecules from the circulation.

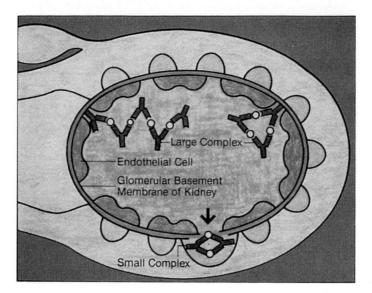

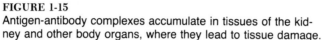

FIGURE 1-15
Antigen-antibody complexes accumulate in tissues of the kidney and other body organs, where they lead to tissue damage.

IMMUNE COMPLEX DISEASES

Immune complexes are clusters of interlocking antigens and antibodies (Figure 1-15). Under normal conditions immune complexes are rapidly removed from the bloodstream by macrophages in the spleen and Kupffer cells in the liver. In some circumstances, however, immune complexes continue to circulate. Eventually they become trapped in the tissues of the kidneys, lung, skin, joints, or blood vessels. Just where they end up probably depends on the nature of the antigen, the class of antibody—IgG, for instance, instead of IgM—and the size of the complex. There they set off reactions that lead to inflammation and tissue damage.

Immune complexes work their damage in many diseases. Sometimes, as is the case with malaria and viral hepatitis, they reflect persistent low-grade infections. Sometimes they arise in response to environmental antigens, such as the moldy hay that causes the disease known as farmer's lung. Frequently, immune complexes develop in autoimmune disease (see above), where the continuous production of autoantibodies overloads the immune complex removal system.

IMMUNODEFICIENCY DISEASES

Lack of one or more components of the immune system results in immunodeficiency disorders. These can be inherited, acquired through infection or other illness, or produced as an inadvertent side effect of certain drug treatments.

People with advanced cancer may experience immune deficiencies as a result of the disease process or from extensive anticancer therapy. Transient immune deficiencies can develop in the wake of common viral infections, including influenza, infectious mononucleosis, and measles. Immune responsiveness can also be depressed by blood transfusions, surgery, malnutrition, and stress.

Some children are born with defects in their immune systems. Those with flaws in the B cell components are unable to produce antibodies (immunoglobulins). These conditions, known as agammaglobulinemias or hypogammaglobulinemias, leave the children vulnerable to infectious organisms; such disorders can be combatted with injections of immunoglobulins.

Other children, whose thymus is either missing or small and abnormal, lack T cells. The resultant disorders have been treated with thymic transplants.

Very rarely, infants are born lacking all the major immune defenses; this is known as severe combined immunodeficiency disease (SCID). Some children with SCID have lived for years in germ-free rooms and "bubbles." A few SCID patients have been successfully treated with transplants of bone marrow (see the following box).

The devastating immunodeficiency disorder known as the acquired immunodeficiency syndrome (AIDS) is caused by a virus (the human immunodeficiency virus, or HIV) that destroys T4 cells and that is harbored in macrophages as well as T4 cells (Figure 1-16). The actions of HIV on the immune system are discussed in detail in Chapters 2, 3, and 4.

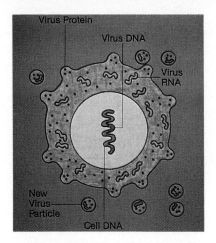

FIGURE 1-16
HIV virus budding from infected T cell.

CANCERS OF THE IMMUNE SYSTEM

Cells of the immune system, like those of other body systems, can proliferate uncontrollably; the result is cancer. *Leukemias* are caused by the proliferation of white blood cells, or leukocytes. The uncontrolled growth of antibody-producing (plasma) cells can lead to *multiple myeloma*. Cancers of the lymphoid organs, known as *lymphomas*, include Hodgkin's disease. These disorders can be treated—some of them very successfully—by drugs and/or irradiation.

IMMUNOLOGY AND TRANSPLANTS

Since organ transplantation was introduced over a quarter of a century ago, it has become a widespread remedy for life-threatening disease. Several thousand kidney transplants are performed each year in the United States alone. In addition, physicians have succeeded in transplanting the heart, lungs, liver, and pancreas.

The success of a transplant—whether it is accepted or rejected—depends on the stubbornness of the immune system. For a transplant to "take," the body of the recipient must be made to suppress its natural tendency to get rid of foreign tissue (see the box below for information on the fetus).

Scientists have tackled this problem in two ways. The first is to make sure that the tissue of the donor and that of the recipient are as similar as possible. Tissue typing, or histocompatibility testing, involves matching the markers of self on body tissues; because the typing is usually done on white blood cells, or leukocytes, the markers are referred to as human leukocyte antigens (HLA) (Figure 1-17). Each cell has a

---

BONE MARROW TRANSPLANTS

When the immune response is severely depressed—as the result of inherited defects, cancer therapy, or AIDS—one possible remedy is a transfer of healthy bone marrow. Bone marrow transplants are also used to treat patients with cancers of the blood, the blood-forming organs, and the lymphoid system—the leukemias and lymphomas.

Once in the circulation, transplanted bone marrow cells travel to the bones where the immature cells grow into functioning B and T cells. Like other transplanted tissue, however, bone marrow from a donor must carry self markers that closely match those of the person intended to receive it. This match is essential not only to prevent the transplant from being rejected, but also to fend off a life-threatening situation known as graft-versus-host disease. In graft-versus-host disease, mature T cells from the donor attack and destroy the tissues of the recipient.

To prevent graft-versus-host disease, scientists have developed techniques to "cleanse" the donor marrow of potentially dangerous mature T cells. These include chemicals and, more recently, a monoclonal antibody (OKT3) that specifically recognizes and eliminates mature T cells.

For cancer patients who face immunosuppressive therapy but who have no readily matched donor, doctors have used "autologous" transplants: the person's bone marrow is removed, frozen, and stored until therapy is complete; then the cells are thawed and reinfused.

BUT A FETUS IS NOT REJECTED

A fetus, which carries foreign antigens from its father as well as immunologically compatible self antigens from its mother, might be expected to trigger a graft rejection. But the uterus is an "immunologically privileged" site where immune responses are subdued. One source of protection appears to be a substance produced by the fetus, perhaps in response to antibodies from the mother; the substance promotes the development of special white blood cells in the uterus, and these cells release a factor that blocks the actions of IL-2. Another substance, produced by the uterus, helps disguise antigens on the fetal surface of the placenta, shielding them from the mother's immune defenses (Figure 1-18).

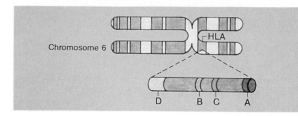

FIGURE 1-17
Human leukocyte antigens. Chromosome 6, site of genes that encode HLA antigens.

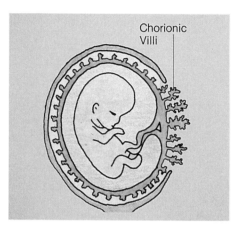

FIGURE 1-18
The fetus is not rejected by the immunologic system. The chorionic villi are the only fetal tissues that come into contact with the mother.

double set of six major antigens, designated HLA-A, B, C, and three types of HLA-D—DR, DP, and DQ. (HLA-A, B, and C are the same as the class I antigens encoded by the genes of the major histocompatibility complex; HLA-D region molecules are the class II MHC antigens.)

Each of the HLA antigens exists—in different individuals—in as many as 20 varieties, so that the number of possible HLA types reaches about 10,000. Histocompatibility testing relies on antibodies to determine if a potential organ donor and recipient share two or more HLA antigens, and thus are likely to make a good "match." The best matches are identical twins; next best are close relatives, especially brothers and sisters.

The second approach to taming rejection is to lull the recipient's immune system. This can be achieved through a variety of powerful immunosuppressive drugs. Steroids suppress lymphocyte function; the drug cyclosporine holds down the production of the lymphokine interleukin-2, which is necessary for T cell growth. When such measures fail, the graft may yet be saved with a new treatment: OKT3 is a monoclonal antibody that seeks out the T3 marker carried on all mature T cells. By either destroying T cells or incapacitating them, OKT3 can bring an acute rejection crisis to a halt.

Not surprisingly, any such all-out assault on the immune system leaves a transplant recipient susceptible to both opportunistic infections and lymphomas. Although such patients need careful medical follow-up, many of them are able to lead active and essentially normal lives.

IMMUNITY AND CANCER

The immune system provides the body's main defense against cancer. When normal cells turn into cancer cells, some of the antigens on their surface change. These new or altered antigens flag immune defenders, including cytotoxic T cells, natural killer cells, and macrophages.

According to one theory, patrolling cells of the immune system provide continuing bodywide surveillance, spying out and eliminating cells that undergo malignant transformation. Tumors develop when the surveillance system breaks down or is overwhelmed. Some tumors may elude the immune defenses by hiding or disguising their tumor antigens. Alternatively, tumors may survive by encouraging the production of suppressor T cells; these T cells act as the tumor's allies, blocking cytotoxic T cells that would normally attack it.

Blood tests show that people can develop antibodies to many types of tumor antigens (although the antibodies may not actually be effective in fighting the tumor). Skin testing (similar to skin testing for tuberculosis) has demonstrated that tumors provoke cellular immunity as well. Furthermore, studies indicate that cancer patients have a better prognosis when their tumors are infiltrated with many immune cells. Immune responses may underlie the spontaneous disappearance of some cancers.

Tests using antibodies derived from batches of human serum can detect various tumor-associated antigens—including carcinoembryonic antigen (CEA) and alpha-fetoprotein (AFP)—in blood samples. Because such antigens develop not only in cancer but in other diseases as well, the antibody tests are not useful for cancer screening in the general population. They are, however, valuable in monitoring the course of disease and the effectiveness of treatment in patients known to have cancer.

More recently, scientists have developed monoclonal antibodies (see Hybridoma Technology, p. 22) that are targeted specifically at tumor antigens. Linked to radioactive substances, these antibodies can be used to track down and reveal hidden cancer metastases within the body. Monoclonal antitumor antibodies are also being used experimentally to treat cancer—either in

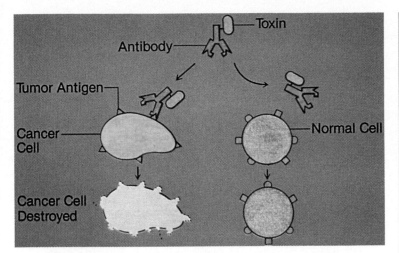

FIGURE 1-19
Immunotoxins. Antibodies targeted against cancer cells can be coupled with toxins, drugs, or radioactive substances, which they deliver directly to the cancer cell.

their native form or as immunotoxins (Figure 1-19), linked to natural toxins, anticancer drugs, or radioactive substances.

Other efforts to attack cancer through the immune system center on stimulating or replenishing the patient's immune responses with substances known as *biological response modifiers*. Among these are interferons (now obtained through genetic engineering) and interleukins. In some cases biological response modifiers are injected directly into the patient; in other cases they are used in the laboratory to transform some of the patient's own lymphocytes into tumor-hungry cells known as lymphokine-activated killer (LAK) cells, and, more recently, the even more potent tumor-infiltrating lymphocytes (TILS), which are then injected back into the patient.

THE IMMUNE SYSTEM AND THE NERVOUS SYSTEM

A new field of research, known as psychoneuroimmunology, is exploring how the immune system and the brain may interact to influence health. For years stress has been suspected of increasing susceptibility to various infectious diseases or cancer. Now evidence is mounting that the immune system and the nervous system may be inextricably interconnected.

Research has shown that a wide range of stresses, from losing a spouse to facing a tough examination, can deplete immune resources, causing levels of B and T cells to drop, natural killer cells to become less responsive, and fewer IgA antibodies to be secreted in the saliva.

Biological links between the immune system and

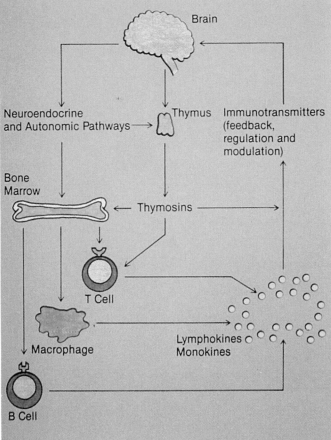

FIGURE 1-20
The immune system and the nervous system communicate through a variety of pathways.

the central nervous system exist at several levels (Figure 1-20). One well-known pathway involves the adrenal glands, which, in response to stress messages from the brain, release corticosteroid hormones into the blood. In addition to helping a person respond to emergencies by mobilizing the body's energy reserves, these "stress hormones" decrease antibodies and reduce lymphocytes in both number and strength.

More recently it has become apparent that hormones and neuropeptides (hormone-like chemicals released by nerve cells), which convey messages to other cells of the nervous system and organs throughout the body, also "speak" to cells of the immune system. Macrophages and T cells carry receptors for certain neuropeptides; natural killer cells, too, respond to them. Even more surprising, some macrophages and activated lymphocytes actually manufacture typical neuropeptides. At the same time, some lymphokines secreted by activated lymphocytes, such as interferon and the interleukins, can transmit information to the nervous system. Hormones produced by the thymus, too, act on cells in the brain.

In addition, the brain may directly influence the immune system by sending messages down nerve cells. Networks of nerve fibers have been found that connect to the thymus gland, spleen, lymph nodes, and bone marrow. Moreover, experiments show that immune function can be altered by actions that destroy specific brain areas.

The image that is emerging is of closely interlocked systems facilitating a two-way flow of information, primarily through the language of hormones. Immune cells, it has been suggested, may function in a sensory capacity, detecting the arrival of foreign invaders and relaying chemical signals to alert the brain. The brain, for its part, may send signals that guide the traffic of cells through the lymphoid organs.

FRONTIERS IN IMMUNOLOGY

HYBRIDOMA TECHNOLOGY

Through a stratagem known as hybridoma technology, scientists are now able to obtain, in quantity, substances secreted by cells of the immune system—both antibodies and lymphokines (Figure 1-21). The ready supply of these materials has not only revolutionized immunology but has also created a resounding impact throughout medicine and industry.

A hybridoma is created by fusing two cells, a secreting cell from the immune system and a long-lived cancerous immune cell, within a single membrane. The resulting hybrid cell can be cloned, producing many identical offspring. Each of these daughter clones will secrete, over a long period of time, the immune cell product. A B-cell hybridoma secretes a single specific antibody.

Such monoclonal antibodies, as they are known, have opened remarkable new approaches to preventing, diagnosing, and treating disease. Monoclonal antibodies are used, for instance, to distinguish subsets of B cells and T cells. This knowledge is helpful not only for basic research but also for identifying different types of leukemias and lymphomas and allowing physicians to tailor treatment accordingly. Quantitating the numbers of B cells and helper T cells is all-important in immune disorders such as AIDS. Monoclonal antibodies are being used to track cancer antigens and, alone or linked to anti-cancer agents, to attack cancer metastases. The monoclonal antibody known as OKT3 is saving organ transplants threatened with rejection, and preventing bone marrow transplants from setting off graft-versus-host disease.

Monoclonal antibodies are essential to the manufacture of genetically engineered proteins (see Genetic Engineering, p. 25); they single out the desired protein product so it can be separated from the jumble of molecules surrounding it. Monoclonal antibodies are also the key to developing new types of vaccines (see Vaccines through Biotechnology).

With growing experience, scientists have devised several sophisticated variants on the monoclonal antibody. For instance, they have created some monoclonal antibodies of human rather than mouse origin; human monoclonal antibodies can be used for therapy without risking an immune reaction to mouse proteins. They have also succeeded in "humanizing" mouse antibodies by splicing the mouse genes for the highly specific antigen-recognizing portion of the antibody into the human genes that encode the rest of the antibody molecule.

Other monoclonal antibodies have been designed to behave like enzymes; these so-called catalytic antibodies or abzymes speed up, or catalyze, selected chemical reactions by binding to a chemical reactant and holding it in a highly unstable "transition state." By in fact cutting the proteins they bind to, such antibodies may be useful for such things as dissolving blood clots or destroying tumor cells. Yet other researchers, by fusing two hybridoma cells that produce two different antibodies, have created hybrid hybridomas that secrete artificial antibodies made up of two nonidentical halves: while one arm of the bispecific antibody binds to one antigen the second arm binds to another. One may bind to a marker molecule, for instance, and the second to a target cell, creating an entirely new way to stain cells. Or, one arm of a chimeric antibody may bind to a killer cell while the other locks to a tumor cell, creating a lethal bridge between the two.

THE SCID MOUSE

Research in immunology took a giant step forward with the development and manipulation of the SCID mouse (Figure 1-22). Lacking an enzyme necessary to fashion a functional immune system of their own, SCID mice—like their human counterparts with Severe Combined Immunodeficiency Disease (see Immunodeficiency Diseases)—are helpless not only to fight infection but also to reject transplanted tissue.

In the late 1980s, scientists transformed the SCID mouse into an in vivo model of the human immune system. One group of researchers painstakingly transplanted a human fetal thymus gland and lymph nodes into the adult SCID mouse, then injected them with embryonic human immune cells. Some of these cells traveled to the human thymus, where they matured into T cells; others developed into working B cells and macrophages, circulating through the lymph nodes. A

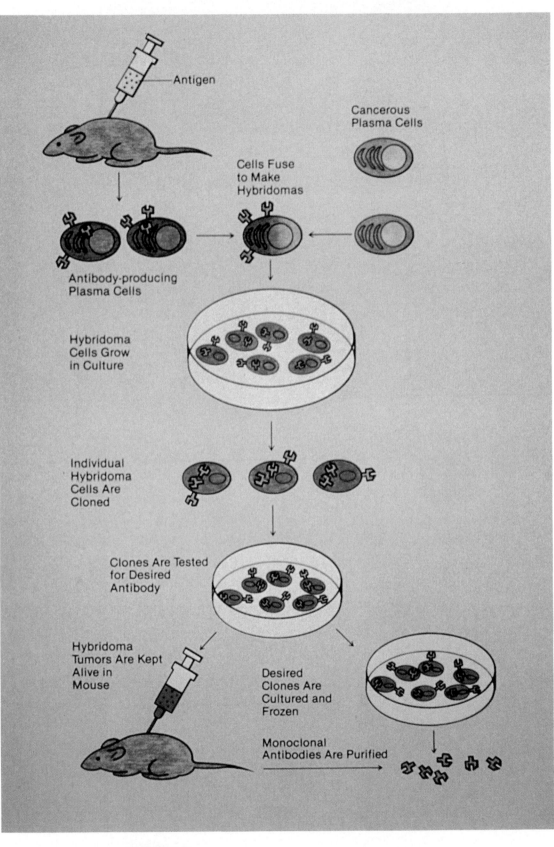

FIGURE 1-21
Using hybridoma technology to make monoclonal antibodies.

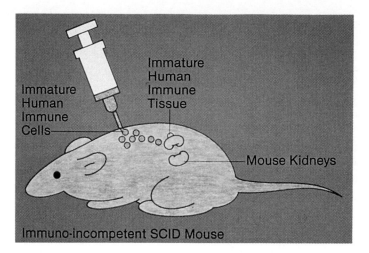

FIGURE 1-22
The severe combined immunodeficiency disease (SCID)
mouse provides a living model of the human immune system.

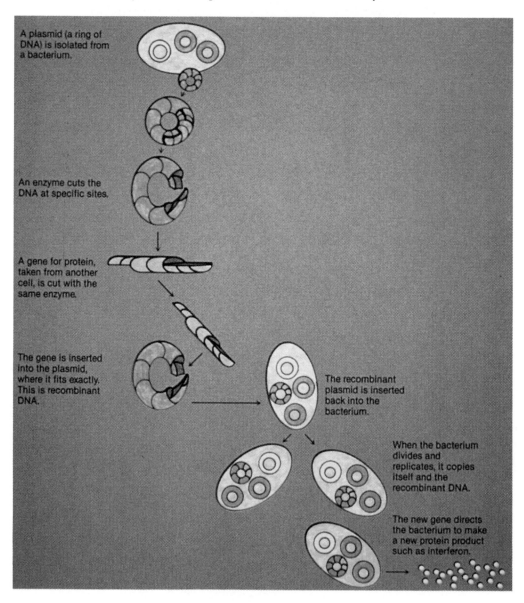

A plasmid (a ring of
DNA) is isolated from
a bacterium.

An enzyme cuts the
DNA at specific sites.

A gene for protein,
taken from another
cell, is cut with the
same enzyme.

The gene is inserted
into the plasmid,
where it fits exactly.
This is recombinant
DNA.

The recombinant
plasmid is inserted
back into the
bacterium.

When the bacterium
divides and
replicates, it copies
itself and the
recombinant DNA.

The new gene directs
the bacterium to make
a new protein product
such as interferon.

FIGURE 1-23
Recombinant DNA.

second group of researchers implanted mature human T cells in the SCID mouse. Such systems amount to a living test tube, making it possible to study the effects of drugs and of viruses, including HIV, in an intact mammalian immune system.

GENETIC ENGINEERING

Genetic engineering, more formally known as recombinant DNA technology, allows scientists to pluck genes (segments of DNA) from one type of organism and combine them with the genes of a second organism. In this way relatively simple organisms such as bacteria or yeast, or even mammalian cells in culture, can be induced to make quantities of human proteins, including interferons or interleukins. Tobacco plants are producing monoclonal antibodies, and goats are secreting the clot-dissolving heart attack drug tPA (tissue plasminogen activator) in their milk.

Another facet of recombinant DNA technology involves gene therapy (Figure 1-23). The idea is to replace defective genes with normal genes, or to endow a cell with new capabilities. The feasibility and safety of gene transfer were demonstrated when, in 1989, tumor-infiltrating lymphocytes, or TILs (see Immunity and Cancer), were equipped with a marker gene (so they could be tracked and monitored), then reinjected into patients with advanced cancer. To deliver the gene into the TIL, the scientists used a virus, exploiting its natural tendency to invade cells; before being used as a "vector," the virus was altered so that it could not reproduce or cause disease. This experiment demonstrated that gene-modified cells could survive for long periods in the bloodstream and in tumor deposits without harm to the patient.

The earliest attempts to use genes therapeutically focused on a form of severe combined immunodeficiency disease, or SCID (see Immunodeficiency Diseases), which is caused by lack of an enzyme due to a single abnormal gene. The gene for this enzyme—adenosine deaminase (ADA)—is delivered into the patient's T cells by a modified retrovirus. When the virus splices its genes into those of the T cells, it simultaneously introduces the gene for the missing enzyme. After the treated T cells begin to produce the missing enzyme, they are injected back into the patient.

Gene therapy is also being tried in cancer patients. TILs reinforced with a gene for the antitumor cytokine known as tumor necrosis factor (TNF) have been administered to patients with advanced melanoma, a deadly form of skin cancer. Plans are under way to engineer a cancer "vaccine" designed to improve anticancer immune responses by taking small bits of tumor from patients with cancer, outfitting the tumor cells with genes for immune cell activating cytokines such as IL-2, and reinjecting these gene-modified tumors into the patient. The enhanced immune response triggered by this technique may help prevent the recurrence of cancer, or may permit the recovery of potent TILs from tumor types which ordinarily do not cause a strong immune response.

THE STEM CELL

Scientists have long sought the stem cell, the precursor cell that continuously replenishes the body's whole panoply of blood cells, both red and white. Using monoclonal antibodies to sort through the cells of the bone marrow, researchers in the late 1980s succeeded in isolating the stem cell of the mouse. Although stem cells represent a small portion of all bone marrow cells (perhaps one in 2000), implanting just a few of them completely restored immune function in mice whose immune systems had been experimentally destroyed. The human stem cell, once it is successfully isolated and purified, holds great promise for streamlining bone marrow transplants as well as for gene therapy.

IMMUNOREGULATION

Research into the delicate and complex checks and balances that regulate the immune response is leading not only to an appreciation of the events involved in normal immunity, but also to abnormalities of immune functions. Eventually it may be possible to treat diseases such as systemic lupus erythematosus by selectively suppressing parts of the immune system that are overactive and selectively stimulating those that are underactive.

CHAPTER 2

HIV Infection: Progression and Management

AIDS is an acronym for the term acquired immunodeficiency syndrome. This syndrome is a set of defined clinical conditions that are the final result of infection with human immunodeficiency virus (HIV). This chapter will focus on HIV infection, with a review of (1) phases of HIV infection, (2) pathophysiology, (3) epidemiology, and (4) management of HIV infection. An overview of AIDS will be presented in Chapter 4.

PHASES OF HIV INFECTION

Infection with HIV initiates a process of gradual and accelerating destruction of the body's immune system. This process can be described as having five phases (Figure 2-1). Transmission of the virus is possible during all five phases. The *first phase* of the infection is an asymptomatic incubation period, which may be as short as 4 weeks or as long as 6 months. It is sometimes referred to as the *window period.* During this phase, HIV replicates in the blood, but the infected person exhibits no detectable physiologic response. Also during this phase, the virus can be detected by laboratory tests used to detect HIV antigen. These tests are rarely relied on because they elicit many false negative results.

The *second phase* of the infection is a short, symptomatic period early in the infection, called *acute primary HIV infection.* Infected people experience symptoms that are flu-like, with fever, lymphadenopathy, skin rash, and malaise. A few people experience more

acute symptoms, e.g., meningoencephalitis with headache, stiff neck, high fever, convulsions, and alterations in consciousness and cognition. Although not all HIV-infected people remember experiencing symptoms, experts believe that the symptoms coincide with the body's production of sufficient detectable antibodies. Ideally, HIV-infected persons should be identified by antibody tests (see Management of HIV Infection in this chapter) during this phase so that they can take precautions to prevent further transmission. Most infected persons view these symptoms as signs of common influenza, however, and do not seek testing.

The *third phase* of the infection is a prolonged asymptomatic period lasting from 1 year to as long as 15 to 20 years, depending on the state of the person's immune system at the time of infection, behaviors to maintain health, and therapeutic interventions. The infected person continues to demonstrate serum antibodies against HIV. These antibodies, however, are not protective. During this period the infected person experiences a progressive decline in immune function associated with a fall in helper T lymphocytes (CD4+ cells). However, because of the asymptomatic nature of this phase, few infected persons realize that they have been infected by HIV and have their immune status evaluated. Recent developments in antiviral therapy have been shown to extend this phase (see Management of HIV Infection in this chapter). Therefore it is extremely important to identify HIV-infected persons during this asymptomatic period if they have not been diagnosed earlier. This third phase is called *asymptomatic HIV infection.*

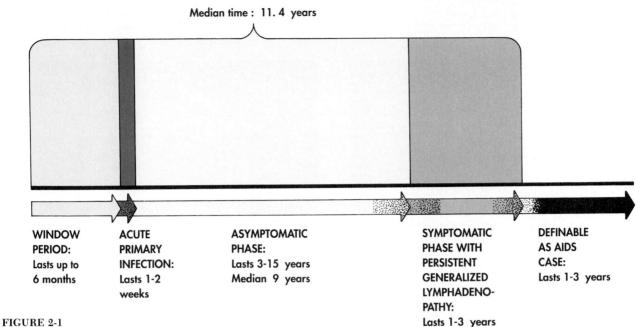

Median time : 11. 4 years

WINDOW PERIOD:	ACUTE PRIMARY INFECTION:	ASYMPTOMATIC PHASE:	SYMPTOMATIC PHASE WITH PERSISTENT GENERALIZED LYMPHADENO-PATHY:	DEFINABLE AS AIDS CASE:
Lasts up to 6 months	Lasts 1-2 weeks	Lasts 3-15 years Median 9 years	Lasts 1-3 years	Lasts 1-3 years

FIGURE 2-1
The five phases of HIV infection.

The *fourth phase* of the infection begins with the onset of symptoms of immune suppression in the infected person and continues until the person develops an AIDS-defining condition. This phase is sometimes referred to as *persistent generalized lymphadenopathy.* The symptoms result from two pathologic processes: (1) failure of the immune system to defend against pathogens and (2) the virus' direct attack on nerve cells. Symptoms vary but may include persistent low-grade fever, night sweats, continuous or intermittent diarrhea, lymphadenopathy, unintended weight loss, oral lesions, fatigue, rashes, cognitive slowing, and peripheral neuropathy. Any of these symptoms are indicators that the disease is likely to progress to diagnosable AIDS within the next 2 to 3 years.

The *fifth phase* of the infection is AIDS. This means that the person has experienced immune suppression and acquired a condition that meets the criteria for definition of an AIDS case, as specified by the Centers for Disease Control (CDC).[29] The criteria for defining an AIDS case were established to ensure uniformity in reporting of AIDS cases. Therefore, a diagnosis of AIDS should be considered an assist in determining the extent of HIV-related disease rather than a diagnosis for clinical management of infected persons. An AIDS diagnosis has important prognostic value, as 80% to 90% of persons with a diagnosis of AIDS die within 3 years of the diagnosis. CDC recently expanded the criteria for the case definition to include all persons with a CD4+ T-lymphocyte count less than 200 cells/mm^3. The expansion includes the addition of three new clinical conditions—pulmonary tuberculosis, recurrent pneumonia, and invasive cervical cancer—and retains the 23 clinical conditions in the AIDS surveillance case definition published in 1987.[29] The new definition became effective January 1, 1993, and is to be used by all states for AIDS case reporting. The CDC Case Definition for AIDS is reproduced in part inside the front cover of this book.

PATHOPHYSIOLOGY OF HIV INFECTION

There are two known types of HIV virus: *HIV-1* and *HIV-2.* HIV-1 is widespread throughout the world and causes AIDS. HIV-2 is mainly found in West Africa and, increasingly, in those countries that are commercially and epidemiologically linked to West Africa and causes a different illness. There may also be other diseases caused by other HIV types.

HIV belongs to a family of viruses called *retroviruses,* so named because they convert their genetic *RNA* (ribonucleic acid) to *DNA* (deoxyribonucleic acid) once they enter the host cell. HIV infects a host target cell by binding to a receptor on the target cell. GP 120, a surface protein on the viral envelope of HIV, binds to the CD4+ receptor on the surface of helper T lymphocytes, monocytes, macrophages, and certain nerve cells. The virus penetrates the cell, and once inside, the virus strips itself of its protective coating, exposing its RNA to the target cell. The virus releases an enzyme, *reverse transcriptase,* which converts the viral RNA to DNA. The viral DNA then enters the target cell's genetic material and integrates with the cellular DNA. The alteration of the cell's genetic material into part virus–part cell (provirus) changes the cell's normal function in favor of the virus. Thus the infected host cell produces more HIV. When sufficient quantities of the virus are produced, the host cell ruptures, destroying the cell and releasing the virus in the blood to seek new target cells with the appropriate receptor (Figure 2-2).

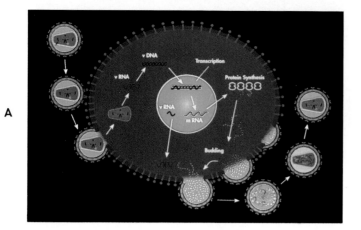

A

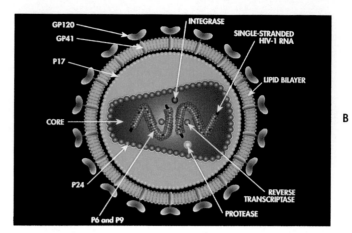

B

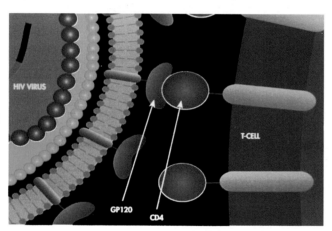

C

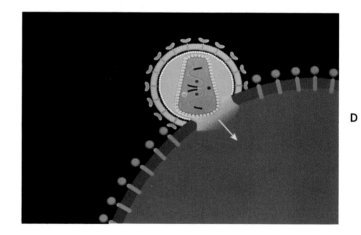

D

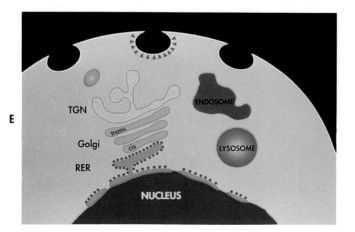

E

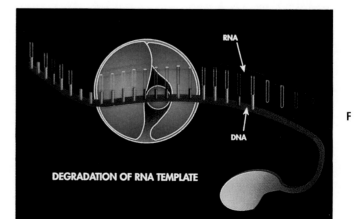

F

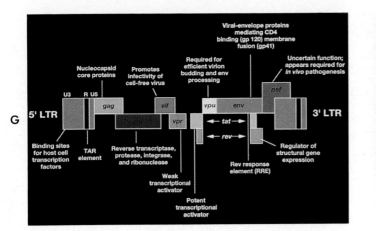

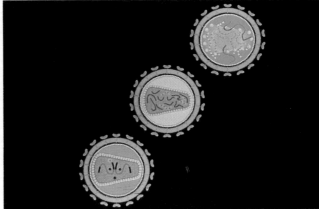

FIGURE 2-2
How the human immunodeficiency virus functions. **A, HIV life cycle. B, Mature HIV virion.** The mature HIV virion has several structures that enable it to penetrate and alter the activity of T cells. These include GP 120 on the surface and a heterodimer containing reverse transcriptase (RT) and RNase, integrase, and protease. **C, Virion T cell binding site.** The binding protein GP 120 on the HIV cell membrane targets the receptor protein CD4+ on the surface of normal T cells. **D, Virion entry into T cell.** Following protein binding, the cell membranes fuse. By endocytosis, the HIV virion enters the T cell. **E, Pathways of endocytosis.** Extracellular proteins enter the cell through a coated or uncoated pit, which delivers it to an endosome. The endosome routes the protein material through the trans-Golgi network into the cytoplasm, where viral DNA is synthesized. **F, Synthesis of viral DNA.** Using the virion's RNA as a template, RT creates an RNA/DNA hybrid containing a single strand of each protein. RNase degrades the RNA strand, and RT synthesizes double-helix, viral DNA from the remaining DNA strand. Integrase inserts the viral DNA into the host genome. **G, HIV genome.** The HIV genome contains codes for every aspect of the viral life cycle: binding segments for host transcription factors; a gag region containing virion core polyproteins; a pol region containing protease, reverse transcriptase, and integrase; vpu, which promotes budding; and an env region, which mediates binding. **H, HIV virion maturation.** Newly budded HIV virions are immature and noninfectious because their proteins are not organized in a functional manner. Protease cleaves the polyproteins into smaller, functional units, producing a mature, infectious virion.

Recent research has demonstrated that HIV virus is chronically produced at low, barely detectable levels throughout asymptomatic infection. Slight changes occur to the virus during each of these replications, allowing the virus to adapt itself to survive in the host. Gradual collapse of the immune system probably permits overt replication of more virulent variations of the virus. See the box on page 30 for other recent research on HIV.

It is interesting to note that the converted DNA, described above, can remain in a state of slowed activity until the CD4+ T cells are activated by invasion of pathogens and other foreign antigens, such as cancer-inducing agents. In the case of HIV-infected CD4+ T cells, activation results in replication of HIV rather than CD4+ T cells. Thus an important defender is not only lost to the immune system, but also adds to the infection burden by creating more HIV. Gradually, through repeated pathogenic invasions, CD4+ T cells become depleted. T cell–mediated immunity is important for control of tumors and for defense against intracellular pathogens such as viruses, mycobacteria, fungi, and protozoa. CD4+ cells also play a key role in stimulating B lymphocytes to produce antibodies necessary to the humoral immune response. Depletion in the CD4+ cells occurs at a rate of approximately 50 cells per year and results in impairment in antibody response, particularly in children who have not yet formed these antibodies. Humoral immunity defects limit the usefulness of serologic antibody tests to diagnose some infections in HIV-infected people. Failure of the immune system results in the pathologic processes associated with symptomatic HIV infection and AIDS.

As mentioned earlier, HIV does not limit its invasion to CD4+ T cells, but the action in other cells is less clear. HIV invades monocytes and macrophages, which probably carry the virus throughout the body. HIV has been found in neurons and glial cells of the brain. Many of the central nervous system (CNS) manifestations of HIV infection are attributed to the direct destruction of these cells by the virus. In addition, many believe that HIV invades some B lymphocytes, the Langerhans' cells, progenitor cells of bone marrow, follicular dendritic reticulum cells of lymph node germinal centers, and natural killer (NK) cells. These are all cells that are involved in different ways in the presentation of antigen to stimulate the immune response,

or, as in the case of NK cells, in destruction of invading antigens.

The pathology resulting from HIV infection and immune suppression is incredibly complex, and the resulting disease manifestations are extremely variable. This is discussed further in Chapter 4.

TRANSMISSION OF HIV INFECTION

HIV is a blood-borne infection, which is known to be transmitted in three ways: sexually (either heterosexual or homosexual), transfer of infected blood, or from mother to infant (in the perinatal process or through infected breast milk). The box below summarizes these routes of transmission.

SEXUAL TRANSMISSION

In the worldwide epidemic, male-to-female and female-to-male transmission is the primary mode of HIV transmission. Experts estimate that 75% of the world's HIV infections have occurred through heterosexual transmission.[172] Both semen and vaginal secretions contain HIV. Menstrual blood also contains HIV. The exact portal(s) of entry of the virus to the bloodstream is not clear. Several plausible explanations have been offered. One is that the HIV virus penetrates mucous membranes directly. Support for this hypothesis comes from research that has shown that uncircumcised males are

---

IDIOPATHIC CD4+ T LYMPHOCYTOPENIA ("THE NEW AIDS VIRUS")

At the 1992 International AIDS Conference in Amsterdam researchers reported a puzzling new discovery. There were reports of individuals who exhibited immunosuppression as measured by abnormally low CD4+ counts but who did not test positive for HIV-1 or HIV-2 and who did *not* have any other immunosuppressive condition. This raised the question of whether there was another organism that could cause destruction of CD4+ T lymphocytes. Extensive follow-up of these cases, however, has not revealed any infectious agent causing the immunodeficiency. Experts presently believe it unlikely that there is a common cause for the reported "atypical" cases of immune suppression. These cases seem to be part of a syndrome, recognized for some time, where some people are susceptible to opportunistic infections with no discernible cause. Even though this phenomenon has been recognized for decades, there were no laboratory tests available until the mid-1980s to permit quantifying the degree of immunosuppression. The ability to count CD4+ T lymphocytes permits this quantification, but has not uncovered a "new virus" or revealed a new disease. For further information on this matter refer to *The New England Journal of Medicine*, Feb. 11, 1993.

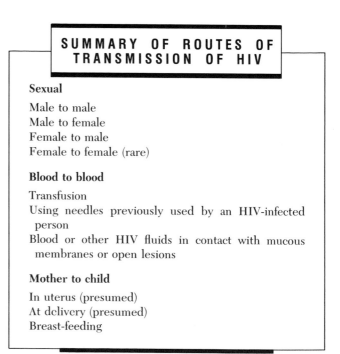

SUMMARY OF ROUTES OF TRANSMISSION OF HIV

Sexual

Male to male
Male to female
Female to male
Female to female (rare)

Blood to blood

Transfusion
Using needles previously used by an HIV-infected person
Blood or other HIV fluids in contact with mucous membranes or open lesions

Mother to child

In uterus (presumed)
At delivery (presumed)
Breast-feeding

RISK OF HIV TRANSMISSION ASSOCIATED WITH SEXUAL PRACTICES

High risk (in descending order of risk)

- Receptive anal intercourse with ejaculation (no condom)
- Receptive vaginal intercourse with ejaculation (no condom)
- Insertive anal intercourse (no condom)
- Insertive vaginal intercourse (no condom)
- Receptive anal intercourse with withdrawal prior to ejaculation
- Insertive anal intercourse with withdrawal prior to ejaculation
- Receptive vaginal intercourse (with spermicidal foam but no condom)
- Insertive vaginal intercourse (with spermicidal foam but no condom)
- Receptive anal or vaginal intercourse (with a condom)*
- Insertive anal or vaginal intercourse (with a condom)*

Some risk (in descending order of risk)

- Oral sex with men with ejaculation
- Oral sex with women
- Oral sex with men with pre-ejaculate fluid (pre-cum)
- Oral sex with men, no ejaculation or pre-cum
- Oral sex with men (with a condom)

Some risk (depending on situation, intactness of mucous membranes, etc.)

- Mutual masturbation with external or internal touching
- Sharing sex toys
- Anal or vaginal fisting

No risk

- Masturbating with another person without touching one another
- Hugging/massage/dry kissing
- Frottage (rubbing genitals while remaining clothed)
- Masturbating alone
- Abstinence

Unresolved issues

- The role of pre-cum in transmission
- The protection offered by covering female genitals with a dental dam during oral sex on the woman
- The risk of transmission from wet kissing

Modified from Schram.[144]
*Risk lower if no ejaculation and/or if spermicidal foam is used.

more likely to be infected. These findings suggest that the foreskin holds infected fluids against the glans penis, allowing an extended opportunity for the virus to penetrate. A second explanation is that the tissue-to-tissue friction associated with vaginal or anal intercourse produces lesions that allow points of entry for the virus. This belief is supported by data that show that anal intercourse, with its higher probability of tissue damage, is the most risky sexual practice. Further evidence for lesions to enhance transmission comes from epidemiologic studies that show that individuals with a history of genital ulcerative diseases (e.g., syphilis, herpes, chancroid) are more likely to be HIV infected.

Regardless of the exact mechanism of penetration of the virus, it is clear that contact with the sexual fluids of an HIV-infected person presents a risk of transmission of the virus. While it is impossible to quantify exactly the risk of transmission for various sexual practices, there is evidence that some practices are more risky than others. The box above compares the risk of HIV

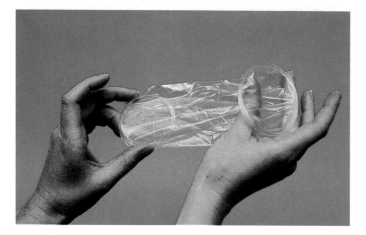

FIGURE 2-3
Female condom.

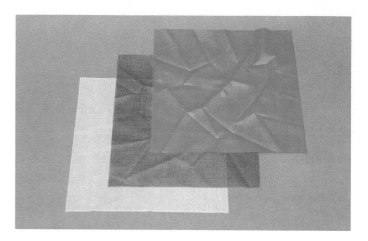

FIGURE 2-4
Latex dental dam.

transmission associated with different sexual practices. One must note that appropriate barrier protection can substantially reduce, *but not eliminate*, the risk of transmission. A properly utilized male condom (see Patient Teaching Guide, p. 246) may reduce the risk of male-to-female transmission by as much as 90%. While there are no data on the recently introduced female condom (Figure 2-3), there is no reason to believe that it will not be effective in reducing transmission. Experts believe that the virus can pass between mucous membrane lesions anywhere on the body or from genital fluids and mucous membrane lesions. For this reason, barrier precautions should be used also for oral sex. A condom on a male and an impermeable cover on a female, such as a latex dental dam (Figure 2-4) or plastic wrap, are recommended.

BLOOD-TO-BLOOD TRANSMISSION

Direct injection of HIV-infected blood into the circulatory system of another person seems to be a highly efficient mechanism for transmission. In all cases, transfusion with infected blood seems to transmit the virus. Using a syringe contaminated with HIV-infected blood also is an effective mode of transmission. A large proportion of current and former injection drug users (IDUs) who have shared needles and syringes with others are HIV infected. It is not clear whether their infections result from use of contaminated drug-taking equipment or sexual behaviors associated with drug use. There are, however, two case reports where HIV-contaminated syringes were inadvertently used in diagnostic procedures and both patients seroconverted.

Transmission of HIV through transfusion with blood

and blood products is very rare in developed countries. Clotting factors are now heat treated and recombinant factors are genetically engineered so as to eliminate these products as a means of transmission. Blood donors are screened by questionnaire so as to eliminate high-risk donors. Blood taken for transfusion is screened for HIV antibodies. Because some donors may have been recently infected and not yet produced antibodies, there is a risk that some infected blood will not be detected. Current estimates suggest that somewhere between 1 in 88,000 units and 1 in 300,000 units are infected.[52]

It is potentially possible to prevent HIV transmission among IDUs. This requires a ready supply of clean equipment and continual education of injection drug users. Obtaining clean equipment is difficult in many states where possession of a needle without a doctor's prescription is illegal. Even when needles can be obtained legally, they can be too expensive or inaccessible at the time the user wishes to inject. Drug addicts are highly compulsive in their drug-taking behavior and are unlikely to significantly postpone gratification while waiting for clean injection equipment. Programs to teach IDUs about the necessity of clean needles and syringes and how to clean with bleach are being conducted in many places (Figure 2-5). Education is often supplemented with programs to exchange clean needles for previously used ones. These programs have reported some success.

PERINATAL TRANSMISSION

Authorities realized very early in the AIDS epidemic that children born to HIV-infected women could de-

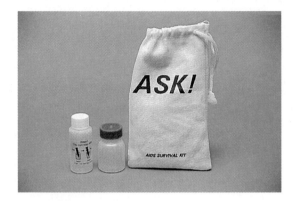

FIGURE 2-5
Needle cleaning kit.

velop AIDS. They quickly recognized this because HIV infection in neonates rapidly progresses to AIDS, usually within 2 years. What authorities still do not understand is why only 20% to 25% of neonates born to infected mothers are infected with the virus. This is a major mystery of HIV transmission, as it is not clear why the virus passes to only some neonates. It is also not known whether the virus is transmitted in utero or at the time of birth or at both times. There seems to be no difference in neonatal infection rates by form of delivery. Infants who are delivered by cesarean section have the same likelihood of being infected as infants delivered vaginally. This, together with the finding that HIV can be found in the tissue of aborted fetuses at 20 weeks' gestation, may suggest that transmission occurs across the placenta. Attempts to relate infant infection rates to the clinical state of the mother have been unsuccessful. Infants born to asymptomatic HIV-positive women have the same infection rates as infants born to mothers with full-blown AIDS.

Until this phenomenon is better understood, the only prevention of perinatal HIV transmission seems to be prevention of pregnancy in HIV-positive women. Unfortunately, many women do not know they are HIV positive and, often, only discover their serostatus when their children are discovered to be positive. Screening women and their sexual partners prior to the women

becoming pregnant has the potential for reducing the number of HIV-positive children. Screening during pregnancy with available abortion could reduce further the number of HIV-infected children. Many HIV-infected women who know their serostatus, however, choose to become pregnant and to carry their children to term. For further discussion of these issues please refer to the section on women in Chapter 12.

The matter of children born to HIV-infected women is further complicated by postpartum events. All neonates of HIV-positive mothers will be born with HIV antibodies. In 75% to 80% of these children the antibodies are maternal antibodies and will disappear in 12 to 15 months after birth. These infants are not infected with the virus. Those infants who are truly infected will continue to test positive for the HIV antibody for the remainder of their lives. Infected children generally progress rapidly to symptomatic AIDS and die by 2 or 3 years of age.

All children, even those uninfected, born to HIV-infected mothers are likely to be severely impacted by the disease. They are the children of parents with a lethal disease, and they are likely to be orphaned during their childhood. The potential size of this problem is illustrated by the World Health Organization estimate that the HIV epidemic will create as many as 10 million orphans in Africa during the 1990s.[172]

Table 2-1

CONCENTRATION OF CELL-FREE HIV IN BODY FLUIDS

Serum-derived fluid	Percent of specimens yielding HIV	Infectious particles per milliliter of fluid
Plasma	100	1-500
Tears	40	<1
Saliva	6	<1
Urine	20	<1
Vaginal/cervical secretions	31	<1
Semen	33	10-50
Breast milk	20	<1
Cerebrospinal fluid	53	10-1000

Adapted from Levy.[107]

Another form of maternal-to-child transmission is possible through breast-feeding. HIV has been demonstrated in breast milk. In addition, AIDS has been reported in breast-fed children of women who were infected by postpartum blood transfusions. The risk of transmission by means of breast-feeding is not well understood. It seems to be of sufficient magnitude that authorities recommend that HIV-positive women in developed countries should not breast-feed their children. This recommendation also holds for developing countries where there is access to a sufficient quantity of safe substitutes for breast milk.

Research has shown that HIV can be found at different concentrations in different body fluids. These findings are summarized in Table 2-1.

HEALTH CARE WORKER RISK

A special area of concern for blood-to-blood transmission is the risk to health care workers from exposure to contaminated blood while delivering care to HIV-infected persons. The Centers for Disease Control has been conducting an ongoing study to determine the risk following such exposure. See Figure 2-6 for results of this study, "Surveillance of Health Care Workers Exposed to the Blood of Persons Infected with Human Immunodeficiency Virus (HIV): United States." At the time of this writing there have been over 1500 cases investigated where a health care worker has been exposed to the blood of a known HIV-infected individual

---

OBJECTIVES

- Estimate the risk to health care workers of acquiring HIV infection after exposure to HIV-infected blood.
- Describe the circumstances of exposures sustained by health care workers.
- Collect information on post-exposure use and toxicity of chemotherapeutic agents.

METHODS

Eligibility	HCWs who sustain a percutaneous (e.g., needlestick, cut), mucous membrane, or nonintact skin exposure to HIV-infected blood.
Data collection, HIV serology	Performed at baseline, 6 weeks, 3, 6, and 12 months post-exposure.
Information on AZT use, toxicity	Obtained from the cooperating invesigator by telephone interview or completion of questionnaire.

AZT USE IN CDC SURVEILLANCE PROJECT, OCTOBER 1988 TO JUNE 1991

- 630 new workers enrolled
- 166 (26%) workers initiated AZT therapy
- 133 workers: follow-up information available:
    96 (72%) experienced one or more symptoms—nausea (59); malaise/fatigue (43); headache (27); vomiting (14)
    30% discontinued AZT use due to adverse events before completing the prescribed course

FIGURE 2-6
Surveillance of health care workers exposed to the blood of persons infected with human immunodeficiency virus (HIV): United States.

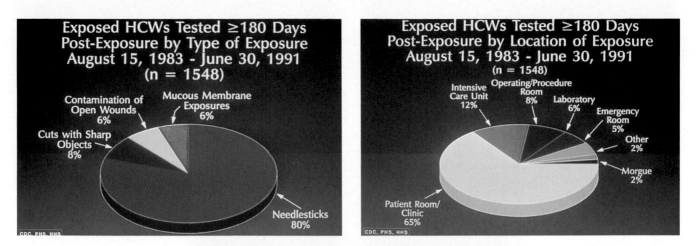

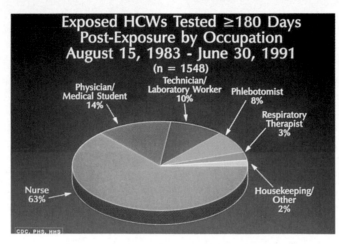

HIV SEROPREVALENCE* AMONG ENROLLED HEALTH CARE WORKERS, AUGUST 1983 TO JUNE 1991

Exposure type	Number positive	Number tested	Infection rate per 100 HCWs (upper limit of 95% CI)
Percutaneous	4	1366	0.29 (0.67)
Mucous membrane/nonintact skin	0	182	0.00 (1.62)
TOTAL	4	1548	0.26 (0.59)

*Serum tested ≥ 180 days after exposure.

CONCLUSIONS

- The average occupational risk of acquiring HIV infection after percutaneous exposure to HIV-infected blood is 0.3%.
- The risk after mucous membrane or nonintact skin exposure is lower than 0.3%, but not well quantified.
- Symptoms occurred in 72% of those taking AZT.
- Efficacy and safety of AZT prophylaxis after occupational HIV exposure are currently unknown.

FIGURE 2-6
For legend see opposite page.

through a needle stick, a cut with a sharp instrument, or a splash to the mucous membranes or open lesion. The health care workers entered into the study if they were negative for HIV antibodies at the time of the exposure. They were followed for 1 year after exposure. Only 4 persons (0.3%) of the 1500 health care workers have seroconverted. All seroconverters had experienced their exposure through a needle stick.

In another CDC study, 85 health care workers, who deny any other risk except occupational risk, have been diagnosed with AIDS. About 62% of these individuals remember incidents of exposure to the blood and body fluids of patients. The HIV status of the patient was not known, however, and the HIV status of the health care worker was not determined at the time of exposure.

One can conclude that there is a small, but real, risk of occupational exposure for health care workers. The risk can be minimized by careful adherence to universal precautions and avoidance of certain high-risk practices such as recapping needles and failing to use proper procedures for disposing of sharps. In addition, proper use of barriers, such as gloves, gowns, and goggles, can reduce the potential for exposure to HIV. Health care workers must be cautious so as to protect themselves, and they have an absolute duty to avoid behaving in a way that puts co-workers at risk. The box below delineates body fluids to which universal precautions apply and do not apply. Also see Infection Control in Chapter 14.

An additional potential blood-to-blood transmission risk is associated with an infected health care worker passing the infection to patients. There has been one case report of a dentist who seems to have transmitted his HIV infection to six of his patients, although the mechanism of transmission is unclear.[35] Follow-up studies of thousands of patients who have been treated by HIV-infected health care workers have not revealed any other transmissions.[35] Thus, this mode of transmission is possible but extremely unlikely.

DISTRIBUTION OF HIV INFECTION

Epidemiologists have had great difficulty tracking the course of the HIV epidemic. One reason is that it has been difficult to track the progression of infection in individuals. Most HIV infections are unrecognized until symptoms appear during the last stages of the infection. Frequently this is 8 to 12 years after onset of infection in adults. Consequently, the current data on the epidemic come from diagnosed cases of AIDS that represent infections that probably occurred 8 to 12 years prior to diagnosis. Thus, the best and most current data describe the HIV epidemic as it was, on the average, 10 years ago.

UNIVERSAL PRECAUTIONS FOR PREVENTION OF TRANSMISSION OF HIV AND HBV IN HEALTH CARE SETTINGS

Universal precautions apply to:

Blood	Pleural fluid
Semen	Peritoneal fluid
Vaginal secretions	Pericardial fluid
Cerebrospinal fluid	Amniotic fluid
Synovial fluid	

Universal precautions do not apply to the following fluids (unless they contain visible blood):

Feces	Tears
Nasal secretions	Urine
Sputum	Vomitus
Sweat	Breast milk
Saliva	

From CDC.[37]

Another problem in understanding the epidemic is that not all cases of AIDS have been diagnosed or reported. People may become ill and die without encountering the medical care system, physicians may not have recognized all cases of AIDS, or disease reporting systems may have been inadequate. While these problems are present in developed countries, they are particularly acute in developing countries. For example, as of the end of 1992, African countries have reported approximately 160,000 cases of AIDS, while the World Health Organization (WHO) estimates AIDS cases in Africa to be in excess of 1,500,000.[172] Therefore, this review of the epidemiology of HIV infection must rely on reported cases of AIDS, recognizing that the numbers may or may not reflect present HIV infections or transmission rates.

From the documentation of the first case of AIDS in 1981 until the end of 1992, over 250,000 cases of AIDS have been reported in the United States alone. From 1990 to 1992, between 40,000 and 45,000 cases were been reported per year in the United States.[27] See Figure 2-7 for maps of the distribution of the cumulative AIDS cases in the United States in 1988, 1990, and 1992. Worldwide, there have been over 500,000 cases reported since the start of the epidemic.[172] This is considered to be a substantial underestimate of the numbers of cases, because of the lack of reporting in many developing countries. The WHO estimates that approximately 2,000,000 cases of AIDS have occurred in the world. They also estimate that 500,000 of these cases occurred in children, over 90% in sub-Saharan Africa.

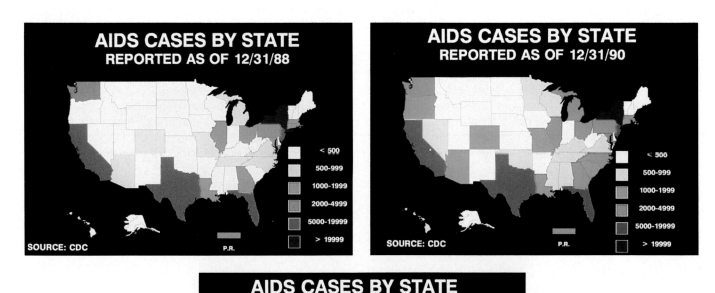

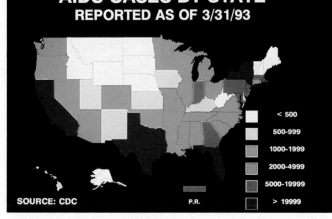

FIGURE 2-7
Distribution of cumulative AIDS cases in U.S.— 1988, 1990, and March 1993.

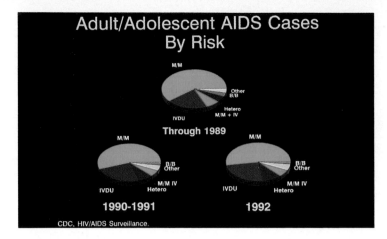

FIGURE 2-8
Exposure categories for people over 13 years of age and diagnosed with AIDS in the U.S.—1980-1989, 1990-1991, 1992.

The reported AIDS cases reflect very different patterns of transmission of HIV in different geographic areas. In the major industrialized countries of the world (i.e., North America, Australia, and Western Europe) transmission has occurred primarily from male-to-male sexual contact and by intravenous drug users sharing contaminated equipment. Within these geographic areas there is substantial variation in the proportion of cases attributable to each method of transmission. For example, in Scandinavia the vast majority of cases are in homosexual men, while in Italy and Spain fewer than one half of the cases are in homosexuals. The majority of cases in those countries have been associated with IV drug use. Variation in transmission patterns can be seen by geographic area in the United States as well. California still reports that four of five AIDS cases are in men with a history of male-to-male sex, while New Jersey reports only one out of four of its recent cases from this risk group.

Because male-to-male sex and IV drug use are the predominant modes of transmission in industrialized nations, the vast majority of AIDS cases have been in males in these countries. Typically, 90% of cases have been in men. However, this seems to be changing as the epidemic reaches into new groups. Some states in the United States are now reporting that 15% to 20% of their new cases result from heterosexual transmission. In 1991, the male-to-female ratio in Florida was 5:1; in New York it was 4:1; and it was 3:1 in New Jersey. All of these ratios are much closer than they were in the 1980s. The pie charts in Figure 2-8 illustrate the changes in risk categories of those diagnosed with AIDS over time. The increase in the proportion of cases in heterosexual males and females is matched by the increasing proportion of cases found in IV drug users. As

a result of the increases in the proportions in these groups, the percent of cases attributable to male-to-male transmission has declined sharply in the 1990s. This is because the total number of cases due to male-to-male transmission has remained relatively stable while the total number in the other risk categories has increased.

Outside the industrialized countries, the predominant modes of transmission are male-to-female and female-to-male sexual activity and perinatal transmission. Perhaps 80% to 90% of HIV infection in the developing countries is transmitted in these ways. As a result, the male-to-female ratio in these countries is 1:1. Some estimate that there are 1.2 infected women for every infected man in some areas of Africa. This high rate of heterosexual transmission results in a very high rate of pediatric AIDS in the developing countries. See Figure 2-9 for the estimation of the global distribution of HIV infection by gender.

While the true rates of HIV infection are not known, seroprevalence studies are done to estimate the prevalence (amount at any one time) of infection in the population. In these studies, blood samples from selected population groups are examined for evidence of HIV infection. The blood samples usually have come from groups, such as military recruits, hospitalized patients, prostitutes, women attending prenatal clinics, or persons attending sexually transmitted disease (STD) clinics, who are being examined for other purposes. No matter how accurate the estimates of current infections, the numbers do not tell us about the rate of new infections. The best estimates of the growth in the infection rate in the United States come from seroprevalence studies that are repeated year after year on the same type of population, such as military recruits. In the pe-

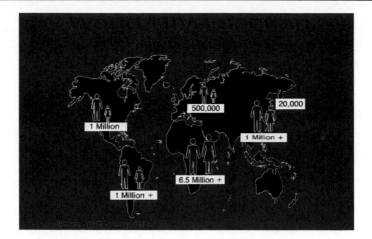

FIGURE 2-9
Estimates of global distribution of HIV infection by gender.

Table 2-2

NUMBER AND PERCENT OF HIV-POSITIVE TESTS BY RISK GROUP: TESTING AT PUBLICLY FUNDED SITES, 1991

Risk group	Number of tests	Percent positive
Heterosexual males and females with reported risk*	489,014	1.9%
Homosexual/bisexual	162,833	11.8%
Heterosexual IDU	141,756	8.3%
Homosexual/bisexual/IDU	12,197	17.4%
Blood recipients	30,495	2.0%
Other/no acknowledged risk	1,161,120	1.2%
TOTAL	1,997,415	2.8%

Data from CDC.[32]

*Heterosexual males and females whose sex partners are infected with HIV or are at risk for infection; heterosexuals with multiple sex partners.

riod 1985 to 1990, 12 out of 10,000 recruits tested positive for HIV. This has been essentially stable since 1988. The CDC reported that 2.8% of 1,997,415 HIV tests, performed at publicly funded HIV testing and counseling sites, were positive. The rates of positive tests by risk group are shown in Table 2-2. With regard to ethnicity, 1.9% of whites, 2.8% of Native Americans, 3.6% of African Americans, and 4.6% of Hispanics were positive. By gender, 4.2% of males and 1.3% of females were positive. HIV-positive tests increased with age, as 0.5% of persons 13 to 19 years old, 2.2% of persons 20 to 29 years old, and 4.3% of persons 30 to 39 years old were positive. This type of data, together with sero-

prevalence studies of hospitalized patients, has led the CDC to estimate that over 1,000,000 Americans are infected with HIV.

Based on similar types of seroprevalence studies, the WHO estimates that 9 to 11 million people are infected with HIV.[172] Two thirds of these infected people reside in Africa. The remainder reside in Latin America, North America, Western Europe, and South Asia. WHO further estimates that there will be at least 15 to 20 million HIV infections by the mid- to late 1990s, as new infections seem to be occurring at a rate of greater than 1,000,000 per year. Figure 2-9 shows the WHO estimates of infection as of 1992 and illustrates the relative proportions of males and females who are infected worldwide.

MANAGEMENT OF HIV INFECTION

Because of HIV's direct attack on CD4+ T lymphocytes and the subsequent vulnerability of the body to infections and cancers, medical management is two-pronged. The physician attempts to retard the destruction of the immune system and to prevent or treat the sequelae of the destruction. This section of the book will present management of the HIV infection itself, while subsequent chapters will be concerned with treatment of the various infections and malignancies associated with immunosuppression. Management of the HIV infection is important because HIV demonstrates a particular affinity for entering, replicating within, and, eventually, destroying CD4+ T lymphocytes. Therefore the important elements of management of HIV-infected persons are to recognize that HIV infection has occurred, to monitor its effect on the immune system, to administer pharmacotherapeutic agents to reduce or eliminate the effect of the virus on the immune system, and to preserve the general health of HIV-infected persons.

DIAGNOSTIC TESTS FOR HIV

The presence of HIV infection in a person is usually recognized by analysis of the blood for the presence of the antibody to HIV. The primary screening test for this is the enzyme-linked immunosorbent assay (ELISA). The ELISA is considered to be a very sensitive test, meaning that it is exceptionally accurate for ruling out the presence of antibody. If the test is negative, there is no antibody present. Because there are virtually no false-negative results, a single negative ELISA test is considered definitive in determining the lack of antibodies. Unfortunately, the ELISA may indicate the presence of antibodies when they are not actually present. Therefore, the test elicits a large number of false-positive results. If an ELISA test is repeated on a blood sample, that has previously been shown to be ELISA positive, the repeat test will be negative 70% of the time. Even if the second ELISA is positive, there is still a chance that the result is a false positive. A blood sample that tests positive twice with the ELISA is retested with more confirmatory laboratory tests such as the Western Blot. Other serologic tests used for confirmation include the indirect immunofluorescent antibody (IFA) test, HIVAGEN, polymerase chain-reaction (PCR), radioimmunoassay (RIA), and radioimmunoprecipitation assay (RIPA). See the following box. These tests are much more specific than the ELISA and elicit very few false-positive results. They are also more expensive to administer, making them less desirable for screening purposes.

LABORATORY TESTS FOR HIV ANTIBODIES OR ANTIGEN

Enzyme-linked immunosorbent assay (ELISA)
Western Blot
Indirect immunofluorescent antibody (IFA)
HIVAGEN
Polymerase chain-reaction (PCR)
Radioimmunoassay (RIA)
Radioimmunoprecipitation assay (RIPA)
p24 antigen
Viral culture

The recommended sequence for testing for HIV antibodies is as follows: (1) Perform an ELISA on a blood sample. If negative, the person is considered to be negative for HIV antibodies (the person may still have the virus but have not yet produced antibodies). (2) If the ELISA is positive, an ELISA test is repeated on the same blood sample. Again, a negative result indicates that the person does not have antibodies (but still may have the virus). (3) If the person is positive on the second ELISA, a Western Blot test is done on the same blood sample. Either a positive or a negative result is considered definitive for HIV antibodies. This testing sequence is exceptionally accurate, with false-positive results occurring as few as 7 times per million assays. There are times, however, when the Western Blot cannot be interpreted as either positive or negative. Such cases can be the result of laboratory artifact, the influence of other infections on the blood, or the fact that the infected person is sufficiently early in the infection so as to have an antibody production below the threshold for determining a positive test result. Persons with an indeterminate result on the Western Blot are generally retested in 1 to 2 months. Because there is some probability that such persons may be infected, they should be instructed to behave as if they were infected (practice abstinence or safer sex, avoid pregnancy and donating blood, etc.).

This three-step testing process avoids the possibility of falsely informing people that they are positive. The social, psychological, and legal implications can be profound. It is also important to not give any results until a positive, a negative, or an indeterminate result can be definitively given, to avoid needlessly alarming the person. The psychological reaction to a positive HIV antibody test is often severe. Upon hearing that the test is positive, individuals may do or say things that have life-altering effects on their jobs, health, families, and personal relations. If they must react to a test result, it should be a definitive result.

While the three-step test sequence is excellent at determining the presence of HIV antibodies, it does not directly detect the presence of the virus. This is an important consideration early in infection, when the virus is present but the body has not begun producing antibodies. This period, called the "window period," may last from as little as 4 weeks to as long as 6 months after infection. Tests have been developed to detect the presence of the virus in the blood (see the box on this page). The p24 antigen test detects p24, an antigen present in the blood very early in HIV infection. This antigen essentially disappears about the time that detectable antibody production begins (seroconversion). The p24 antigen, undetectable during the long asymptomatic phase of infection, reemerges in the blood about the time that symptoms of immune suppression appear. Blood levels rise until they approximate the levels of early infection. Some physicians monitor the blood levels of p24 antigen as a possible predictor of severe disease onset.

Another method for detecting HIV is through viral culture. Cultures take from 2 to 6 weeks, are labor intensive to perform, and are subject to error. While a positive test result is an almost certain diagnosis of HIV infection, a negative result may indicate a true negative or a false negative resulting from error in the culture process.

PRE-TEST AND POST-TEST COUNSELING

A person may seek or be offered an HIV test for a variety of reasons. Either the health care provider or the client may suspect that there is some likelihood of HIV positivity. Health care provider suspicion may arise from client symptoms that suggest either immune deficiency (e.g., lymphadenopathy) or potential exposure (e.g., contracting a sexually transmitted disease or having needle tracks on the arm). The index of suspicion will be heightened if the person describes a history of high-risk behaviors or symptoms suggesting immune suppression or has active tubercular disease (either new infection or reactivation of a latent infection). In like manner, the client may know of potential exposures that have placed him or her at risk for HIV infection. Some persons also seek HIV testing before beginning a new sexual relationship.

No matter what the origin of the concern that gives rise to testing, HIV testing should be preceded by a thorough explanation of the testing process, including names of the tests and interpretation and significance of their results. At a minimum, *pre-test counseling* should cover all the items listed here, which are excerpted from Grimes.[83] Also see the Patient Teaching Guide on HIV Testing, p. 251.

1. The tests for HIV are not tests for AIDS, but rather for presence of antibodies to HIV.
2. It may take as long as 6 months from infection with HIV until the body produces a level of antibodies that can be detected through presently available tests. Therefore, testing will only reveal the state of infection as of 6 months before the test. If the person has engaged in high-risk behavior over the past 6 months and tests negative today, he or she will require retesting. The client who is anxious about a potential exposure can be tested earlier than 6 months and be retested at 6 months if the first test was negative.
3. The blood is first tested with the ELISA test. This test is very sensitive and will detect all antibody that is present. Because of its sensitivity, the ELISA has many false-positive results and no false-negative results for people who have actually produced antibodies. Therefore, a negative test result for a person whose exposure was longer than 6 months prior to testing is a true negative result. A positive test result may be a true positive or a false positive. If the result is positive, the test will be run a second time on the same sample of blood. A second positive result suggests that the blood be tested with a second blood test, the Western Blot. This is a highly specific test, which rarely elicits false-positive results. The probability of a false-positive result with both ELISA tests and one Western Blot is less than 1 in 100,000 people tested. A person who has a positive Western Blot test is considered to be positive for HIV.
4. There is a possibility of an indeterminate result with the Western Blot. This occurs when a diagnostic band on the test cannot be clearly interpreted. The person with an indeterminate result is asked to return for retesting in a few months to determine if there had been a laboratory artifact or if he or she needed more time to produce a sufficient number of antibodies.
5. Clients should be informed as to whether the test results will be anonymous (i.e., names are not linked to the results) or confidential. In the latter case, the client should be informed about the safeguards that will be employed to preserve confidentiality.
6. People being tested should be prepared for the eventuality that their test may be positive. They need a plan for what they will do in such an eventuality. They need to have considered: Who will be available to offer support? Whom will they tell? How will they tell them?
7. They should also be prepared for how they will prevent transmission to others. Health care providers must discuss, before testing, the need to inform sexual and needle-sharing partners if the result is positive. Those being tested must be informed of their responsibility to prevent transmission by ensuring that past partners are tested and instructed on how to prevent transmission.
8. It is common for people being tested to become stressed between the time the blood is drawn and test results are available. This is normal and expected. They should be given guidance as to how to manage the stress.
9. After discussing the above points, the client must be given the opportunity to decide whether

he or she wishes to be tested. In many states, the client cannot be tested for HIV without giving permission.

Pre-test counseling is an excellent opportunity to discuss with people the need to change or avoid behaviors which put them at risk for HIV infection. People who are aware that their health care provider believes them to be at risk for HIV are very attentive to health education messages. This education, however, needs to be provided in a nonjudgmental manner. The "paying for your sins" approach is counterproductive. It is a turnoff, and people stop listening when they sense a moralizing attitude. When the client stops listening, a valuable opportunity to prevent further spread of this deadly virus may be lost.

An appointment for providing test results should be established when blood is drawn for the test. *Post-test counseling* is essential and must be done in person with the client. *Test results should never be given over the phone.* Positive results are devastating and need to be dealt with in an empathetic, personal manner. Negative results should be explained in light of the tests' inability to identify recent infection. Because both the ELISA and the Western Blot are tests for the presence of the HIV antibody, they will not be positive until the infected person begins to produce antibodies against HIV, sometimes as long as 6 months after infection. Clients need to be told this so that they can be retested later if it has been less than 6 months since they engaged in high-risk behavior.

The content of the post-test counseling appointment will be guided by the test result. Both positive and negative results should be given to the client immediately to avoid prolonging the client's anxiety. The health care provider can expect an emotional reaction to either result, and should provide enough time for the client to express it. In addition, the client's potential for a suicidal response should be evaluated. Appropriate psychiatric consultation or referral should be sought when necessary.

The HIV-positive person should be told the following:

1. The test result indicates that the person is infected with the virus, not that the person has AIDS. The best data available suggest that the median length of time between infection and the diagnosis of AIDS in adults may be as long as 11 years; much of this time is without symptoms.
2. New treatments have been shown to delay onset of serious symptoms and to prolong life, even for those who already have symptoms. Scientists regularly are discovering new treatments and new uses for existing treatments. Many health care providers view HIV infection as a chronic disease, which is becoming more and more manageable. People who are HIV positive must not give up hope.
3. A person who is HIV positive must avoid transmitting the virus by:
   - Not donating blood, semen, or body organs
   - Practicing sexual abstinence
   - Using "safer" sex practices if abstinence is impossible. This includes using condoms or nonpenetrating sex that avoids exposure of partners to one's body fluids
   - Not sharing personal hygiene items (razors, toothbrushes, etc.)
   - Informing health care providers of his or her HIV status
   - Encouraging all sexual or needle-sharing partners to obtain HIV testing
   - Not sharing needles with another person
   - Taking all necessary steps to avoid pregnancy (for women)
4. The health care provider will not abandon the HIV-positive client and will help find appropriate specialists and social services for the client as the need arises.

News of a positive test result usually is so devastating that people often do not hear or remember any other information. Therefore, a follow-up counseling and education session should be scheduled to repeat the information discussed here and to allow the client to ask questions.

In the case of a negative result, the emotional content of the counseling session is less difficult. However, the educational component of the session is no less important. Except in cases of testing that is required because the person is applying for insurance, has had an occupational exposure, or received a potential exposure through a blood transfusion, there was some past behavior that led the client and health care provider to decide testing was necessary. This behavior, until stopped, will continue to put the client at risk for infection. The sense of relief experienced by people hearing that they are negative makes them attentive and full of resolve to avoid these circumstances in the future. This is an excellent opportunity for the health care provider to communicate clear messages about avoidance of IV drug use, unsafe sexual practices, use of condoms, and avoidance of multiple sexual partners.

There are other implications to HIV testing. HIV is a disease that greatly stigmatizes people. HIV-infected people are thought to engage in behaviors considered by many to be morally reprehensible. These same behaviors are against the law in many states. In addition, many people incorrectly believe that HIV infection can be spread through casual contact and, therefore, will cut off interaction with someone who is infected. Testing positive can result in job loss, loss of medical insurance, and rupture in family and social relations. Therefore, the health care provider and the client must carefully determine who will have access to the records of test results or who will know a test has been ordered. While all medical information should be confidential, special precautions may be necessary in the case of HIV infection. This special need was recognized by several state legislatures, which have made the unauthorized release of HIV test results subject to civil and criminal penalties. All health care providers should appreciate the moral and legal implications of unauthorized release of HIV results.

MONITORING IMMUNE STATUS
Measurement of CD4+ Cells

Because one of the major impacts of HIV infection is gradual destruction of the body's CD4+ T cells, continual monitoring of the level of these cells is a basic tool for management of persons with HIV infection. Individuals who are not HIV infected will typically have 800 to 1000 CD4+ cells per cubic millimeter of blood, with a range from 600/mm^3 to 1200/mm^3. CD4+ counts can vary greatly for the same individual, with the presence of infection, or even with the time of day that the blood sample is taken. A CD4+ count is performed as soon as a person is known to be positive, in order to establish a baseline for the person and to establish where the person is in the disease process. An HIV-infected person with a CD4+ count in the normal range will probably have several years of symptom-free life ahead of him or her. Individuals with CD4+ counts between 200 and 500 will be quite likely to have generalized symptoms (night sweats, lymphadenopathy, etc.) and may also experience some opportunistic infections. With CD4+ counts below 200, an HIV-infected person is likely to contract any of the infections or malignancies associated with AIDS. Recognizing that CD4+ counts below 200 are markers of severe immunosuppression in HIV-positive persons, the Centers for Disease Control decided to include a CD4+ count of less than 200 in the case definition of AIDS. Persons with CD4+ counts of less than 50 are highly likely to have, or be at risk for, multiple opportunistic diseases. They are also at risk for progression to death.

Thus the CD4+ count is an extremely good surrogate marker of the state of the immune system and a good predictor of HIV-related disease. Table 2-3 shows the rates of people progressing to an AIDS-defining condition within 18 months by their CD4+ counts. The count also has been shown to be a good predictor of the

Table 2-3

RATES OF PEOPLE PROGRESSING TO AN AIDS-DEFINING CONDITION WITHIN 18 MONTHS BY CD4+ COUNT

CD4+ count/mm^3	Probability of receiving an AIDS-defining diagnosis
100	60%
200	30%
300	15%
400	8%
500	3%

Data from Bartlett.[8]

Table 2-4

PERCENT OF PERSONS WITH A SPECIFIC CD4+ COUNT SURVIVING FOR 1 YEAR

CD4+ count/mm^3	Percent surviving for 1 year
200-499	92
100-199	79
60-99	71
40-59	62
20-39	51
10-19	48
5-09	44
1-04	17

Data from Nightingale and Cal.[122]

likelihood of survival. Table 2-4 shows the 1-year survival of a large cohort of HIV-infected persons by their CD4+ counts.

Many HIV-infected persons view the CD4+ count as the most important information they receive about their condition. They are often knowledgeable about the meaning of this test and its relationship to progression of their infection. When providing information on test results, health care workers should remind their patients that CD4+ counts fluctuate as much as 20% within the same laboratory, and more between laboratories, due to multiple patient and laboratory factors. Therefore, health care workers should caution patients against reading too much meaning into any single CD4+ count, particularly if it is being compared with a test performed at a different laboratory.

Table 2-5

HEMATOLOGIC TESTS USED IN PREDICTING HIV PROGRESSION

Test	Common term	Value above which is considered abnormal*
Serum p24 antigen	p24 ag	40 (pg/ml)
Beta-2 microglobulin	β_2 M	10^{-6} (g/L)
Neopterin level	None	10 (nmol/L)
Erythrocyte sedimentation rate	ESR	50 (mm)
Immunoglobulin G	IgG	17 (g/L)
Immunoglobulin A	IgA	4 (g/L)

Note: Serum anti-p24 and serum anti-p18 determinations also are used for predictive purposes. They are reported as positive or negative. In HIV-infected persons, negative values are considered to predict more rapid progression to severe disease.
*Data for these values are from Chevret, Roquin, Ganne, and Lefrere.[41]

CD8+ Suppressor Cell Assay

Another test utilized to monitor HIV-positive persons is the CD8+ suppressor cell assay. This test measures the level of CD8+ T suppressor cells, which normally range between 300 and 600/mm³ of blood. The result of this test is used in conjunction with a CD4+ cell count performed on the same sample of blood to determine the ratio of CD4+ cells to CD8+ cells. The normal value for this ratio is in the range of 1.8-2.0 to 1. In HIV-infected persons the difference between the measures progressively declines until it approaches zero. This is a result of both increasing CD8+ counts early in the infection and declining CD4+ counts. Later in the infection the CD8+ count also tends to decline.

The role of the CD8+ suppressor cell in HIV infection is not well understood. One research study has shown that CD8+ cells inhibit replication of HIV *in vitro*.[160] Several studies have attempted to evaluate the T4/T8 ratio as a predictor of the future course of HIV infection, with wide variation in results. There is no evidence that the T4/T8 ratio is a better predictor of disease course than is the absolute CD4+ count by itself.

Other Laboratory Tests for Monitoring

Several other laboratory tests utilized to predict the likelihood of progression to severe immunosuppression

are presented in Table 2-5. All have been evaluated in research studies for their ability to predict disease progression. None have been found to be superior to others in all circumstances. In addition, most of the studies on these laboratory tests have been conducted on male cohorts. Therefore, the ability of the tests to predict disease progression for women is not known. Finally, one should recognize that laboratory findings are only indicators of underlying physiologic processes in HIV infection. The findings do not dictate the types and severity of opportunistic diseases that an infected person may experience or the person's ability to recover from these diseases. None of the tests in Table 2-5 have been shown to have any clinical significance. Only the CD4+ count has been used for making clinical decisions.

ANTIRETROVIRAL THERAPY

Antiretroviral therapy is one of the most rapidly developing areas of pharmacotherapy. New compounds are now being tested and are likely to be on the market by the time this book is published. At this moment, dozens of studies of antiretrovirals are being conducted. These studies are evaluating various dosage levels of different drugs and combination therapies that are being administered at different stages of HIV infection and immunosuppression. As a result, this book will only cover the standard therapies now in use. Different therapies and different approaches to therapy most likely will be in use by the time this book is published. Readers are encouraged to consult knowledgeable colleagues and pharmacology books. The principal antiretroviral drugs in current use, dosages, and known side effects are presented here.

Zidovudine (AZT, Retrovir). This drug is a nucleoside analog whose function is to inhibit the reverse transcriptase of the HIV virus. It has been demonstrated to prolong survival, reduce the number of opportunistic infections, and slow the rate of immunosuppression when given to persons whose CD4+ counts are less than 500/mm³. Clinicians recommend that all persons with CD4+ counts below that level receive zidovudine. The recommended dosage is 500 to 600 mg per day, usually given at 100 mg every 4 hours during waking hours. Some physicians believe that compliance improves when the dosage is 200 mg every 8 hours. There is no evidence that one regimen is therapeutically superior to another. People are maintained on the recommended dosage until they experience side effects or until zidovudine appears to lose its effectiveness (as evidenced by rapid decline in CD4+ counts or onset of new opportunistic disease). Many persons report side effects that include nausea, insomnia, headache, flu-like symptoms, fatigue, and/or myalgia during the first weeks of therapy. Almost all persons are relieved of these symptoms after 6 to 8 weeks. The major side effects, however, are macrocytic anemia (unaffected by folic acid, vitamin B_{12}) and granulocytopenia. These are relatively infrequent (1% to 2% of persons per year) in asymptomatic persons on 500 to 600 mg/day. These side effects increase to as high as 40% of persons with a diagnosis of AIDS or those who are long-term users of zidovudine.[8] Hemoglobin values of <7.5 g/dl or an absolute neutrophil count (ANC) of <500/mm^3 suggests need for intervention. Medical management includes discontinuing zidovudine, reducing the dosage, adding other antiretroviral drugs, transfusing blood, or administering recombinant human erythropoietin, G-CSF (Neupogen), GM-CSF (Prokine, Leukine), or some combination of these approaches. Recent efficacy studies suggest that reducing the dosage to 300 mg/day or switching to ddI may be the preferred options.

Dideoxyinosine (ddI, Videx). This drug is another nucleoside analog, which inhibits reverse transcriptase. Clinical studies have established its value in treating persons with advanced HIV infection, defined as asymptomatic persons with CD4+ counts of less than 200/mm^3 or symptomatic persons with counts less than 300/mm^3. For persons with these characteristics ddI slows the decline in CD4+ counts and the onset of opportunistic infections and other AIDS-defining conditions. Persons with an AIDS-defining condition prior to receiving ddI benefit less. ddI is also recommended for those who have toxic events while taking zidovudine or who experience clinical or immunologic deterioration while on zidovudine. The definitions of clinical and immunologic deterioration have not been established but commonly include recurrent or refractory opportunistic infections and unexpectedly rapid decline in CD4+ counts.

The recommended dosage schedule for ddI is based on body weight as outlined here:

Weight in Pounds	Weight in Kilograms	Dosage in Tablets	Dosage in Buffered Powder
>132	>60	200 mg bid	250 mg bid
<132	<60	125 mg bid	167 mg bid

ddI is difficult to take. The drug is poorly absorbed in an acid medium, so a major component of the medication is an antacid buffer that has a chalky, metallic taste. The chewable tablets are quite hard and some persons, particularly those with oral lesions or dental problems, have difficulty chewing them. The drug must be taken on an empty stomach to prevent destruction by gastric acid. Buffered tablets are supplied in dosages of 25 mg, 50 mg, 100 mg, and 150 mg. At least two tablets must be taken at a time to maximize the amount of buffering ingested while achieving the proper dose of ddI. The drug also is available as a buffered powder. This is added to at least 1 ounce of water and is stirred or shaken for 3 to 6 minutes. Because of the buffering of ddI, drugs that require an acid pH (such as ketoconazole, quinolones, tetracycline, and dapsone) cannot be taken within 2 hours of taking ddI. Careful instruction and follow-up monitoring must be provided to the person receiving ddI.

Both minor and major side effects have been associated with use of ddI. The minor ones include confusion, leukopenia (5% of patients), rash, and diarrhea (35% of patients). Diarrhea is probably due to the alkaline buffer added to the drug. The major side effects are peripheral neuropathy, pancreatitis, and, rarely, hepatic failure and/or cardiomyopathy. Peripheral neuropathy in hands and feet is seen in 5% to 12% of patients within 9 months of onset of therapy, with the rate higher in persons who already have HIV-related neuropathy or who are taking other neurotoxic drugs. People experiencing neuropathy should discontinue ddI immediately to avoid permanent neurologic damage. Pancreatitis occurs in 5% to 9% of persons taking ddI, and is sometimes fatal. Serum amylase should be monitored and patients should be instructed to report abdominal pain, nausea, or vomiting to their health care providers. Persons with a history of pancreatitis, alcoholism, or elevated triglycerides should avoid ddI.

Dideoxycytidine (ddC, Hivid). This is another nucleoside analog that inhibits reverse transcriptase. Presently, it is approved only for use in combination with zidovudine in treatment of advanced HIV disease (CD4+ count less than 300/mm^3) or when the person is experiencing clinical or immunologic deterioration while on zidovudine. Clinical or immunologic deterioration is presumed when the person is experiencing recurring or refractory opportunistic infection or a decline in CD4+ more rapid than the expected decline of around 50 CD4+ cells per year.

The recommended dosage for ddC is 0.75 mg every 8 hours together with 200 mg zidovudine every 8 hours. If the person experiences zidovudine toxicity, zidovudine can be reduced to 100 mg every 8 hours. The major toxicity of ddC is peripheral neuropathy, which may occur in as many as one sixth to one third of persons taking the drug. Mild neuropathy can often be resolved by reducing the dosage to 0.375 mg every 8 hours. Moderate to severe peripheral neuropathy may be cause for withdrawal of ddC. Other side effects include pancreatitis (<1%, but higher in persons with a history of pancreatitis), nausea, vomiting, rash, diarrhea, oral or esophageal ulcers, headache, fever, fatigue, arthralgia, pruritus, myocardiopathy, and myalgia.

Combination and alternating therapy. A number of studies are being conducted to test whether zidovudine and ddI taken together are more effective against HIV than is zidovudine alone. If these drugs have synergistic effects, treatment will be improved with combination therapy because the toxicities of the drugs do not overlap. Researchers also are investigating the effects of alternating antiretroviral drugs to avoid drug resistance.

New drugs. The most successful approach to HIV treatment has been the use of reverse transcriptase inhibitors such as AZT, ddI, and ddC. At least two new compounds, D4T and 3TC, are being tested. In addition, other drugs have been developed that purport to attack HIV at different stages of its life cycle. Also, therapeutic vaccines, which are intended to produce HIV-destroying antibodies in already infected persons, are being tested. Preventive vaccines, aimed at preventing the virus from successfully colonizing in a person when infected, are being developed. Such vaccines, if effective, would act like measles or hepatitis B vaccines.

Immune Suppression: Stages and Associated Conditions

As discussed in Chapter 2, HIV preferentially attacks CD4+ lymphocytes, destroying them and reducing their number. Consequently, the cellular immune response, and eventually the humoral immune response, becomes impaired. Previously nonpathogenic, normal flora organisms multiply unchecked. In addition, the body's normal defenses against externally transmitted organisms are weakened. Organisms that would have caused no disease or mild, self-limiting disease take hold and produce severe, nonresolving infections. The loss of CD4+ lymphocytes is also associated with loss of the natural killer (NK) cells that normally control the proliferation of malignant cells, such as those associated with lymphomas and Kaposi's sarcoma.

As a result, an HIV-infected person is subjected to a broad variety of infections and unusual pathologies. In general, the appearance of these infections is related to the state of the immune system as measured by serum CD4+ counts. The various stages of immunosuppression and associated illness can be somewhat arbitrarily divided into four parts based on CD4+ counts (see p. 48). These four stages and the general issues for health management during each stage of immune suppression will be described. Information on specific pathologies will be discussed in subsequent chapters.

Generalized* Disease Manifestations with CD4+ T Lymphocyte Depletion

>500 CD4+ cells

* Decline in CD4+ cells
* Loss of energy
* Lymphadenopathy
* Low-grade fever
* Night sweats

• Hairy Leukoplakia
▪ KS lesions
▪ Shingles
▫ Psychologic reaction to decline in CD4+ cells

200 to 500 CD4+ cells

* Idiopathic thrombocytopenia
* Anemia (AZT side effect)
* Granulocytopenia (from AZT)
* Progressive, disseminated histoplasmosis
• Oral thrush
• Intermittent diarrhea (due to *Giardia lamblia, E. histolytica, Campylobacter jejuni, Salmonella, Shigella*)
▪ Folliculitis
▪ Seborrhea
▪ Psoriasis

▪ Dry skin
▪ Skin breakdown
▪ Anal and genital herpes
▪ Vulvovaginal thrush
° Bacterial pneumonia (due to *S. pneumoniae, H. influenzae, S. aureus*)
° *Pneumocystis carinii* pneumonia
° Pulmonary tuberculosis
+ Mild cognitive slowing
+ Peripheral neuropathy
▫ Psychologic reaction to starting zidovudine (AZT)

50 to 200 CD4+ cells

* Extrapulmonary TB
* Lymphoma
* HIV wasting syndrome
• HIV gingivitis
• HIV periodontitis
• Oral aphthous ulcers
• Esophageal candidiasis
• Esophageal herpes
• Severe diarrhea (due to *M. avium* complex, cytomegalovirus, *Cryptosporidium*, CMV, HSV, *Microspordium*)
• Pancreatitis (ddI side effect)
▪ Rectal and cervical dysplasia
▪ Molluscum contagiosum
▪ Human papillomavirus (warts)

▪ Decubiti
▪ Dermatologic drug reactions
° Cryptococcal pneumonia
° Pulmonary lymphoma
° Pulmonary Kaposi's sarcoma
° CMV or HSV pneumonia
+ Cytomegalovirus retinitis
+ Meningitis due to toxoplasmosis, *Cryptococcus*
+ Cytomegalovirus encephalitis
+ Progressive multifocal leukoencephalopathy
+ Advanced loss of motor control
+ Peripheral neuropathy
+ AIDS dementia complex

<50 CD4+ cells

All previous conditions may occur, often in combination, usually without relief.
* Constant pain

* Systemic drug reactions
* Loss of mobility
+ Blindness
▫ Social isolation
▫ Response to dying

*There is a great deal of variation in the manifestations that any one person may experience.
Code for manifestations: *Systemic • Oral and GI ▪ Skin ° Pulmonary + CNS/neurologic ▫ Psychologic

GENERALIZED DISEASE MANIFESTATIONS
WITH CD4+ T LYMPHOCYTE DEPLETION

Disease manifestations are listed for the CD4+ cell count level where they first occur.
Once they are present, the manifestations may continue to occur throughout the course
of declining CD4+ levels. There may be a great deal of variation in the manifestations
that any one person may experience.

>500 CD4+ cells

* Decline in CD4+ cells
* Loss of energy
* Lymphadenopathy
* Low-grade fever
* Night sweats
- Hairy leukoplakia
■ KS lesions
■ Shingles
□ Psychologic reaction to decline in CD4+ cells

200 to 500 CD4+ cells

* Idiopathic thrombocytopenia
* Anemia (AZT side effect)
* Granulocytopenia (from AZT)
* Progressive, disseminated histoplasmosis
- Oral thrush
- Intermittent diarrhea (due to *Giardia lamblia, E. histolytica, Campylobacter jejuni, Salmonella, Shigella*)
■ Folliculitis
■ Seborrhea
■ Psoriasis
■ Dry skin
■ Skin breakdown
■ Anal and genital herpes
■ Vulvovaginal thrush
° Bacterial pneumonia (due to *S. pneumoniae, H. influenzae, S. aureus*)
° *Pneumocystis carinii* pneumonia
° Pulmonary tuberculosis
+ Mild cognitive slowing
+ Peripheral neuropathy
□ Psychologic reaction to starting zidovudine (AZT)

50 to 200 CD4+ cells

* Extrapulmonary TB
* Lymphoma
* HIV wasting syndrome
- HIV gingivitis
- HIV periodontitis
- Oral aphthous ulcers
- Esophageal candidiasis
- Esophageal herpes
- Severe diarrhea (due to *M. avium* complex, cytomegalovirus, *Cryptosporidium*, HSV, *Microsporidium*)
- Pancreatitis (ddI side effect)
■ Rectal and cervical dysplasia
■ Molluscum contagiosum
■ Human papillomavirus (warts)
■ Decubiti
■ Dermatologic drug reactions
° Cryptococcal pneumonia
° Pulmonary lymphoma
° Pulmonary Kaposi's sarcoma
° CMV or HSV pneumonia
+ Cytomegalovirus retinitis
+ Meningitis due to toxoplasma gondii, *Cryptococcus neoformans*
+ Cytomegalovirus encephalitis
+ Progressive multifocal leukoencephalopathy
+ Advanced loss of motor control
+ Peripheral neuropathy
+ AIDS dementia complex

<50 CD4+ cells

All previous conditions may occur, often in combination, usually without relief.
* Constant pain
* Systemic drug reactions
* Loss of mobility
+ Blindness
□ Social isolation
□ Response to dying

Disease manifestations are cumulative over time

Code for manifestations:
* Systemic
- Oral and GI
° Pulmonary
■ Skin
□ Psychologic
+ CNS/neurologic

From Grimes DE and Grimes RM: AIDS and HIV infection, St. Louis, 1994, Mosby.

The publisher regrets that the content on p. 48 was not printed as clearly as the authors had intended. We are providing you with a revised copy of this content and hope that you find this copy helpful.

NO SYMPTOMS OR EARLY SYMPTOMS: CD4+ T LYMPHOCYTES GREATER THAN 500/mm³

The first, and longest, stage can be considered to be a time of normal immune function and coincides with the time when CD4+ counts are greater than 500/mm³ of blood. The only HIV-related symptom at this stage is an acute, flu-like illness, lasting 1 to 2 weeks, accompanied by a temporary sharp drop in CD4+ counts. Most HIV-infected people experience this symptom within 6 months of being infected. Many believe that this symptom coincides with the body's production of antibodies. Often, the illness is not recognized as being related to infection with HIV; it is seen as a simple viral illness. Because normal CD4+ counts average 800 to 1000/mm³ and range from 600 to 1200/mm³, most people are free of any further symptoms related to HIV. Although a person is HIV infected during this stage, the immune system is sufficiently intact to ward off both normal flora and environmental organisms. Such individuals, like those who are not HIV infected, will maintain a nonpathogenic balance with their normal flora organisms. They also experience either subclinical or mild, self-limiting disease when infected with environmental pathogens. If they acquire a disease that is not self-limiting, the disease generally responds to treatment. Kaposi's sarcoma is an occasional exception to this general rule. Kaposi's can be found in individuals with CD4+ counts as high as 600 to 700/mm³. As the CD4+ count approaches 500/mm³, HIV-infected people begin to experience constitutional symptoms such as night sweats, lymphadenopathy, and low-grade fevers of unknown origin. Refer to Table 3-1 for a summary of the infected person's problems and the health caregiver's responses that are helpful during this stage.

EARLY DISEASE: CD4+ T LYMPHOCYTES BETWEEN 200 AND 500/mm³

Decline in the CD4+ count to between 200 and 500/mm³ heralds the onset of early symptomatic disease. Constitutional symptoms are common. In addition, unusual oral lesions, such as hairy leukoplakia (seen only in immunocompromised persons), begin to appear. Other oral diseases found at this time include oral thrush and herpes. At this stage of the disease individuals may experience early signs of neuropathologies, including mild loss of motor control and mild depression of reflexes. People report occasional peripheral numbness or tingling sensations. There also may be early signs of cognitive slowing at this stage of the infection. Because these signs may be subtle and because there is often an overlay of psychological stress, these signs are often recognized in retrospect when the disease is more advanced. Obtaining good baseline data on mental and neurologic status (see Chapter 5) helps the health care provider monitor progression of these changes.

As the CD4+ count approaches 200/mm³, HIV-infected persons are likely to experience opportunistic infections. For this reason, the CDC has revised the definition of an AIDS case to include anyone who is HIV positive and has a CD4+ T lymphocyte count of 200/mm³ or less.[29] (See inside front cover for the case definition of AIDS.) The opportunistic infections frequently manifest as gastrointestinal, pulmonary, and dermatologic problems. Because the immune system is moderately impaired, these infections will deteriorate into severe disease if not promptly diagnosed and treated. Most of these infections will respond to conventional treatments with antiinfective drugs if treated early. People who have been thoroughly educated about potential signs and symptoms of infection will be able to detect and report them for early diagnosis and treatment. Readily available telephone consultation and easy access to a health care provider are important for timely intervention.

Patient education is very important at this stage of the immunosuppression, particularly with regard to prevention of physical and emotional stress and infections that may further impair the immune system. HIV-infected people need instruction about the influence of stress on immune function, as described in Chapter 1. Some also need help with minimizing stress in their lives and may require referral for counseling to handle stress. Patients should be instructed also on the influence of each episode of infection on precipitating further decline in immune function (see Chapter 2). Therefore, they need to know how to avoid contact with sexually transmitted, environmental, and food-borne pathogens. For example, simple instruction about safe food preparation, avoiding raw shellfish, or skin care to prevent infections should be provided. (See Patient Teaching Guide, p. 260.)

People at this stage of immunosuppression frequently experience loss of energy and stamina. They find it harder to maintain adequate nutrition and caloric intake because of difficulty in shopping for and preparing food. Education on ways to simplify food preparation and referral to a dietician may be helpful.

Clinicians recommend that people with a CD4+ count below 500/mm³ begin taking the antiretroviral drug zidovudine (AZT) and return to see their physicians every 2 weeks to 3 months for drug monitoring. This has significant psychological implications for most patients. They will be reminded of their HIV status three to five times a day, when they take the medication. As a result, they have difficulty denying that they are infected, and HIV positivity may dominate thinking

Table 3-1

CONDITIONS, PATIENT NEEDS, AND HEALTH CAREGIVER RESPONSES ASSOCIATED WITH CD4+ T LYMPHOCYTES GREATER THAN 500/mm^3

Conditions/symptoms	Patient needs	Caregiver response
Non-HIV-related chronic and acute diseases	Prevent or treat these conditions	Treat, as for anyone with a similar condition; teach patient about nature of the health condition, treatment regimen, and ways to prevent recurrence
Decline in CD4+ cells	Retard CD4+ depletion	Educate patient on importance of health promotion practices, such as diet, exercise, avoiding substance abuse and sources of infection; update immunizations
Loss of energy	Continue with activities of life	Evaluate for anemia, depression, and inadequate nutritional intake, and treat; help client to plan living circumstances in order to reduce energy demand
Lymphadenopathy	Assurance that symptoms are not caused by something other than HIV	Rule out lymphomas and masses caused by treatable infections
Low-grade fevers	Minimize impact on daily life	Teach importance of increasing caloric intake to compensate for increased metabolism with fever; rule out other potential infections unrelated to HIV
Night sweats	Minimize impact on sleeping	Teach importance of fluid replacement; teach skin care
Oral hairy leukoplakia	Assurance that this condition is not pathologic	Reassure that condition is nonpathogenic and will not cause problems with eating or oral hygiene
KS lesions (see also Chapter 10)	Avoid disfigurement	Excise surgically; use radiation therapy, antineoplastic agents, or inject alpha interferon
Shingles (see also Chapter 6)	Control pain; prevent secondary infections	Provide analgesics of sufficient strength to relieve pain; teach skin care to avoid secondary infections; administer acyclovir; consider use of steroids
Psychological reactions to decline in CD4+ cells (see also Psychological Manifestations in this chapter)	Be free of anxiety and depression	Educate client about normal CD4+ cell range and relative accuracy of the test; refer for counseling or support groups; treat with antidepressants or antianxiety drugs

processes. This can induce depression, which may make it hard for the patient to comply with the treatment regimen. Conversely, some people experience a sense of relief when they begin taking zidovudine. It is as if they are finally taking steps to actively combat the disease in a tangible way. Others will cycle back and forth between positive and negative reactions after they have begun antiretroviral drugs. Some type of psychological reaction can be expected at this time. Health care providers can help the patient adjust to this stage of the illness by encouraging him or her to freely discuss feelings, even about treatment. Statements like "How does it feel to begin taking AZT?" may open communication. Also important is the need to assess and discuss side effects that the patient may be having to the drug. The person who is depressed or having trouble adhering to the regimen may use side effects as an excuse to go off the drug. See Table 3-2 for a summary of potential problems that an infected person may experience and health caregiver responses that are helpful during this stage.

Table 3-2

CONDITIONS, PATIENT NEEDS, AND HEALTH CAREGIVER RESPONSES ASSOCIATED WITH CD4+ T LYMPHOCYTES BETWEEN 200 AND 500/mm³

Conditions/symptoms	Patient needs	Caregiver response
Alteration in immune response	Prevent exposure to pathogens; early diagnosis and treatment of infections	Instruct client on: signs and symptoms of infection; what to do when a change or symptoms occur; importance of avoiding unnecessary exposure to pathogens, including STDs; food preparation and diet behaviors to prevent exposure to food-borne infections (see Patient Teaching Guide on Food Safety, p. 260); skin care and personal hygiene to prevent skin infections and to prevent spread of existing lesions; importance of nutrition and ways to simplify food preparation; how to self-administer antiretroviral drugs; side effects of antiretroviral drugs (see Patient Teaching Guide, p. 252); effect of physical and emotional stress on the immune system.
Idiopathic thrombocytopenia	Prevent bleeding	Teach client to avoid mechanical trauma (i.e., use a soft toothbrush and avoid sharp instruments, straining during defecation) and to report bleeding. Stop medication with this side effect. Administer corticosteroids and gamma globulin.
Anemia	Maintain energy level	Stop or reduce zidovudine; administer blood transfusion; administer recombinant human erythropoietin. Instruct client to minimize physical exertion and to eat a diet high in protein and iron.
Granulocytopenia	Eliminate or minimize impact on energy and risk for infection	Stop or reduce zidovudine; administer growth-stimulating factors (G-GSF or GM-GSF). Teach client how to minimize physical exertion to conserve energy. Teach ways to avoid infection.
Oral thrush (see also Chapter 7)	Eliminate oral *Candida;* maintain integrity of mucous membranes for comfort and food intake	Administer and instruct in the use of antifungal mouth rinses. Administer systemic antifungal medications. Teach oral hygiene and how to maintain fluid and food intake while mouth is sore.
Intermittent diarrhea (Chapter 7)	Eliminate causative agent; maintain fluid balance, nutrition, and skin integrity	Assist client to evaluate diet. Teach about fluid replacement and skin care in perianal area. Administer antidiarrheal agents. Obtain stool specimen for culture; administer antiinfective drugs as indicated.
Folliculitis (see also Chapter 6)	Eliminate associated organisms; improve appearance	Administer and instruct in use of topical or systemic antibiotics. Instruct on skin care, use of antibacterial soaps, and avoidance of shaving.
Seborrhea (Chapter 6)	Eliminate causative organism; improve appearance	Instruct how to administer topical corticosteroids, topical moisturizing agents, anti-seborrheic shampoos, and topical antibiotics for secondary infection.
Psoriasis (Chapter 6)	Eliminate cause; improve appearance	Instruct on administering topical corticosteroids, keratolytic agents, antibiotics for secondary infection; use ultraviolet therapy.
Dry skin (Chapter 6)	Moisturize; reduce itching; avoid skin breakdown	Instruct on administering topical moisturizers, avoiding harsh soaps, and the importance of thorough rinsing after use of soap and shampoo.
Skin breakdown (Chapter 6)	Prevent infection	Instruct client to bathe frequently and to dry completely, to administer body powders (antifungal powders, if indicated) and topical antibiotics for secondary infections.
Anal and genital herpes (Chapter 6)	Eliminate lesions; minimize discomfort	Teach skin care to prevent secondary infection; teach self-administration of acyclovir

Continued.

Table 3-2

CONDITIONS, PATIENT NEEDS, AND HEALTH CAREGIVER RESPONSES ASSOCIATED WITH CD4+ T LYMPHOCYTES BETWEEN 200 AND 500/mm³— cont'd

Conditions/symptoms	Patient needs	Caregiver response
Vulvovaginal thrush	Eliminate *Candida*; minimize discomfort	Teach self-administration of systemic and topical antifungals, use of sitz baths and cool compresses for discomfort; teach avoidance of irritants (sprays, douches, etc.)
Bacterial pneumonia due to *S. pneumoniae*, *H. influenzae*, *S. aureus* (see also Chapter 9)	Prevent or eliminate pathogen; maintain oxygenation; manage fatigue	Obtain sputum specimen for culture and sensitivity; administer or teach administration of antibiotics. Administer oxygen; maintain adequate hydration. Instruct client to minimize activity and conserve energy. Provide immunization for other respiratory organisms.
Pulmonary tuberculosis (Chapter 9)	Eliminate pathogen; prevent transmission to others; restore breathing function	Obtain sputum specimen for culture and sensitivity. Administer appropriate antimycobacterial therapy and monitor for compliance. Investigate contacts for diagnosis and treatment. Instruct client and family about the importance of continuation of therapy until discontinued. Prevent transmission by applying AFB isolation (see Chapter 14) and by instructing client (see Patient Teaching Guide on Tuberculosis, p. 259, and Chapters 9 and 11). Monitor for evidence of extrapulmonary tuberculosis.
Mild cognitive slowing (see also Chapter 8)	Eliminate cause if possible; minimize and/or manage effects	Evaluate whether condition is pharmacologically induced or due to depression; change medications or treat for depression, if indicated. Refer for or teach stress reduction and memory techniques (see Chapters 9 and 11).
Peripheral neuropathy (Chapter 8)	Reverse the disorder or slow its progress; eliminate pain	Suspend use of DDI, DDC, or AZT. Administer analgesics and/or lidocaine ointment; teach client safety measures to avoid injury when sensations are altered (see Chapter 11). Refer for physical and occupational therapies, as indicated.
Psychological reaction to beginning zidovudine (AZT) (see also Psychological Reactions in this chapter)	Assistance with the crisis	Evaluate for anxiety, depression, and suicidal ideation; refer for counseling; teach self-administration of antianxiety drugs or antidepressants.

SERIOUS DISEASE: CD4+ T LYMPHOCYTES BETWEEN 50 AND 200/mm³

Once the CD4+ count falls into the range of 50 to 200/mm³, the person is highly prone to experience debilitating and life-threatening disease. He or she may never be symptom free from this point on in the infection. Symptoms may range from constant fatigue to intractable infections and/or serious neurologic and cognitive disorders. Almost every organ system can become involved. Therapeutic interventions are likely to be very complex and prolonged, with many serious side effects. Anti-*Pneumocystis* prophylaxis is begun at this time. Like the beginning of antiretroviral therapy, this is seen by some HIV-infected people as an important marker of progression of the disease. Consequently, some have difficulty adjusting to anti-*Pneumocystis* therapy as well as to this period of the disease process. First-line anti-*Pneumocystis* prophylactic therapies have significant side effects for up to 50% of those being treated, and several may be tried before satisfactory prophylaxis can be found. Some receive aerosolized pentamidine (Pentam), which is administered on a regular schedule through a nebulizer (see Chapter 9). The treatment is time consuming and awkward for some people.

Under the CDC revised case definition for AIDS, any person with HIV infection and a CD4+ count of less than 200/mm^3 is defined as an AIDS case. It is not clear what psychological effect will be experienced by HIV-infected individuals as they approach CD4+ counts of 200/mm^3. Under the previous case definition people often experienced depression when diagnosed with AIDS. It is, therefore, likely that this automatic case definition will trigger depression in people once they measure 200 CD4+ cells/mm^3. It may be necessary to reassure people that the new definition is arbitrary and has no relationship to the progression of actual disease in any one person.

People at this stage may become less able to assist in managing their illnesses and may become more reliant on caregivers. Hospitalization for advanced care and treatment is more frequent and more likely. Social problems commonly accompany this stage. People often lose their jobs, are at risk of losing their health insurance, and have difficulty maintaining their living situations, obtaining care, paying for prescriptions,

maintaining adequate diet, etc. Close coordination between health care providers and social service agencies becomes important. Assisting individuals to access income maintenance programs, such as Social Security Disability (SSD), may be as important as any diagnostic or treatment procedure. Patients will not be able to comply with medical treatments without the financial means or transportation to obtain them.

Compliance with numerous treatment regimens and seeking social service assistance can be extremely time consuming for the person. Waiting for appointments; waiting for prescriptions to be filled; traveling to multiple locations to see medical specialists, to obtain diagnostic procedures, or to receive benefits; filling out paperwork, etc., can consume many hours per week. Unfortunately, this is occurring at the same time that the person is energy depleted and likely to be ill or cognitively impaired, confined to bed, or hospitalized. As one person with AIDS succinctly stated, "Having AIDS is a full-time job." Refer to Table 3-3 for a summary of patient problems and health caregiver responses that are helpful during this stage.

Table 3-3

CONDITIONS, PATIENT NEEDS, AND HEALTH CAREGIVER RESPONSES ASSOCIATED WITH CD4+ T LYMPHOCYTES BETWEEN 50 AND 200/mm^3

Conditions/symptoms	Patient needs	Caregiver response
Advanced immunodeficiency; AIDS diagnosis	Prevent or limit progression of opportunistic disease	Aggressively diagnose and treat opportunistic disease. Instruct client to report changes immediately.
Extrapulmonary TB	Eliminate the pathogen	Aggressively diagnose and treat the infection (see also Chapter 9).
Lymphoma (see also Chapter 10)	Prevent damage to organ systems where lymphomas are found; prevent spread to other areas	Administer antineoplastic drugs and/or radiation therapy. Provide symptomatic relief of side effects of therapy. Monitor lymph nodes for incidence of spread. Biopsy potential new sites. Instruct client to increase fluid intake.
HIV wasting syndrome (see also Chapter 7)	Maintain weight or slow the weight loss; maintain energy	Manage infections that are preventing eating or absorption. Instruct on calorie replacement, maintaining oral hygiene, use of dietary supplements; refer to dietician. Administer total parenteral nutrition (TPN) if indicated. (See Patient Teaching Guide, p. 263.)
HIV gingivitis (Chapter 7)	Eliminate condition; maintain food intake	Refer to dentist for care. Teach client to use a soft toothbrush, to brush and floss frequently during the day, and to use chlorhexidine rinse. Work with client to find foods that can be eaten without oral pain so that nutrition can be maintained.
HIV periodontitis (Chapter 7)	Eliminate condition; reduce the risk of tooth loss; maintain food intake	Refer to dentist for scaling of teeth, debridement, and antibiotic therapy. Teach client to use a soft toothbrush, to brush and floss frequently during the day, and to use chlorhexidine rinse. Work with client to find foods that can be eaten without oral pain so that nutrition can be maintained.

Continued.

Table 3-3

CONDITIONS, PATIENT NEEDS, AND HEALTH CAREGIVER RESPONSES ASSOCIATED WITH CD4+ T LYMPHOCYTES BETWEEN 50 AND 200/mm³—cont'd

Conditions/symptoms	Patient needs	Caregiver response
Oral aphthous ulcers (Chapter 7)	Eliminate pain with eating	Administer and teach use of mouth rinses (Miles solution, Dyclone, Benadryl, or viscous lidocaine), intralesional or topical corticosteroids (prednisone in severe cases). Work with client to find foods that can be eaten without oral pain so that nutrition can be maintained.
Esophageal candidiasis or herpes infections (Chapter 7)	Eliminate infection; swallow without pain	Administer or teach client to self-administer antifungals or acyclovir, as appropriate. Counsel client on foods and fluids that can be swallowed without pain.
Severe diarrhea due to *M. avium* complex, *Giardia lamblia*, *E. histolytica*, CMV, *Cryptosporidium*, *Campylobacter jejuni*, *Salmonella*, *Shigella* (Chapter 7)	Eliminate causative organism; minimize fluid and nutritional loss; prevent perianal skin breakdown	Collect stool specimen for culture; diagnose and treat with appropriate antimicrobial agent. Teach client to self-administer antidiarrheal medications. Evaluate as to whether diarrhea is due to side effects of medications (particularly ddC). Teach client or home caregiver to increase hydration and calorie intake to compensate for loss of fluid and nutrients. Teach cleansing of perianal area, sanitary handling of feces, and thorough handwashing to prevent transmission of organisms. Teach safe food handling. (See Patient Teaching Guide, p. 260.)
Pancreatitis	Eliminate cause; minimize damage; relieve pain	Stop medications that have adverse effects on the pancreas. Evaluate and counsel client to avoid intake of alcohol. Correct metabolic, fluid, and electrolyte imbalances. Monitor and assist breathing, if indicated. Administer analgesics.
Rectal and cervical dysplasia (see also Chapter 10)	Prevent progression to cancer	Regular Pap smears; surgery as indicated.
Molluscum contagiosum (see also Chapter 6)	Reduce number and severity of lesions; prevent autoinoculation	Mechanically remove lesions by curettage or freezing. Teach client to avoid scratching lesions so that they are not spread to other parts of body. Teach client to avoid sexual contact that would transmit lesions.
Human papillomavirus (warts) (Chapter 6)	Eliminate lesions; prevent invasive malignancies	Monitor (with routine Pap smears) for conversion to malignancy. There is controversy as to whether removal of warts increases the risk for malignant conversion of cells.
Decubiti (Chapter 6)	*Prevent;* promote healing; prevent septicemia	Monitor skin and vascular status regularly. Promote nutrition and hydration to prevent loss of skin integrity. Avoid continuous pressure, friction, or injury to compromised tissue; change position hourly; position to avoid pressure on bony prominences; use pressure-relieving mattress; maintain skin hygiene; manage decubiti according to the stage of breakdown (see Chapter 11).
Dermatologic drug reactions (Chapter 6)	Prevent anaphylaxis; eliminate or reduce pain, itching, and disfigurement	Recognize reactions and stop drug; review drug history and find substitute drugs. Administer antihistamine or topical medications as indicated to relieve symptoms. Teach client about skin care.

Table 3-3

CONDITIONS, PATIENT NEEDS, AND HEALTH CAREGIVER RESPONSES ASSOCIATED WITH CD4+ T LYMPHOCYTES BETWEEN 50 AND 200/mm³—cont'd

Conditions/symptoms	Patient needs	Caregiver response
Cryptococcal pneumonia, CMV or HSV pneumonia (see also Chapter 9)	Eliminate pathogen; maintain oxygenation; manage fatigue	Obtain sputum specimen for culture and sensitivity; administer antiinfectives. Administer oxygen; maintain adequate hydration. Instruct client to minimize activity and conserve energy. (See Chapter 11).
Cytomegalovirus (CMV) retinitis (see also Chapter 8)	Eliminate pathogen; prevent blindness	Diagnose and treat with ganciclovir or foscarnet early to prevent permanent blindness.
Meningitis/encephalitis due to *Toxoplasma gondii, Cryptococcus neoformans,* CMV (Chapter 8)	Eliminate pathogen; control pain; maintain support of physical function to prevent death or permanent disability	Administer IV antiinfective therapy; administer analgesics. Provide life support (fluids and electrolytes, breathing) as indicated. Provide all care as indicated by client's level of consciousness. (See Chapter 11).
Progressive multifocal leukoencephalopathy (Chapter 8)	Adapt daily life to symptoms (altered consciousness or cognition, aphasia, blindness, hemiparesis, and/or ataxia); control pain	Provide support for activities of daily living for symptomatic client. Ensure safety. Administer analgesics.
Advanced loss of motor control (Chapter 8)	Adapt activities of daily living to alterations in walking, standing, position, balance, grabbing, and holding	Provide assistance with activities of daily living, transportation, etc. Provide assistive devices and equipment, such as walkers. (See Chapter 11).
Peripheral neuropathy (Chapter 8)	Adapt life to cope with constant pain and paresthesia; control pain	Provide analgesics and safety equipment and help with ADLs. (See Chapter 11).
AIDS dementia complex (Chapter 8)	Strategies for coping with forgetfulness, loss of concentration, slowed cognition, dysphasia; assistance with decisions and legal affairs	Depends on severity: help structure home environment to minimize stimuli and to promote safety, teach client to focus on one task at a time and to make lists and schedules, provide for guardianship, home care, and assistance with all ADLs, as indicated. (See Chapter 11).
Psychological reaction to being diagnosed as an AIDS case; reaction to starting anti-*Pneumocystis* therapy	Relief of anxiety and/or depression	Reinstruct client on disease progression, available treatment, and value of prophylaxis. Monitor suicide potential. Provide support, counseling, and/or psychopharmacologic interventions.

ADVANCED DISEASE: CD4+ T LYMPHOCYTES BELOW 50/mm³

The person with a CD4+ count below 50/mm³ is probably experiencing at least one AIDS-related disease at any point in time. He or she is taking multiple medications to counteract both the effect of an immunocompromised state and the side effects of the medications. The number of different prescribed drugs tends to accumulate during this time due to the need to use a combination of antiretroviral therapies, multiple prophylactic treatments, and multiple therapeutic drugs. Many clinicians believe that opportunistic organisms cannot be eliminated, only suppressed, by antimicrobial drugs during this stage. Therefore, once a person is treated for an infection and the symptoms are resolved,

he or she will continue to take a maintenance dose of the antiinfective.

The need to constantly deal with symptoms and chronic, severe discomfort causes psychological, as well as physical, stress. Symptoms, such as an emaciated appearance, disfiguring lesions, and uncontrollable diarrhea, are often visible and embarrassing. People at this stage frequently fear that others will be repulsed by their presence and, therefore, suppress their natural desire for social interaction. Social interaction is also made difficult because of fatigue, inability to find transportation, time required for treatments, and loss of cognitive skills. Sometimes the most significant interactions in the person's life are visits to health care providers and social service agencies. As a result, the patient may demand more time and attention from caregivers, both in the care setting and by telephone.

At this point in the illness, almost every person will have needs for multiple social services to help with basic activities of daily living, such as income maintenance, housing, transportation, meal preparation, shopping assistance, household chores, financial management, and paying bills. Every person requires either a case manager or a significant other to coordinate the multiple services that are needed. Significant others generally perform this function more easily and effectively if they have the assistance of a health care provider or case manager who is knowledgeable about community resources.

People at this stage of the disease generally want to complete the "unfinished business" of their lives. They will need to consider issues such as power of attorney, living wills, burial plans, and disposal of property (see Chapter 13). They may wish to reconcile with estranged family members and repair broken relationships. These concerns are all part of dealing with impending death. Health care providers must listen for these concerns and even initiate discussion of these issues when the patient is still cognitively able to make decisions. Although it may be difficult for a health care provider to initiate such a discussion, many have discovered that patients welcome the opportunity to talk about and plan for their death. They look to the health care provider to give them permission to talk about

their concerns. Health care providers also benefit from such a discussion, as they need to know who will be making decisions for the patient when he or she is no longer competent to do so. Providers need to know the patient's wishes regarding how vigorously to pursue diagnostic and therapeutic interventions. Furthermore, it may be time for referral to a nursing home or a hospice. These arrangements are best made in advance and with the patient's knowledge. Advance planning is necessary because it is sometimes difficult to find institutions that will accept HIV-infected patients or that have openings.

This time in the disease process also heralds the time when the provider has to begin the process of saying good-bye. This can be difficult because the relationship between provider and patient may have been long term and intense. If the patient has been significant to the provider, he or she should be told this. Reaching closure is important both for the patient and for the caregiver. The death of a patient is always difficult, but it can be made easier when there are no regrets related to unspoken words. Those who care for persons with HIV have a special burden because all their patients, many in the same age group as the provider, die. Easing the burden by letting go is a duty that caregivers owe to themselves as well as their patients. Refer to Table 3-4 for a summary of patient problems and health caregiver responses that are helpful during this stage.

Table 3-4

CONDITIONS, PATIENT NEEDS, AND HEALTH CAREGIVER RESPONSES ASSOCIATED WITH CD4+ T LYMPHOCYTES LESS THAN 50/mm^3

Conditions/symptoms	Patient needs	Caregiver response
All previous conditions occur, often without relief		
Constant pain	Relief	Administer analgesics and other comfort measures for pain relief. (See Patient Teaching Guide, p. 254.)
Systemic drug reactions	Relief of symptoms	Review drug history; eliminate as many drugs as possible; substitute for drugs causing symptoms. Provide symptomatic relief.
Loss of mobility	Strategies for coping with daily life	Provide assistive devices and equipment. Help with simplifying client's living arrangements and provide assistance with ADLs. (See Chapter 11.)
Blindness	Strategies for coping with daily life	Arrange for protective living, live-in assistance, help with ADLs, and auditory stimulation, such as radio and tapes. (See Chapter 11.)
Social isolation	Increased interaction	Contact volunteer groups who provide visitors, telephone reassurance, or recreation; encourage use of telephone and joining support groups.
Response to dying	Reassurance that one won't be alone at time of death; assistance in managing legal and personal affairs	Reassure client that he or she will not be abandoned; refer to hospice program if client desires. Help client find appropriate legal advice and a power of attorney. Discuss living wills, client's desires about funeral arrangements, and desires to see clergy. Keep client informed about changes in his or her condition. *Accept that person is dying, and prepare to "let go."*

PSYCHOLOGICAL MANIFESTATIONS

The psychological progression of HIV disease does not follow the somewhat orderly process of physical disease and its relationship to CD4+ count. Psychological impact begins with discovery that one is HIV positive, which may occur at almost any CD4+ level. Some people's HIV positivity is not discovered until they have been hospitalized with a severe opportunistic infection at under 200 CD4+ cells/mm³. Others will have been recently infected. These people may have been found to be HIV positive when they donated blood or because they deliberately sought testing. The psychological progression will be dependent on where the person is in the disease process, the state of the person's mental health when diagnosed, and a host of behavioral and personality traits, coping mechanisms, etc. Being diagnosed with HIV is a severe stressor, leading to crisis for most people. Crises tend to exacerbate any existing or underlying psychiatric problems.

Nichols[121] described a number of potential reactions and phases that a person experiences after testing positive for HIV infection. These reactions follow the situational distress model of *crisis, transitional state,* and *deficiency/acceptance state,* frequently followed by a *death preparatory state.* The progression of reactions is frequently interspersed with repeated crises, so common in HIV disease. The *initial crisis* coincides with learning the test result. This phase is characterized by reactions experienced by others in crisis, i.e., affective numbing and acute denial alternating with intense anxiety. The denial may be so complete that the person disregards all health care advice. Intense anxiety leads to loss of ability to focus attention on one's environment or personal needs. It is because of the narrowing of perceptual focus during crisis that people in crisis do not hear or understand what is being told to them. For this reason, post-test counseling must be provided to the HIV-positive person at a visit subsequent to when the test result is given, as discussed in Chapter 2.

It is not difficult to understand why the diagnosis of HIV precipitates crisis, as the diagnosis heralds the realization of social stigma, excruciating and prolonged suffering, and significant losses along the way to a premature death. Even the person who is in denial is cognizant of the types of losses that other HIV-positive people have experienced, such as loss of job, health insurance, friends, sex life, ability to bear children, privacy, and all aspects of control over life. Depending on one's life situation, an infected person may also be preoccupied with concerns about how to tell family or friends that he or she is infected or gay. Infected people may also have the burden of telling their children that they are infected. One is not surprised, then, that people with a recent diagnosis of HIV may spend weeks or months when HIV positivity dominates their thinking.

In addition to denial, the person may experience either extreme anxiety or depression. Anxiety can be a functional behavior if it helps one summon the energy and resolve to face the problems associated with HIV positivity. Paralyzing anxiety may be temporarily relieved by antianxiety pharmacologic agents. Antianxiety drugs, however, must be monitored closely and withdrawn before they interfere with the person's ability to productively adapt to his or her situation. Depression can become disabling and even life threatening if severe and accompanied by thoughts of (or attempts at) suicide. Some HIV-positive people report being so distraught that they give away all belongings or quit their jobs only to realize, too late, that they had 10 to 20 more years to live. Antidepressant medications and counseling may be temporarily needed.

The *transitional state,* according to Nichols, begins when alternating feelings of anger, guilt, self-pity, and anxiety overcome denial. This is a period of disruption and confusion. In this stage, people begin thinking of themselves as having HIV infection. This may be viewed as acceptance of the reality of the infection and the need to deal with its consequences. Having HIV is, in effect, an addition to one's self-image. This stage may be the time when counseling for "plan making" can be best utilized and when the HIV-infected individual is willing to seek social services or support groups. Acceptance of one's HIV status may give rise to feelings of guilt about previous behaviors. The reality of the future may also induce despondency and suicidal ideation. While thoughts of suicide arise periodically throughout the course of HIV infection (as with any other fatal illness), occurrence of such thoughts is very high during this transitional stage. Health care providers should monitor and manage the underlying depression when this occurs.

Health care providers can provide education and assistance to help the person solve the problems that confront him or her. One important intervention is to review with the patient the nature of HIV infection, including its long incubation period, the nature of treatments for prevention of opportunistic infections, the partial success of current antiretroviral treatments in retarding disease progression, and the hope of better treatments in the future. This is not meant to falsely reassure the person but to give a realistic picture of the person's future. Knowing that one may have extended periods of time to prepare for and deal with problems can prevent a person from taking the precipitous actions described above. Hope in a future can be a marvelous antidepressant.

People in this transitional phase are helped by participating in support groups with other HIV-positive people. This seems to reduce the sense of isolation often felt by the newly diagnosed. In addition, other HIV-positive people can often provide sound advice on what works and what does not work when coping with HIV. These people, through their experiences with problem solving, act as role models for the newly diagnosed. They provide examples, upon which the newly diagnosed can base their own problem-solving efforts. Being shown how to live with HIV can reduce anxiety and uncertainty of the unknown. Short-term psychotherapy, which is aimed at clarifying choices and making plans, can also be beneficial.

The third stage described by Nichols is *acceptance* of the consequences of HIV infection. The change to this phase often coincides with some significant occurrence in the person's laboratory values, symptoms, or therapy. For some people, the occurrence is a sharp drop in CD4+ count. For others it is an episode of an opportunistic infection followed by a diagnosis of AIDS. Still others accept their status when antiretroviral or anti-*Pneumocystis* therapy is initiated.

This period is often marked by resolve to take more responsibility for life and the progress of the disease by changing health habits, life-style, and sexual behaviors. A person in this stage may be receptive to health education messages, particularly about nutrition, exercise, stress reduction, treatment for substance abuse, prevention of exposure to infection, and the value of positive thinking.

The person also may be vulnerable to fads and quackery, such as macrobiotic diets, coffee enemas, megadosing with vitamins, use of herbs, crystals, etc. The person's desire to actively fight the disease and to find a "cure" is so strong that he or she believes claims about so-called "alternative therapies." Many of these unconventional therapies, such as positive imagery, may be helpful; others, such as wearing crystals, are harmless. Some, like macrobiotic diets and megadosing on some vitamins, can be harmful; while others, such as blood heating, can be expensive as well as useless. Health care providers, who recognize the person's need for control over the illness, will be sensitive to discussion about alternative therapies. Patients will acknowledge their use of these remedies and will be open to discussion of safe alternatives if their health care providers are nonjudgmental. Otherwise, the person who senses disapproval will continue to experiment with alternative therapies without informing the provider. Side effects to these therapies may be mistaken for side effects or failure of prescribed treatments. For example, weight loss may be interpreted as the beginning of wasting syndrome when its real cause might be inadequate protein and calorie intake associated with a mac-robiotic diet. It is, therefore, to the advantage of the health care provider and the patient to have open communication about all the person's health-seeking behaviors. The provider can reinforce the beneficial and neutral behaviors while educating about alternatives to the harmful practices. In any event, the final decision about using any therapy does rest with the infected person.

Some people, during this stage, begin "shopping" for another doctor as a means of finding the "cure." A person may have heard that another provider does things differently or better. Switching physicians in an effort to find someone who is more compatible is not necessarily bad. However, it can disrupt continuity of care, particularly if medical records are not sent to the new provider. Often this is the case because a person does not wish to offend the original physician or may want to be able to return if the new provider does not work out. Sometimes, infected people see multiple physicians at the same time. This creates risks for drug interactions when multiple physicians, unaware of the drugs being prescribed by the others, prescribe multiple drugs. Smart health care providers will communicate with the patient in an accepting, nonjudgmental manner about the person's use of other providers. This will encourage the patient to provide critical information about other medications he or she is taking.

The last phase is called the *preparatory* stage, which is characterized by concerns about becoming totally dependent on others and about preparing for death. Nichols says that one's concern about total dependency supersedes concern about death. Fear of dependency seems to induce suicidal ideation in many late-stage AIDS patients. However, most continue to struggle for life. The concern about death leads individuals to tie up the loose ends of their lives. They complete their "unfinished business." They are anxious for reconciliations with estranged friends and family. In addition, estranged friends and family are apt to seek out the person with AIDS as death nears. Completing unfinished business may also take the form of finishing projects—writing papers or reports, building, mastering a challenge, taking a long awaited trip, etc. Almost all of these actions are healthy reactions to impending death, and health care workers can facilitate these actions.

The infected person may also wish to exert some control over the nature of his or her death through such actions as writing a living will or choosing the place (home, hospice, or hospital) to die. He or she may also wish to give "power of attorney" and control over his or her care to a trusted friend or family member. This can be a good plan, as it gives health caregivers a single person with whom to communicate. These issues are important to discuss, and patients generally welcome the opportunity to talk about them. Discussion can be

PSYCHOLOGICAL REACTION TO HIV INFECTION

Reactions to learning that one is HIV positive
Crisis

Denial
Affective numbing
Persistent anxiety
Depression and suicidal ideation

Transitional state

Alternating reactions of:
   Anger
   Guilt
   Self-blame
   Anxiety
   Depression and self-pity
Self-isolation and difficulty in interacting with others
Fear of loss of sex life
Fear of contaminating others
Fear of rejection and stigmatization
Fear of loss of job and health insurance
Fear of loss of financial independence
Preoccupation with life-style changes and measures to protect immune system and to avoid infection
Preoccupation with issues of confidentiality and fear of stigmatization
Summary: HIV infection dominates the infected person's thinking, often to the exclusion of other major life concerns.

Reactions to becoming symptomatic
Acceptance or acknowledging consequences

Resolve to take responsibility for disease progression
Seek cures; preoccupation with medical treatments and alternative therapies
Focus on health-promoting behaviors
Preoccupation with maintaining normalcy of life and meeting basic needs for food, shelter, etc.
Preoccupation with symptom control
Grief over losses: health, physical attractiveness, job, ability to care for self, etc.
Hopelessness and suicidal ideation
Emotional exhaustion
Stress reaction to dealing with demands of medical treatment, pain, and medical expenses
Embarrassment because of physical symptoms (e.g., lesions and diarrhea)
Loneliness
Uncontrollable expressions of anger related to neurologic effects of the disease
Summary: Symptom management dominates one's life. Medical treatment and maintaining basic activities of daily living are all consuming. Living with AIDS is a full-time job.

Preparing for dying

Concern with resolving the business of one's life (e.g., reconciliations, disposing of property)
Preoccupation with pain and pain control
Preoccupation with other disease symptoms
Fear of abandonment before death
Concern with planning for death with care providers
Fear of dying; fear of dying alone
Summary: Dying becomes a full-time job.

initiated through questions such as "Who would you like to make decisions about your care, if you are unable to do so?" Such a question will often lead to other discussions relating to death, living wills, and so forth. These legal issues are presented in Chapter 13.

People may also be concerned about disposing of their property, and directing them to an attorney may put their minds at ease. Dispersing all that one owns, even if small, is important because it provides a sense of completion to life. If the client cannot afford an attorney, there are often local volunteer programs to assist in these matters. AIDS service programs and/or a case manager can help in locating such resources.

A particular area of concern for parents facing death is making arrangements for care of their children after death. This is extremely important for them and can dominate thinking and behavior until it is resolved. Even after arrangements have been made, parents will vacillate in their thinking as to whether they have made the right choice. The problem of child placement becomes even more complex if the child is also HIV positive. Placement becomes far more difficult because the parent has fewer or no choices. HIV-positive individuals with children should be encouraged to make ar-

rangements for their children as soon as possible after diagnosis. This will put their minds more at ease and can help avoid very difficult legal complications later in the illness. Parents also need help in finding child care during visits to health care providers, during hospitalization, and when they are bed-bound during their illness.

These psychological stages, summarized in the preceding box, have been described as if they were orderly processes, occurring at fixed intervals, and experienced by all people in the same way. Reality is not that simple. People with HIV respond with great variation to events in their lives as well as to events caused by HIV. Normal life events may force them into crisis at any time, just as would occur with people without HIV. Each new milestone of the disease may also precipitate crisis. Some people have coping skills that enable them to manage each new crisis, thus reducing its intensity and effect on their lives. Others reexperience severe anxiety or depression with each new struggle. Having a framework, however, may help health care providers understand and respond therapeutically to the psychological needs of HIV-infected persons. This is a necessary part of HIV care.

Opportunistic Organisms in Immune Suppression: An Overview

HIV-infected people, because of immune suppression, are susceptible to infectious diseases caused by a wide variety of microorganisms. Some of these organisms, such as *Candida albicans,* are part of the normal flora of the body and become pathogenic only in an immuno-compromised host. Other organisms, such as *Toxo-plasma gondii,* are ubiquitous in the environment and regularly invade human hosts. When invaded by these organisms, an immunocompetent host either fights off the pathogen or sustains a subclinical infection. An im-munosuppressed person exposed to these organisms becomes overwhelmed by them. Still other organisms, such as herpes virus or *Mycobacterium tuberculosis,* are regularly pathogenic (disease producing) to humans. The acute infection that they cause, however, is gener-ally self-limiting or easily treatable in the immunocom-petent host. These organisms can remain viable and in a quiescent state in their human host until the host's immune system becomes impaired. At this point the organism can reassert itself, causing disease. Because of the complexity of infections associated with immuno-suppression, professionals providing care to HIV-in-fected clients must be familiar with a broad variety of

Bacteria

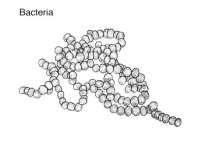

Parasite

Fungus

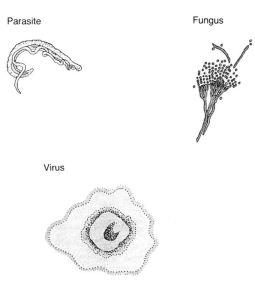

Virus

organisms and their diagnosis and treatment. This chapter will summarize critical information on microorganisms that are commonly pathogenic to those infected with HIV. The microorganisms included here are bacteria and mycobacteria (Table 4-1), protozoa (Table 4-2), fungi (Table 4-3), and viruses (Table 4-4). These microbiologic classifications are based on distinguishing characteristics of the organisms, such as their morphology, chemical composition, growth requirements, and viability outside host cells. A general understanding of microorganism characteristics is helpful to understanding diagnosis and antiinfective treatment of these pathogens.

BACTERIA

Bacteria exhibit characteristics of both plant and animal cells in that they can grow and replicate outside living cells. This makes it possible for bacteria to be transmitted indirectly from one host to another through the environment. Bacteria are divided into 19 categories, differentiated by their morphology (size and shape), staining characteristics, motility, colony formation, nutritional requirements, biochemical activity, and antigenic makeup (Table 4-1). Laboratory tests, such as culture, microscopy, and serum testing for antigens and antibodies, are based on knowledge of these characteristics. For example, mycobacteria, one of the 19 categories of bacteria, can be distinguished from other bacteria because of their acid-fast characteristic. Some bacteria have the ability to develop an encysted or resting stage known as a spore. These bacterial spores are remarkably resistant to heat, drying, and the action of disinfectants. Spore-forming bacteria can remain viable indefinitely in the environment. Most bacteria obtain nutrients from organic matter, either living or dead. In addition, the majority (aerobes) require oxygen to sustain life, while a few (anaerobes) thrive in oxygen-free environments. Most bacteria grow best at ambient or body temperatures; they are either killed or unable to replicate at temperature extremes.

Bacteria differ as to how they cause disease in a host. Some produce enzymes that attack and kill cells directly. Others release toxins that can spread through host tissue, causing cell damage. Bacteria also differ as to whether they are antigenic (i.e., elicit an immune response) and whether the immune response is protective or not. Antigenicity is important in diagnosing the presence of some bacterial infections by serum antibody tests (e.g., *Legionella*) and in developing vaccines against others (i.e., *Streptococcus pneumoniae*).

The goal of antimicrobial therapy against bacteria is to eradicate the organism, if possible, or to suppress its replication until body defenses can take over. Because defenses are impaired in HIV infection, drug therapy to eradicate a specific organism is not always curative. Dosages and routes of administration depend on the sensitivity of the bacteria to a particular antibacterial drug and the location and severity of the infection. Drug therapies for specific infections are discussed in the Medical Management sections, Chapters 6 through 9.

While many bacteria can potentially cause respiratory disease in HIV-infected people, two organisms are particularly common. These are *Streptococcus pneumoniae*, the cause of pneumococcal pneumonia, and *Haemophilus influenzae*, the organism that causes meningitis and upper respiratory infections in newborns and small children. Vaccines are available for both of these pathogens and should be administered to clients early in HIV infection. In addition, conventional antiinfective therapy is effective against these organisms.

A person with HIV may also acquire or have latent sexually transmitted diseases (STDs) caused by bacteria, such as chlamydia, gonorrhea, and syphilis. Other bacterial STDs, such as chancroid and lymphogranuloma venereum, are rare in the United States and are, therefore, rare in HIV-infected people in the United States. Antiinfective treatments for gonorrhea and chlamydia in HIV-infected persons are not different from treatment in noninfected persons. However, follow-up to ensure cure from treatment is exceedingly important for HIV-infected persons. Incompletely treated gonorrhea or chlamydia infections not only encourage spread of these diseases but may place an extra burden on a person's already stressed immune system.

Treatment of syphilis is more complicated in HIV-infected people because of rapid progression of the infection to neurosyphilis. Persons coinfected with syphilis and HIV must be monitored closely for changes in serum antibodies against syphilis. Failure of the serum titers to decline at an expected rate following treatment indicates treatment failure (see Chapter 6).

Bacteria causing acute diarrhea in the HIV infected include *Campylobacter*, *Shigella*, and *Salmonella*, all of which are transmitted by food, water, hands, or articles contaminated with the bacteria. Infection with these organisms can be prevented by proper food handling, water sanitation, and handwashing following defecation. Antibacterial agents are effective against these organisms (see Chapter 7).

Another bacterium, *Clostridium difficile*, flourishes when normal intestinal flora are disturbed. This is the principal organism implicated with diarrhea following antibiotic therapy.

HIV-infected individuals are subject to infections with three mycobacteria, *M. tuberculosis*, *M. avium*

Table 4-1

BACTERIA AND MYCOBACTERIA IN IMMUNOSUPPRESSION

Pathogen (disease name/body site where found)	Diagnostic studies: results	Primary//secondary drugs for treatment	Notes
Bacteria			
Streptococcus pneumoniae (pneumococcal pneumonia/bronchopulmonary)	Gram's stain of sputum: positive for organism; culture of sputum: positive; quellung reaction: positive	Penicillin G//cephalosporin, clindamycin, vancomycin, erythromycin	Common at all stages of HIV; vaccine recommended
Haemophilus influenzae (pneumonia/bronchopulmonary)	Culture or Gram's stain of sputum or respiratory specimen: positive for organism	Ampicillin, amoxicillin-clavulanate, sulfamethoxazole-trimethoprim, second- and third-generation cephalosporins	Somewhat common in all stages of HIV; vaccine is considered to be useful
Clostridium difficile (antibiotic-associated colitis/GI tract)	Toxin assay: positive; endoscopy: visible pseudomembranous colitis; culture of specimen: positive	Metronidazole, vancomycin//bacitracin, cholestyramine, lactobacilli, vancomycin plus rifampin	Somewhat common in HIV infected due to extensive antibiotic use
Salmonella, many species (salmonellosis/GI tract)	Culture of blood, stool, or bone marrow: positive for organism	Ampicillin, amoxicillin, sulfamethoxazole-trimethoprim//second- and third-generation cephalosporins, ciprofloxacin, cefoperazone, cefotaxime, ceftriaxone	Occurrence is 20 times more likely in HIV; occurs at all stages of infection
Campylobacter jejuni (campylobacteriosis, acute gastroenteritis/GI tract, systemic)	Culture of stool specimen: positive for organism	Erythromycin//tetracycline, doxycycline, minocycline, furazolidine, ciprofloxacin	Somewhat common in HIV infected
Shigella spp. (shigellosis, acute gastroenteritis/GI tract)	Culture of stool specimen: positive for *Shigella*	Sulfamethoxazole-trimethoprim//ciprofloxacin, tetracycline, ampicillin, doxycycline, minocycline, nalidixic acid	Occurs in 1% of HIV infected with acute diarrhea
Staphylococcus aureus (folliculitis/skin)	Gram's stain and culture of lesion exudate: positive for gram-positive cocci	Topical antibiotics; if fever or midfacial involvement: penicillinase-resistant penicillin, vancomycin, cephalosporin, clindamycin	Occurs in 70% of HIV infected; mild cases can be controlled with compresses
Chlamydia trachomatis (chlamydia/genitourinary)	Tissue culture of urethral, cervical, or rectal exudate: positive for organism; direct immunofluorescence antibody (DFA) test of exudate or enzyme immune assay (EIA) of exudate: positive for organism; DNA probe technique on exudate: positive for nucleic acid of organism	Tetracycline//erythromycin, azithromycin	Common in sexually active

Continued.

Table 4-1

BACTERIA AND MYCOBACTERIA IN IMMUNOSUPPRESSION—cont'd

Pathogen: (disease name/body site where found)	Diagnostic studies: results	Primary//secondary drugs for treatment	Notes
Treponema pallidum (syphilis/genital)	Depends on duration of infection: darkfield microscopic examination of specimen from lesion: positive for *T. pallidum;* direct fluorescent antibody or silver stain of biopsy specimen: positive for *T. pallidum;* nontreponemal serologic tests (e.g., VDRL, RPR): fourfold or greater increase in serum antibodies; treponemal serologic tests (e.g., FTA-ABS, MHA-TP): reactive; serologic tests are used for screening only	Penicillin//ceftriaxone	Syphilis progresses more rapidly and is difficult to treat in HIV infected
Treponema pallidum (neurosyphilis/central nervous system)	VDRL of CSF: positive; darkfield microscopic examination of CSF: positive for *T. pallidum*	Penicillin, ceftriaxone	
Neisseria gonorrhoeae (gonorrhea/genital, rectal, pharyngeal, urinary, and, rarely, blood)	Culture or Gram's stain of exudate: positive for *N. gonorrhoeae*	Ceftriaxone//cefotaxime, amoxicillin and probenecid, cefuroxime axetil, ceftizoxime	Common in sexually active
Mycobacteria			
Mycobacterium tuberculosis (tuberculosis, TB/pulmonary, may disseminate to other sites)	Infection: Mantoux skin test: >5 mm induration 48-72 hours after testing (see Chapter 9); active disease: culture/microscopic exam of sputum or biopsy specimen: presence of acid-fast bacilli (AFB); chest x-ray: consistent with tuberculosis	Combinations of following: (see Chapter 9): INH, rifampin, pyrazinamide, ethambutol//streptomycin, PAS, cycloserine, ethionamide, kanamycin, capreomycin	Infections increasing in HIV infected and others
Mycobacterium avium-intracellulare (*Mycobacterium avium* complex [MAI, MAC]/pulmonary, GI tract)	Culture of sputum or bronchoscopy specimen to differentiate from *M. tuberculosis;* microscopic examination or culture of stool, blood, or bone marrow specimen: positive for AFB	Rifabutin for prophylaxis; polydrug therapy for treatment: ciprofloxacin, clarithromycin, azithromycin, INH, rifampin, rifabutin, clofazimine, ethambutol, amikacin	Very common in late stages of immunosuppression
Mycobacterium kansasii (atypical tuberculosis, mycobacteria other than TB, MOTT/pulmonary)	Culture of sputum or bronchoscopy specimen: positive	Polydrug therapy: INH, ethambutol, rifampin, ethionamide, cycloserine	Uncommon; occurs in late stages of immunosuppression

complex, and *M. kansasii*. The latter two organisms rarely cause infection in people who are not immunosuppressed. Active disease with *M. tuberculosis* in the HIV infected may be the result of activation of previously acquired *M. tuberculosis*, or it may be newly acquired (see Chapter 9).

Organisms of the *M. avium* complex are widely found in the environment. These organisms are benign in the immunocompetent but can cause severe, life-threatening diarrhea and septicemia in the HIV infected with CD4+ counts less than 50 to 100 cells/mm^3. Recent studies have shown that prophylactic use of rifabutin prevents septicemia (see Chapter 7).

M. kansasii is being diagnosed with increasing frequency in the HIV infected. The organism responds to conventional antituberculosis therapy.

PROTOZOA

Protozoa are single-celled microorganisms that are classified as the lowest form of animal life. Like bacteria, they can live outside a living host. Protozoa can be observed by microscopic examination of specimens containing the organism. About 30 different protozoa have been shown to be pathogenic to humans. Seven of these are of particular importance in immunosuppression (Table 4-2). The most important of these protozoa is *Pneumocystis carinii*, an organism that is ubiquitous in the environment and commonly found as part of the normal flora of immunocompetent people. *P. carinii*, however, becomes an aggressive pathogen and causes severe, life-threatening pneumonia in even the moderately immunosuppressed. *P. carinii* pneumonia (PCP) is often one of the first, severe clinical signs of HIV infection. Prior to availability of PCP prophylactic drugs, PCP was the AIDS-defining condition for about 75% of AIDS cases. Presently it accounts for about 50% of cases defined as AIDS. PCP is also one of the leading causes of death for people with AIDS. See Chapter 9 for further discussion of PCP.

Toxoplasma gondii, another protozoan, causes encephalitis in up to 15% of people with AIDS. The organism also uncommonly causes pulmonary infection in the HIV infected. *T. gondii* is widespread in the environment and is found regularly in cat and bird feces. It causes frequent, subclinical infections in humans. Seroprevalence surveys in the United States show that, depending on the area of the country, 10% to 40% of the population have antibodies against *T. gondii*, suggesting previous infections.

Other protozoa of significance in HIV infection are *Entamoeba histolytica, Isospora belli, Giardia lamblia, Microsporidium* spp. and *Cryptosporidium* spp. These are all frequent causes of diarrhea in the immunocompromised. Antiinfective therapy is reasonably effective against the first three of these protozoa. There is no curative therapy against *Microsporidium* or *Cryptosporidium*. Infection with these protozoa is a severe threat to HIV-infected persons. Diet, fluid replacement, nutrition supplements and education, etc., are important therapies.

FUNGI

Fungi are plant-like organisms that include yeasts and molds. Because they do not produce chlorophyll, they are parasitic to other organic matter for nutrients. Many are parasitic to humans, becoming pathogenic when uncontrolled by normal defenses. Fungi can be detected by microscopic examination of a body specimen containing the organisms. A limited number of systemic and local antifungal drugs are available for therapy (Table 4-3).

Candida albicans is the most common fungus causing pathology in HIV-infected persons. *C. albicans* is a normal flora organism that is not pathogenic under ordinary conditions in immunocompetent hosts. However, under conditions of stress to areas of the body (e.g., skin breakdown), disruption to normal flora (e.g., following antibiotic therapy), invasion to unusual sites (e.g., through indwelling venous catheters), or in immunodeficiency, *C. albicans* can multiply out of control and become aggressive. *C. albicans* infections are common in the mouth, esophagus, and vagina of HIV-infected people. The infections are uncomfortable and, in the case of oral and esophageal candidiasis, can be so painful that hydration and nutrition can become compromised.

Another important fungus is *Cryptococcus neoformans*, commonly found in the soil. The organism is inhaled and rapidly disseminates to the brain. It can cause both meningitis (in 8% to 12% of people with AIDS) and pulmonary disease. Pulmonary infection without concurrent meningitis is unusual. Antifungal therapy is available for both conditions.

Histoplasma capsulatum and *Coccidioides immitis* are two endemic fungi of significance in HIV. The frequency with which they occur varies by geographic location. Histoplasmosis is more likely to be found in people who have lived some of their lives in the central United States and along the northeast U.S.-Canadian border. Coccidiomycosis is much more common in the southwest United States in a band of desert stretching from southern Texas to southern California. Both fungi first manifest as pulmonary disease, becoming systemic and affecting almost all body systems. Sepsis is a poten-

Table 4-2

PROTOZOA IN IMMUNOSUPPRESSION

Pathogen (disease name/body site where found)	Diagnostic studies: results	Primary//secondary drugs for treatment	Notes
Entamoeba histolytica (amebiasis, amebic dysentery/GI tract, cysts in liver)	Microscopic examination of stool specimen: positive for motile amoeba	Metronidazole, dehydroemetine, diloxanide furoate	More common in travelers and gay men
Pneumocystis carinii (Pneumocystis carinii pneumonia/pulmonary, sometimes disseminates to other body sites)	Microscopic examination of sputum or specimen obtained by bronchoscopy or bronchoalveolar lavage: positive for PCP; gallium scan: >3; diffusing capacity of carbon monoxide: <75% of expected; chest x-ray: observable interstitial infiltrates	Trimethoprim-sulfamethoxazole, dapsone, or pentamidine for prophylaxis; for treatment: TMP/SMX, or dapsone and trimethaprim; corticosteroids for severe disease// clindamycin, atovaquone, or pentamidine	Very common in persons with HIV; prophylaxis is given to anyone with history of PCP or with a CD4+ count less than 200/mm^3
Toxoplasma gondii (toxoplasmosis/central nervous system and, rarely, pulmonary)	Immunofluorescent antibody (IFA) test: elevated IgM or IgA in previously negative person; CT scan or MRI: findings positive for neurologic lesions	Pyrimethamine plus folinic acid plus sulfadiazine for acute disease and for suppressive therapy	Once treated, patients will be maintained on suppressive therapy for remainder of life
Cryptosporidium spp. (cryptosporidiosis/GI tract)	Microscopic examination of acid-fast stain of stool specimen: positive for *Cryptosporidium*	No specific therapy approved at this time; supportive therapy includes dietary supplements and antidiarrheal drugs	Very common in HIV-infected persons; 20% to 30% of diarrheas in HIV are caused by this organism
Isospora belli (isosporiasis/GI tract)	Microscopic examination of acid-fast stain of stool specimen: positive for *Isospora*	Trimethoprim plus sulfamethoxazole used for acute disease and for suppressive therapy	Somewhat common in HIV-infected persons
Giardia lamblia (giardiasis/GI tract)	Microscopic examination of stool specimen: positive for *G. lamblia*	Quinacrine//metronidazole, furazolidone	Somewhat common in HIV infected; most common in gay men and travelers
Microsporidium spp. (microsporidiosis/GI tract)	Electron microscopy of biopsy specimen from small intestine; positive for *Microspordium*	No specific therapy approved at this time; supportive therapy includes dietary supplements and antidiarrheal drugs	About 25% of all diarrhea in HIV infected is due to *Microsporidium*

tial complication. In addition, *Aspergillus* species, which are among the most common fungi in the environment, sometimes cause bronchopulmonary and/or systemic aspergillosis in the immunocompromised.

Another group of fungal infections, called mucormycoses, are relatively rare and difficult to treat. In the rhinocerebral form, mucormycosis causes progressive ulceration of the nose and sinuses. The ulcers eventually penetrate through the hard palate and into the brain and carotid artery. Surgical debridement slows the progression of this infection.

Table 4-3

FUNGI IN IMMUNOSUPPRESSION

Pathogen (disease name/body site where found)	Diagnostic studies: results	Primary//secondary drugs for treatment	Notes
Candida albicans (candidiasis, thrush/mouth, esophagus, pulmonary system, vagina, skin; may also infect wounds, catheters, and IV sites)	Culture or microscopic examination of specimen: positive; because *Candida* is a normal flora organism, identification is not necessarily diagnostic	Prophylaxis and treatment with amphotericin B, ketoconazole, fluconazole; vaginitis treated with clotrimazole, miconazole, or nystatin cream; oral rinses of chlorhexidine gluconate or nystatin	Oral, vaginal, and esophageal pathologies are very common; pathogenic infections in other sites are rare
Cryptococcus neoformans (cryptococcosis/pulmonary and central nervous systems)	CNS infection: CT scan or MRI: positive findings; serum or CSF cryptococcal antigen: >1:2; India ink stain of CSF specimen: positive; culture of blood or CSF specimen: positive Pulmonary infection: culture of specimen from bronchoscopy or bronchoalveolar lavage: positive; chest x-ray: positive	Amphotericin B alone or with 5-flucytosine or fluconazole; fluconazole for suppressive therapy	Meningitis is very common in HIV infection; pulmonary infection is less common and coincides with meningitis when it occurs; suppressive therapy is maintained for life
Histoplasma capsulatum (histoplasmosis/systemic and pulmonary infections)	Culture of blood, sputum, or bone marrow specimen: positive; microscopic examination of specimen obtained from biopsy or bronchoalveolar lavage; positive	Amphotericin B for acute disease; suppressive therapy with itraconazole	More common in HIV infected who live in areas where the organism is endemic in the environment (Ohio, Mississippi, and St. Lawrence river valleys) and in advanced HIV infection
Coccidioides immitis (coccidioidomycosis, valley fever, desert fever, San Joaquin fever, coccidioidal granuloma/systemic, CNS, and pulmonary infections)	Culture of blood or CSF: positive; microscopic examination of sputum or specimen obtained from biopsy or bronchoalveolar lavage: positive	Amphotericin B//fluconazole or amphotericin B with 5-flucytosine; fluconazole for suppressive therapy	Found in advanced HIV infection and in those who live in or have travelled to the desert in southwestern U.S.; survival is poor
Mucor (mucormycosis, zygomycosis/pulmonary and rhinocerebral)	Microscopic examination and culture of biopsied specimen: positive	Amphotericin B; irrigations with amphotericin	Relatively rare, but it is severe when it occurs; surgical debridement may be necessary
Aspergillus (aspergillosis/pulmonary and systemic)	Biopsy of pulmonary tissue culture: positive	Amphotericin B, itraconazole	Seen in patients with leukopenia

VIRUSES

Viruses are tiny particles that are neither animal nor plant life forms. They lack the ability to produce energy, and are, therefore, dependent on living cells for all of their metabolic and reproductive needs. Viruses cannot be seen by ordinary light microscopy but can be observed by electron microscopy. They consist of a single or double strand of either deoxyribonucleic acid (DNA) or ribonucleic acid (RNA), but not both, covered by a protein cover (capsid). More than 300 different viruses have been isolated from animals, some of which appear to be harmless to humans. Viruses are classified by many different schemes, which include their type of RNA or DNA, their origin (e.g., reovirus), the type of disease they produce (e.g., poliovirus), or the area of the body that they invade (e.g., rhinovirus) (Table 4-4).

The mode of action of viruses is to interfere with host cell metabolism so as to either kill the cell directly or alter its replication in some way. Because of their dependence on living cells, viruses cannot survive outside host cells or in the environment as can other microorganisms. Some viruses are antigenic, eliciting an immune response in their host. Vaccines have been developed to protect against many of these viruses, such as measles, mumps, rubella, polio, rabies, and influenza. Attempts to develop antiviral drugs have had mixed success. Once inside a cell, the viruses' genetic material becomes incorporated into that of the host cell. No drugs have yet been developed to extract this bit of genetic material from the host cell so that the cell will not reproduce the virus when it makes other cell proteins. Therefore, although some antiviral agents do act to suppress replication of the virus, none exists to kill the virus.

The most important virus causing pathogenic processes in HIV infection is HIV itself. HIV attacks not only lymphocytes but also nerve cells and cells within the gastrointestinal tract. Its effects are discussed in Chapter 2. Other viruses of importance are hepatitis viruses, herpesviruses, human papillomavirus, molluscipoxvirus, and cytomegalovirus.

Hepatitis A infections can occur in HIV-infected people for the same reasons as in non-HIV-infected people—exposure through contaminated food, improper food handling, poor control of sewage, inad-equate handwashing, and oral/anal sexual practices. Hepatitis A infection is common in a subclinical form in the general population, with 50% to 75% of the population carrying antibodies against hepatitis A virus (HAV). It is not clear whether hepatitis A is more common in HIV-infected people or just more severe. Hepatitis B virus (HBV) is known to be (and hepatitis C is thought to be) transmitted in the same ways as HIV—sexually, parenterally, and mother to child at birth. Therefore, HIV-infected people are more likely to be infected with and/or carriers of HBV than is the general population. HIV-infected individuals who are seronegative for HBV should receive the hepatitis B vaccine. All health care workers who have a potential exposure to the blood or body fluids of their patients should also be immunized against HBV. The probability of a health care worker contracting hepatitis B following exposure to blood of a HBV-infected patient is 100 times higher than the risk associated with the same exposure to HIV.

Herpes zoster infections in the form of shingles or central nervous system symptoms are common in HIV-infected persons. These manifestations are a result of the inflammatory response in the infected host cells in the spinal cord ganglia. The original virus infection caused chickenpox. It is estimated that 95% of adult Americans harbor this virus, which only becomes pathogenic under periods of extreme stress, severe disease, immunosuppressive therapy, or HIV infection. Herpes simplex virus (HSV) infections are also quite common in the HIV infected, with 10% to 25% of such persons having mucocutaneous manifestations. A very small number (<1%) of HIV-infected people develop herpes simplex pneumonia or meningitis.

Cytomegalovirus (CMV) is present in 80% to 90% of HIV-infected persons and causes serious infections in 30% of them. The most dramatic CMV-related presentation is CMV retinitis, which occurs in 5% to 10% of HIV-infected people. Also, CMV is the cause of 10% to 40% of diarrheas and occasionally causes pneumonia and encephalitis.

Molluscipoxvirus and human papillomavirus (HPV) can cause disfiguring skin lesions in the HIV infected. Certain subtypes of HPV have been linked to development of malignancies. The appearance of the characteristic dermal, genital, or anal/rectal warts should be monitored with Pap smears, colposcopy, and/or sigmoidoscopy.

Table 4-4

VIRUSES IN IMMUNOSUPPRESSION

Pathogen (disease name/body site where found)	Diagnostic studies: results	Primary//secondary drugs for treatment	Notes
Herpes zoster (V-Z virus, shingles/skin, nerves, and, rarely, pulmonary and central nervous systems)	Electron microscopy and N-cell culture: positive	Acyclovir//vidarabine; analgesics for pain; foscarnet	Fairly common in HIV-infected persons; extremely painful
Herpes simplex virus (HSV, herpes/mouth, esophagus, anus, rectum, visceral and, rarely, in pulmonary and central nervous systems)	Viral culture: positive	Acyclovir//foscarnet for treatment of resistant organisms and suppression	Very common; foscarnet is extremely expensive
Cytomegalovirus (CMV/eye, colon, esophagus, and, rarely, in hepatobiliary and pulmonary systems)	Culture of biopsied specimen: positive	Foscarnet or ganciclovir for treatment and suppression	Foscarnet may act synergistically with AZT to inhibit HIV; foscarnet is very expensive; lifetime suppression is needed
Molluscipoxvirus (molluscum contagiosum/skin)	Microscopic or histologic examination of lesion core: positive	No approved drug therapy	Fairly common in HIV-infected persons; may be treated with curettage or freezing
Human papillomavirus (HPV, warts, condylomata acuminata/external genitalia, vagina, cervix, anus, urethra)	Microscopic examination of biopsied specimen: positive	Topical application of podofilox, podophyllin, or trichloroacetic acid; evidence suggests that removal may increase risk for cancer	Freezing and curettage sometimes used but removal may increase risk for cancer
Hepatitis A virus (HAV, hepatitis/liver)	Serology: elevation of IgM or IgA; IgA may be elevated from previous infection	Immune globulin given within 2 months of exposure; no specific treatment against virus	Uncommon, except to those who are exposed to a person with HAV, eat raw shellfish, travel to areas with poor sanitation, or practice oral/anal sex
Hepatitis B virus (HBV, serum hepatitis/liver)	Serology: positive for HBeAg and HBsAg or anti-HBe	HB immune globulin for postexposure prophylaxis; hepatitis B vaccine preexposure; no specific treatment against HBV	Uncommon, except to those with multiple sex partners or IV drug users; carrier state exists in 5% to 10% of cases; immunization recommended for HIV infected who are seronegative
Hepatitis C virus (non-A, non-B hepatitis/liver)	Serology: positive hepatitis C antibody	No specific treatment	Associated with blood transfusion; not clear whether it can be transmitted by sexual or other means; carrier state possible
Papovavirus JC (PML, progressive multifocal leukoencephalopathy/CNS)	CT scan: characteristic PML lesions (presumptive)	No specific treatment	Occurs in 1% to 3% of HIV-infected persons

CHAPTER 5

Assessment and Diagnostic Procedures

During the long course of HIV infection, infected people are subject to all of the normal ills that affect people of their age and life circumstances. They have the same needs for health education and for preventive, curative, psychosocial, and rehabilitative services as noninfected people. In addition, because of their present or potential immunocompromised state, HIV-infected people need health care unique to their disease. Also, they may be taking antiretroviral drugs, antiinfective drugs, and a wide variety of prescribed medications, over-the-counter (OTC) drugs, and nutritional supplements for relief of symptoms. As a result, HIV-infected people require special monitoring for side effects of treatments in addition to monitoring for disease progress. This chapter presents the critical elements of monitoring HIV-infected persons throughout the course of HIV infection and will include health history, physical examination, laboratory testing for immunosuppression, collecting and handling specimens, and diagnostic tests for infectious diseases. This latter topic will present information on laboratory tests to identify pathogens, skin tests, gallium scans, antibiotic sensitivity testing, and hematologic tests. Monitoring of specific body systems for HIV-related diseases will be discussed in Chapters 6 through 10.

HEALTH HISTORY

A thorough health history from a person who is newly diagnosed with HIV or is seeing a health care provider for the first time is essential (Table 5-1). The history establishes baseline information about concurrent risks and health problems the person may have, life stresses, immunization status, high-risk practices, availability of support systems, need for referrals for counseling or social services, and need for health education. Taking the history begins a professional-client relationship that may last for many years. Because HIV infection is a progressive, chronic disease, the health history must be updated periodically to reflect changes, such as the person's living circumstances, health practices, immunization status, functional abilities, and mental status. Medication use should be reviewed each time an HIV-infected person is seen by a health care provider. Those infected with HIV are frequently taking many medications, some of which are very toxic. They take medications prescribed by more than one physician as well as OTC drugs, all of which may interact to their detriment.

PHYSICAL EXAMINATION

The initial and subsequent physical examinations for the HIV-positive person are also comprehensive (Table 5-2). People with HIV are at risk for all health problems affecting others of their age and gender. In addition, they are at high risk for all of the sequelae of HIV infection, which can affect every body system. Consequently, a comprehensive physical examination is performed at the initial encounter with a health care pro-

Text continued on p.74.

Table 5-1

HEALTH HISTORY FOR THE PERSON WITH HIV

History items	Rationale
Previous infections, particularly tuberculosis, hepatitis B, syphilis, fungal infections, herpes, condyloma	These infections may resurface as immune status becomes compromised; educate client about symptoms to monitor in future
Previous sexually transmitted diseases (gonorrhea, syphilis, chlamydia, etc.); sexual orientation, practices, or number of partners	To educate client about risks, safer sexual practices; to discuss need to inform sexual partners about HIV status of client
Environmental exposures because of travel, occupation, or residence; circumstances of exposure to organisms	To determine the likelihood of latent infections that may become symptomatic later, such as tuberculosis, tropical diseases, fungal diseases (coccidioidomycosis, histoplasmosis, cryptosporidiosis, etc.)
Immunizations	To update old immunizations and administer new ones such as hepatitis B, pneumococcal, MMR, polio, tetanus, influenza
Pulmonary history, including smoking, asthma, bronchitis, allergies, recent-onset dyspnea or shortness of breath	Institute care for lung-damaging conditions that may increase the risk for HIV-related pulmonary diseases; to educate client about additional risk to lungs from smoking; begin therapy to prevent allergies and sinusitis
Psychiatric illnesses, hospitalizations, and medications for psychiatric symptoms; patterns of alcohol and drug use; coping mechanisms; present level of social interaction; presence of supportive people in the person's life; reaction to news of being HIV positive; suicidal ideation; plans for dealing with HIV disease	Determine need for crisis intervention, referral for psychiatric consultation, drug or alcohol treatment, psychotropic medications and/or referral to support groups; establish baseline against which changes can be compared
Medication review: all prescribed and OTC drugs; allergies	Evaluate impact of prescribed drugs on immune system (e.g., corticosteroids), potential for drug interactions between prescribed and OTC drugs, and client's behaviors regarding medication use; in addition, recently prescribed drugs provide information about treatment of pathology that may have been unrecognized as being related to HIV status
Previously diagnosed non-HIV-related diseases, surgeries, hospitalizations	Previous medical history can affect course and treatment of HIV-related diseases; client may require concurrent treatment of these conditions
Social and living conditions: exposure to pets and other animals, employment, adequacy of income for needs, living arrangements, recreation, availability of significant others	Determine risk for exposure to opportunistic organisms and need for referral to community social service agencies
Health habits: smoking; alcohol and drug use; diet, exercise, and sleep practices	Determine need for health education, referral for substance abuse treatment or other types of counseling

Continued.

Table 5-1

HEALTH HISTORY FOR THE PERSON WITH HIV—cont'd

History items	Rationale
Systematic review of recent symptoms: *General:* night sweats, chills, lymphadenopathy, fever, unintended weight loss, fatigue, pain; recurring or refractory illness (e.g., sinusitis)	Detect previously experienced HIV-related pathology; institute therapy for current illness; evaluate need for referral to specialists (dentist, eye care professional, neurologist, etc.)
Oral/gastrointestinal: pain on chewing or swallowing, persistent nausea, vomiting or diarrhea, anorexia, bleeding, cramping; perianal or rectal itching, pain, or bleeding	
Genitourinary: itching, burning, urethral discharge, lesions, incontinence	
Skin: lesions, rashes, dryness	
Sensory: changes in vision, photophobia, double or blurred vision, periorbital pain; tinnitus or hearing loss	
Neurologic: headache, lightheadedness, memory loss, word-finding difficulty, mood swings, gait disturbance, thought pattern disturbance, stiff neck, seizure activity, paresthesia, listlessness or inability to concentrate; peripheral pain, burning, tingling, or numbness	
Respiratory: shortness of breath, wheezing, cough	
Any other symptoms	People with HIV infection are at risk for all the life stresses and pathologies (such as chronic diseases, cancers, pregnancy, etc.) that others of their age and life circumstances experience

Table 5-2

PHYSICAL EXAMINATION FOR THE PERSON WITH HIV

Area of examination	Rationale
Behavior and appearance: Observe posture, gait and movement, dress and personal hygiene, affect, communication patterns; weigh client.	Identify signs of low energy, malaise, weakness, neurologic changes, and depression, all which could indicate systemic disease, neurologic disease, or depression; severe loss of weight (wasting) is a symptom of advancing immune suppression (see wasting in Color Plate 34).
Body temperature: Assess temperature, flushing, and diaphoresis.	Detect fever associated with systemic infection.
Oral cavity: Inspect lips, tongue (dorsal, ventral, and lateral surfaces), gingiva, all areas of buccal mucosa, palate, pharynx, and tonsils for exudate, inflammation, and lesions (Figure 5-1). Palpate all areas that do not elicit gagging for induration and pain; collect specimen for laboratory analysis (pp. 79-80).	Identify lesions and inflammation associated with HIV disease (aphthous ulcers, herpes, hairy leukoplakia, oral candidiasis, gingivitis, periodontitis, Kaposi's sarcoma, oral warts) and assess status of oral hygiene (Color Plates 21-33); establish treatment and education plan; refer client for dental care.

Table 5-2

PHYSICAL EXAMINATION FOR THE PERSON WITH HIV—cont'd

Area of examination	Rationale
Eyes: Inspect eyelids and conjunctiva for inflammation, exudate, or lesions; examine retina; examine visual acuity and fields of vision. Collect specimen of exudate for laboratory analysis (p. 80).	Establish baseline or detect HIV-related pathology (Kaposi's sarcoma or herpes of conjunctiva, CMV retinitis) (Color Plate 35); refer to eye care professional for correction of vision; treat infections.
Nose and sinuses: Inspect nasal passages for inflammation and discharge; inspect frontal and maxillary sinus areas for swelling; palpate sinuses for pain. Collect specimen of discharge for laboratory analysis (p. 80).	Detect and initiate treatment for sinus infections, which are common with HIV infection.
Skin: Inspect exposed and unexposed skin for signs of inflammation, jaundice, dehydration, and lesions. Note lesion location, arrangement, size, shape, color, texture, elevation, and characteristics of any exudate (see Color Plates 39-57). Collect specimen for laboratory analysis (p. 82). Inspect for evidence of needle tracks.	Establish baseline, or detect and treat HIV-related lesions associated with seborrheic dermatitis, *Staphylococcus*, herpes simplex, herpes zoster, *Mycobacterium*, molluscum contagiosum, *Candida albicans*, ringworm, parasites, or drug reactions (see Color Plates 1-5, 7-12, 17, 18, 21-26). The skin is also a good window for many systemic diseases. If needle tracks are present, counsel and refer for treatment for IV drug use.
Lymph nodes: Inspect and palpate (by moving skin over area to be palpated) sites of all lymph nodes (Figure 5-2) for erythema, heat, swelling, texture, movement, and tenderness of any nodules.	Detect and treat localized infections, generalized lymphadenopathy, and lymphomas (Color Plate 38). Superficial, painless, movable nodes less than 1 cm in diameter are common in healthy adults.
Lungs: Check respiratory rate and depth for tachypnea, dyspnea. Palpate thoracic expansion from posterior and anterior positions (limitation in expansion may indicate inflammation and pain); palpate the chest wall for tactile fremitus (increased with pneumonia). Percuss the chest (dull over areas of consolidation associated with pneumonia; resonant with bronchitis); auscultate breath sounds (wheezes or rales associated with opportunistic infections); evaluate characteristics of cough. Collect sputum specimen for culture (pp. 80-81).	Detect and treat non-HIV-related infections; establish baseline, as respiratory disease is common in later stages of HIV infections; detect and treat opportunistic respiratory diseases (e.g., *Pneumocystis carinii* pneumonia, *Candida*, tuberculosis).
Abdomen: Auscultate abdomen for bowel sounds; auscultate over liver and spleen for friction rubs (indicating enlargement); palpate and percuss abdomen to identify organ enlargement and areas of tenderness.	Identify hepatosplenomegaly associated with infection, tumors, chronic alcohol/drug use, or reactions to prescribed medications; identify and treat the many possible gastrointestinal infections due to bacteria, parasites, and viruses; identify and treat GI Kaposi's sarcoma.
Genitourinary: Inspect external genitalia for inflammation, lesions, exudates, and signs of parasites; with gloved hand, palpate lesions for consistency or tenderness. Female: Using a speculum, inspect cervix and vaginal walls for edema, erythema, lesions, and exudate; obtain specimen of exudate for laboratory analysis; obtain specimen of cervical cells for Pap analysis (see Figure 5-3 and pp. 82-83). Male: Inspect testes for asymmetric enlargement; palpate scrotum for tenderness; obtain specimen of urethral discharge for laboratory analysis (see Figure 5-4).	Identify and treat STDs; identify and document for baseline data the presence of untreatable lesions; identify and treat cervical and other genitourinary and pelvic tumors.
Anal/rectal area: Inspect perianal area for inflammation, lesions, exudates, and signs of parasites; insert gloved finger into anal opening to palpate for lesions and tenderness; collect rectal exudates (see Figure 5-5) or fecal specimen for laboratory analysis (pp. 84-85).	

Continued.

Table 5-2

PHYSICAL EXAMINATION FOR THE PERSON WITH HIV—cont'd

Area of examination	Rationale
Neurologic system: Assess for numbness or pain in extremities, hyperreflexia, hypertonia, ataxia, motor weakness, gait disturbance, and hemiparesis.	Identify and treat acute infections and tumors; identify chronic demyelinating polyneuropathy; establish baseline data.
Mental status: Assess for decreased level of consciousness or confusion indicating acute CNS infection or drug reactions; assess changes in cognition, behavior, or emotional responses associated with HIV-related dementia or depression; evaluate orientation, short-term memory, and cognition with simple tests of cognition such as the Mini-Mental State Exam (see the box on p. 77).	Detect and treat acute infection or drug reactions; differentiate symptoms of AIDS dementia from depression or anxiety for treatment of the latter two; establish baseline against which future behavior can be compared.
Other: Assess for pathology in any body system suggested by symptoms the person is experiencing.	People with HIV are still at risk for health problems unrelated to HIV status.

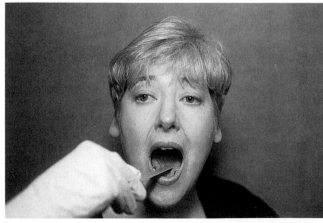

FIGURE 5-1
Examining the oral cavity.

vider and periodically thereafter. This is recommended not only to detect pathology but also to establish baseline information against which future changes can be compared. The physical assessment also presents an opportunity to educate the client about changes to monitor and report to the health care provider. If there is insufficient time at each visit for a complete physical examination, it may be completed in parts over a series of visits. The examination may be performed by a physician in order to initiate treatment and referrals or by a nurse in order to understand the client's condition, identify client problems associated with the pathology, and initiate nursing interventions and referrals. A gentle reminder: *Do not forget to wear examination gloves!*

LABORATORY TESTING FOR IMMUNOSUPPRESSION

Baseline laboratory testing (Table 5-3) is relatively brief. It includes the basic tests performed for all persons regardless of symptomatology or findings from the history or physical. Symptoms or examination and history findings might suggest other testing.

The most important test listed is the CD4+ count, because it reflects progression of infection and is the basis of many interventions. For example, a CD4+ count of less than $500/mm^3$ is the indicator value for commencing antiretroviral therapy, and a value of less than $200/mm^3$ is indication for starting anti-*Pneumocystis* prophylaxis (see Chapter 9).

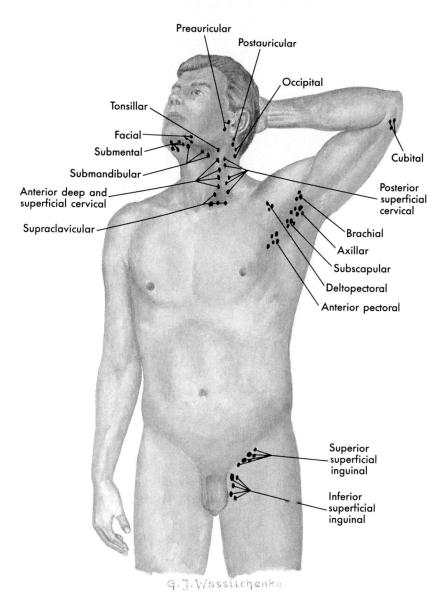

FIGURE 5-2
Location of palpable lymph nodes. (From Grimes.[82])

The CD4+ count also can be the basis for developing teaching plans and counseling for the client. For example, those with CD4+ counts >700/mm³ have no need to arrange a living will or power of attorney, but those with counts of less than 50/mm³ may need to deal with these issues. Persons with high CD4+ counts need instruction on how to maintain general health status with diet, exercise, and stress reduction. The CD4+ count can be an important determinant of the content and priority of health education.

The other tests in the laboratory panel are more often used for establishing baseline information against which future results can be compared than for diagnostic purposes. It must be remembered that positive re-

sults from skin testing for TB exposure and serologic testing for toxoplasmosis antibodies do not necessarily indicate active disease. If, however, either test is negative and later becomes positive, that information provides direction for a diagnostic evaluation.

In summary, the initial history, physical, and laboratory panel provide essential baseline information against which the future can be compared, the basis upon which differential diagnoses can be developed when symptoms appear, and the foundation of health education of the client. This last item is important because it allows the client to become an active participant in the management of a long-term, progressive disease.

Table 5-3

LABORATORY AND DIAGNOSTIC TESTS FOR IMMUNOSUPPRESSION

Test	Rationale
Hematology	
CD4+ count	To stage the disease; determine the need for antiretroviral or antiinfective prophylaxis; provide information and education to client on disease progression
CBC with differential and platelets	To diagnose anemia, neutropenia, and thrombocytopenia, which result from HIV infection and as side effects of antiretroviral therapy.
Skin tests	
Mantoux (with PPD) for TB: with anergy testing with two of the following: *Candida albicans*, tetanus toxoid, mumps	To determine exposure to TB and need for further diagnosis for active disease either now or in future (see Chapter 9). A negative Mantoux (<5 mm induration) may result from inadequate cellular immunity and may be a false negative. Negative results on the anergy tests indicate a possible false negative on the TB test.
Serology	
Toxoplasma antibody titer	To establish negative baseline for comparison if client develops toxoplasmosis later.
Venereal Disease Research Laboratory (VDRL) or rapid plasma reagin (RPR)	To rule out untreated syphilis; treat if present. Establish baseline data in event of relapse at a later time.
Hepatitis B: anti-HBs and HBsAg	To assess hepatitis B status prior to administering hepatitis B vaccine.
Other diagnostic tests	
Chest x-ray	To provide baseline data for later comparison, as respiratory diseases are common in HIV infection.
Pap smear	To detect cervical dysplasia and neoplasia, which coincide with HIV infection in women.
Other	Any other test that may be indicated because of client age, living circumstances, or symptoms to confirm or diagnose health problems unrelated to HIV.

Collecting and Handling Specimens

As was seen in Chapter 4, many different organisms cause infections in immunosuppression. It is crucial to identify the exact organism that is causing a clinical manifestation so that appropriate antiinfective therapy can be initiated rapidly and effectively. The importance of this cannot be overemphasized. Time lost before therapy is begun may mean the difference between life and death for the patient. In addition, ineffective therapy contributes to the development of drug-resistant organisms.

The exact microorganism causing disease generally can be determined in one of three ways: (1) microscopic examination of a specimen of fluids, exudates, secretions, or tissue containing the organism; (2) identification of organism characteristics in a culture of a specimen containing the organism; and (3) identification by

MINI MENTAL STATE EXAMINATION

"MINI-MENTAL STATE"

Maximum
Score Score

ORIENTATION

5 ( ) What is the (year) (season) (date) (day) (month)?

5 ( ) Where are we: (state) (county) (town) (hospital) (floor)?

REGISTRATION

3 ( ) Name 3 objects: 1 second to say each. Then ask the patient all 3 after you have said them. Give 1 point for each correct answer. Then repeat them until he learns all 3. Count trials and record.

Trials

ATTENTION AND CALCULATION

5 ( ) Serial 7's. 1 point for each correct. Stop after 5 answers. Alternatively spell "world" backwards.

RECALL

3 ( ) Ask for the 3 objects repeated above. Give 1 point for each correct.

LANGUAGE

9 ( ) Name a pencil and watch. (2 points)

Repeat the following: "No ifs, ands, or buts." (1 point)

Follow a 3-stage command:

"Take a paper in your right hand, fold it in half, and put it on the floor." (3 points)

Read and obey the following:

CLOSE YOUR EYES. (1 point)

Write a sentence. (1 point)

Copy design. (1 point)

_____ Total score

ASSESS level of consciousness along a continuum _____

Alert   Drowsy   Stupor   Coma

INSTRUCTIONS FOR ADMINISTRATION OF
MINI-MENTAL STATE EXAMINATION

ORIENTATION

(1) Ask for the date. Then ask specifically for parts omitted, e.g., "Can you also tell me what season it is?" One point for each correct.

(2) Ask in turn "Can you tell me the name of this hospital?" (town, country, etc.). One point for each correct.

REGISTRATION

Ask the patient if you may test his memory. Then say the names of 3 unrelated objects, clearly and slowly, about one second for each. After you have said all 3, ask him to repeat them. This first repetition determines his score (0-3) but keep saying them until he can repeat all 3, up to 6 trials. If he does not eventually learn all 3, recall cannot be meaningfully tested.

ATTENTION AND CALCULATION

Ask the patient to begin with 100 and count backwards by 7. Stop after 5 subtractions (93, 86, 79, 72, 65). Score the total number of correct answers.

If the patient cannot or will not perform this task, ask him to spell the word "world" backwards. The score is the number of letters in correct order. E.g., dlrow = 5, dlorw = 3.

RECALL

Ask the patient if he can recall the 3 words you previously asked him to remember. Score 0-3.

LANGUAGE

Naming: Show the patient a wrist watch and ask him what it is. Repeat for pencil. Score 0-2.

Repetition: Ask the patient to repeat the sentence after you. Allow only one trial. Score 0 or 1.

3-Stage command: Give the patient a piece of plain blank paper and repeat the command. Score 1 point for each part correctly executed.

Reading: On a blank piece of paper print the sentence "Close your eyes," in letters large enough for the patient to see clearly. Ask him to read it and do what it says. Score 1 point only if he actually closes his eyes.

Writing: Give the patient a blank piece of paper and ask him to write a sentence for you. Do not dictate a sentence, it is to be written spontaneously. It must contain a subject and verb and be sensible. Correct grammar and punctuation are not necessary.

Copying: On a clean piece of paper, draw intersecting pentagons, each side about 1 in., and ask him to copy it exactly as it is. All 10 angles must be present and 2 must intersect to score 1 point. Tremor and rotation are ignored.

Estimate the patient's level of sensorium along a continuum, from alert on the left to coma on the right.

From Folstein MJ, Folstein ME, McHugh PR: Mini-Mental State, *J Psychol Res*, pp. 189-198, 1975.

test tube antibody-antigen reactions of a specimen or of serum. All of these procedures require a specimen of body fluids, secretions, exudates, or tissue containing the organism, its by-products, or antibodies against the organism.

If pathologic agents responsible for infectious diseases are to be correctly identified, specimens must be collected and handled very carefully. Failure to use proper techniques to obtain a specimen can result in contamination with normal flora, which leads to inaccurate laboratory results. Incorrect handling of the specimen after it is collected may result in killing the organisms before culturing or in spurious overgrowth of the organism in the culture.

The danger inherent in handling specimens (or any body fluids of infected patients) cannot be overemphasized. To protect yourself, your colleagues, and other patients, be compulsive about practicing measures that prevent contamination and spread of infection.

Although procedures differ according to the type of specimen, the following general principles apply to the collection and handling of all fluids and tissues.

OBTAINING ADEQUATE SPECIMENS

- Prevent embarrassment by assuring complete privacy and confidentiality for the patient. This will help the patient relax and facilitate collection of a good specimen.
- Obtain the specimen during the acute stage of infection and before initiating antibiotic therapy, if possible.
- The specimen must be representative of the infectious process. Secretions or excretions from uninvolved areas should be avoided during collection.
- Obtain adequate amount of the specimen necessary for tests. Check with your laboratory if unsure.
- Use the proper collection instruments and containers, and place the specimen in a sterile or clean container, as indicated.
- Label the container to identify the patient, source of the specimen (e.g., sputum, urine, or venous blood), date, time collected, test(s) to be performed, and organism suspected.
- For specimens that must be inoculated directly into culture or transport medium, do not open the container until you have obtained the specimen. This prevents environmental organisms from contaminating the medium.
- If the specimen or collection materials are accidentally contaminated by contact with other secretions, the patient's skin, or nonsterile objects, discard the specimen and obtain another.
- When the patient will collect his or her own specimen, give complete verbal and written instructions.
- Maintain the recommended temperature of the specimen, and deliver it to the laboratory as soon as possible to maintain viability of the pathogen.

PROTECTING YOURSELF AND OTHERS

- Always wash your hands before and after collecting specimens or handling body fluids.
- Always wear gloves while collecting and handling specimens. Sterile gloves are necessary for some procedures.
- Wrap securely and properly dispose of contaminated equipment, gloves, linens, and other contaminated objects.
- Protect yourself against needle-stick injury. Do not recap needles. Dispose of needles in a "sharps" container.
- Clean up any spilled specimen.
- Take care not to contaminate the outside of the container with the specimen. If contamination occurs, transfer specimen to another or place contaminated container inside another container or plastic bag.

BLOOD SPECIMENS

Blood is normally sterile, although mild, transient, asymptomatic bacteremia is common. However, septicemia is a serious, life-threatening event necessitating rapid identification of the causative organism. Organisms may be isolated and identified in the laboratory through cultures, microscopic examination, or a variety of serologic tests. Samples obtained by venipuncture are preferred over sampling from intravenous catheters.

It is preferable that blood samples for cultures be obtained before antibiotic therapy is started, because otherwise culturing may be ineffective. This is not always possible because patients may have already received antibiotics. If so, note this on the specimen sent to the laboratory.

Serial blood cultures are usually necessary. Ideally, three blood samples are obtained over a 24-hour period. When this is not possible because of need to initiate therapy, three samples can be obtained 30 minutes apart, or three specimens from three different sites can be drawn concurrently. In addition, blood samples for cultures may need to be obtained daily to monitor the patient's response to therapy until clinical improvement is demonstrated.

Most organisms will grow within 3 days, but some require 7 days for adequate growth. In rare cases, cultures are maintained up to 28 days if unusually fastidious organisms or anaerobic bacteria are suspected.

In addition, Gram's stains are performed immediately to provide a general guide for initiating antimicrobial therapy before culture results are available.

CONTRAINDICATIONS

Patients with coagulation disorders require special precaution. In addition, venipuncture is contraindicated at sites where there are lesions or infection.

COLLECTION PROCEDURES

Aseptic technique is essential to avoid contaminating the specimen with microorganisms residing on the skin. The following procedure should be followed carefully:

1. Assemble this equipment: culture tubes with the appropriate media, 10- or 20-ml syringes (one for each venipuncture), 21-gauge needle (two for each venipuncture), butterfly needles if they will be used, sterile gloves, antiseptic solution (2% iodine or povidone), alcohol swabs, tourniquet, and labels for identification.
2. After washing your hands, clean the venipuncture area with an alcohol sponge to remove superficial dirt and body oil.
3. Using a sponge saturated with an antiseptic solution, clean the venipuncture site in a widening circle, working from clean to dirty. The cleaned area should be about 5 cm in diameter.
4. Wait about 1 minute for the solution to dry and then wipe off the excess antiseptic with an alcohol swab. (Note: if an iodophor compound has been used as the antiseptic, do not remove with alcohol; allow the iodophor solution to dry completely on the skin before venipuncture.)
5. Apply the tourniquet.
6. Put on sterile gloves before palpating the vein.
7. Perform the venipuncture and draw 10 to 20 ml of blood into the syringe (between 2 and 6 ml for small children, depending on their size).
8. Remove the needle and recap, using either the one-handed technique or a hemostat to avoid needle-stick injury.
9. Apply pressure to the puncture site, using sterile gauze, and cover with a small bandage.
10. Still maintaining aseptic technique, insert a sterile needle into the syringe.

BLOOD SPECIMEN PREPARATION

Special media are used for blood cultures, and the correct procedure for preparing the culture bottles or tubes will depend on laboratory protocols at your institution and the type of pathogen suspected. In general, these basic guidelines for preparing blood specimens should be followed:

- Broth cultures require a blood/broth ratio of 1:5 or 1:10, according to instructions. Thus a 1:5 dilution requires that 10 ml of blood is added to a 50-ml bottle.
- For special resins inject the blood into the specimen container and invert the bottle to mix.
- Lysis-centrifugation technique involves drawing blood directly into a special processing tube that is sent to the laboratory. This requires no further preparation.

---

11. Clean the diaphragm tops of the culture bottles with alcohol or iodine and inject the specified amount of blood (usually 3 to 6 ml) into each of the tubes containing culture media.
12. If concurrent specimens are required, repeat these steps at other venipuncture sites.
13. Label each tube with the following information: the patient's name, exact time the blood was drawn, site from which it was obtained or whether it was taken from an IV catheter, and any antibiotics the patient has received within the past 10 days. Keep the culture tubes at room temperature and transport immediately to the laboratory.

PATIENT TEACHING

Explain the procedure and its purpose. Let the patient know that the needle will "stick." After the needle is withdrawn, patients who are not too ill can hold the pressure gauze in place for a minute to stop the bleeding and prevent a hematoma. Explain to the patient that a hematoma may occur. Culture results are usually available in about 3 days.

THROAT, EYE, EAR, AND NOSE SPECIMENS

Secretions and excretions from mucous membranes invariably contain normal flora as well as pathogens. Therefore the specimen obtained must be representative of the pathologic process rather than the surrounding skin.

Mucous membrane specimens should be collected with a sterile polyester swab, not a cotton swab. Preparation of the specimen will depend on the suspected diagnosis. The appropriate culture medium should be available, and if the specimen will be examined microscopically, you will need a slide with coverslip and the appropriate solution for wet-mount preparations.

COLLECTION PROCEDURES

Throat

1. Assemble this equipment: tongue blade, penlight, sterile polyester swab, gloves, slide and solutions, as indicated, appropriate culture, medium, and labels for identification.
2. Put on gloves. Moisten the tongue blade with warm water. (A moist tongue blade does not stimulate the gag reflex as readily as a dry blade, although most patients will gag to some extent.)
3. With the patient's head tilted back, depress the patient's tongue and insert the sterile polyester swab. (Be careful not to touch the swab to the patient's lips, teeth, or buccal mucosa when entering and exiting the mouth.)

4. Swab both tonsils and the posterior pharynx.
5. Prepare the specimen for laboratory examination.
6. Discard gloves and swab properly. Wash hands thoroughly after the procedure.
7. Label the container as to body source of specimen, with the patient's name, date and time of collection, suspected diagnosis, and whether recent or current antibiotic therapy has been given. Transport the specimen to the laboratory immediately.

Eye

1. Assemble this equipment: sterile polyester swab, gloves, slide and solutions, as indicated, appropriate culture medium, and labels for identification.
2. Put on gloves. With the thumb of one hand, place gentle downward traction below the eye to expose the conjunctiva.
3. Instruct the patient to look up. This will help avoid touching the cornea with the swab.
4. Gently place a sterile polyester swab against the conjunctiva, holding in place for about 10 seconds to allow the exudate to absorb into the swab.
5. See 5, 6, and 7 from Throat.

Ear

A specimen should be obtained when there is drainage from the middle ear from a ruptured tympanic membrane.

1. Assemble this equipment: sterile polyester swab, gloves, slide and solutions, as indicated, appropriate culture medium, and labels for identification.
2. Put on gloves. Have the patient tilt the head forward and slightly to the affected side. This will help move the exudate into the distal canal, where it can be reached more easily.
3. Gently insert a sterile polyester swab just inside the external canal, holding in place for about 10 seconds to allow the swab to absorb the exudate.
4. See 5, 6, and 7 from Throat.

Nose

1. Assemble this equipment: penlight, sterile polyester swab, gloves, slide and solutions, as indicated, appropriate culture medium, and labels for identification.
2. Put on gloves. While steadying the patient's head with one hand, insert a sterile polyester swab into the nose (until you reach the turbinates).
3. Rotate the swab gently against the septum and floor of the nares for about 10 seconds to allow the swab to absorb the exudate (Figure 3-10).
4. See 5, 6, and 7 from Throat.

PATIENT TEACHING

Describe the procedure and its purpose. Assure the patient that it will take only a few seconds to obtain the specimen.

SPUTUM SPECIMENS

All too often, sputum samples sent for culturing are little more than saliva and oropharyngeal secretions, rather than specimens from the lower respiratory tract. Failure to follow the proper techniques for obtaining sputum can result in delayed diagnosis. Most laboratories will perform a Gram's stain on a sputum specimen to determine whether it does indeed represent lung secretions. If the majority of cells are from squamous epithelium, the sample is primarily oropharyngeal secretions, and another specimen will be requested. Specimens from the lower respiratory tract of patients with pulmonary infections contain mostly white blood cells and will be cultured.

The most common method used for sputum collection is expectoration. Other less frequently used methods include bronchial aspiration, tracheal cannulation, and translaryngeal aspiration. With the exception of translaryngeal aspiration, all collection techniques are subject to some contamination with oropharyngeal secretions. Following the expectoration procedure carefully, however, reduces the amount of contamination and should produce a specimen that is representative of pulmonary secretions. This method is also without complications.

COLLECTION PROCEDURES

Expectoration

Expectorated sputum can be obtained from a cooperative patient with a productive cough. The specimen should be collected first thing in the morning because pooling of lung secretions during sleep results in a larger quantity of sputum, which contains a maximum number of pathogens. (See Tuberculosis Precautions, Chapter 14).

1. Assemble this equipment: a wide-mouthed container with identification label, gloves, tissues, water, and mouthwash. Wear a mask.
2. Have the patient blow his or her nose to expel excess nasopharyngeal secretions. The patient should then brush and rinse with mouthwash to reduce the number of oral organisms.
3. Have the patient take a deep breath and cough deeply to bring up sputum. If possible, have the patient hold the container and expectorate directly into it.
4. If this fails to produce sputum, there are several

techniques you can use to loosen thickened secretions. An **aerosol nebulizer** increases the moisture content in the lungs, or **intermittent positive-pressure breathing** with an aerosol may be prescribed. **Chest physiotherapy** also loosens secretions from the airways.

5. While wearing gloves, cap the container, taking care that the outside is not contaminated with sputum.
6. Label the container "sputum specimen," with the patient's name, time of collection, and whether antibiotics have been given. Transport immediately to the laboratory.

NURSING CARE

Describe the procedure and its purpose to the patient. For collection by expectoration, encourage the patient to drink fluids the evening before collection.

After expectoration, provide good mouth care and encourage liquids.

PATIENT TEACHING

For collection by expectoration, explain the procedure carefully to ensure the patient understands that sputum, not saliva, is needed.

BRONCHOSCOPY/BRONCHOALVEOLAR LAVAGE

Bronchoscopy permits direct inspection of the larynx, trachea, and bronchi for diagnostic purposes. It also allows collection of biopsied tissue specimens and secretions for bacteriologic or cytologic examination to identify fungi, acid-fast bacilli, and *Pneumocystis carinii*. A flexible fiberoptic bronchoscope is inserted by a physician under sterile conditions. The bronchoscope contains four channels: two light channels, one vision channel, and one open channel that accommodates biopsy forceps, cytology brush for obtaining samples, suction tube, lavage tube, anesthetic, or oxygen. Forceps and brushes can be advanced beyond the bronchoscope field of vision, with the aid of a fluoroscope, to obtain specimens. Bronchoalveolar lavage involves passing fluid through the scope into the bronchial area and then withdrawing the fluid. This procedure is useful for obtaining a specimen containing adequate microorganisms for examination.

Before the procedure, the patient is given atropine to dry respiratory secretions. The patient may also receive a narcotic for sedation and/or a tranquilizer for muscle relaxation. Rarely, the procedure will be performed under general anesthesia. In most cases, a local anesthetic is sprayed or swabbed over the mouth, tongue, and pharynx. The patient is placed in a supine

---

GALLIUM SCANS

A gallium scan is commonly used in the diagnosis of *Pneumocystis carinii* pneumonia. The patient is given a single IV injection of gallium 67 in a citrate solution, a radionuclide that concentrates in abscesses and areas of inflammation. The patient is scanned 4 to 6 hours after injection. Gallium 67 has a short half-life and decays rapidly. Because it is radioactive, it is necessary to adhere to precautions for handling the substance and to follow institutional and state waste disposal procedures. The procedure is contraindicated for pregnant or lactating women.

---

position with neck hyperextended. An oxygen tube is inserted into one nostril and left in place throughout the procedure. Lidocaine jelly is used to lubricate the bronchoscope and suppress the gag and cough reflexes. The bronchoscope is introduced through the nose or mouth and then guided through the trachea and into the mainstream bronchi.

NURSING CARE

1. Obtain patient's signed consent for the procedure.
2. Maintain patient NPO for 6 to 8 hours before the procedure and until gag reflex returns after the procedure (around 2 hours), as evident by stimulation of the uvula.
3. Remove any dental prostheses and inform the physician about loose teeth that patient may have.
4. Administer sedative as ordered.
5. Maintain patient in semi-Fowler's position after the procedure.
6. Discourage patient from talking until voice returns completely; provide patient with pencil and paper to communicate.
7. Throat discomfort is common following the procedure. Warm drinks, saline gargles, or throat lozenges may help.
8. Patients usually cough vigorously following the procedure and produce copious expectorations. Monitor for and report hemorrhage or changes in respiratory rate, rhythm, or breath sounds. Pink-tinged mucus is common; frank bleeding is a complication.

PATIENT TEACHING

Before the procedure explain:

1. The purpose of the procedure and symptoms to expect, particularly stimulation of the gag reflex
2. That sedation will be used to minimize discomfort and that analgesia will be available after the procedure, as needed
3. That the patient must breathe through the tube,

which initially may produce a feeling of suffocation; reassure the patient that the tube will remain open

4. That the patient will not be able to talk while the tube is in place and may be unable to talk for a short time following the procedure

5. That the procedure may take up to 45 to 60 minutes

WOUNDS AND DECUBITI SPECIMENS

A clean wound or ulcer contains essentially no pathogens. Signs of infection mandate microscopic examination and culturing of a specimen from the lesion to identify the responsible pathogen(s). Specimens for deep wounds and decubitus ulcers are cultured for both aerobic and anaerobic organisms. The technique for collecting specimens for anaerobic cultures must be precise because anaerobic organisms are destroyed quickly when exposed to oxygen and will fail to grow in culture.

COLLECTION PROCEDURES

Aerobic and anaerobic cultures

1. Assemble this equipment: a sterile 21-gauge needle and 10-ml syringe or sterile cotton swab, aerobic and anaerobic culture tubes, antiseptic solution, sterile gauze pads, gloves, and labels for identification.

2. Put on gloves and cleanse the area surrounding the wound with gauze pads soaked in the antiseptic solution to reduce contamination by normal flora nearby. Take care that no solution touches the wound, however, since this may affect culture growth.

3. For aerobic cultures: Express the wound (if necessary) by pressing on skin around the wound with sterile gauze pads to obtain an exudate. With a sterile cotton-tipped swab, collect as much exudate as possible. If the wound is deep, you may need to insert the swab into the wound and rotate gently to collect the specimen. Place the swab immediately in the aerobic culture tube and cap.

   For anaerobic cultures: Insert the needle into the wound and aspirate 1 to 5 ml of exudate or insert the swab deeply into the wound and gently rotate. Depending on instructions from the laboratory, either (1) immediately cover the needle and send the entire syringe to the laboratory or (2) open the stoppers and immediately inject the aspirate into the anaerobic culture tube

and quickly replace the double stoppers. If using an anaerobic culture tube, you must not open the stopper until you are ready to inject the specimen into the tube.

4. Properly discard gloves, swab, and any other objects that have touched the area.

5. Label the tube with the patient's name, time of collection, type of wound (e.g., puncture wound, decubitus ulcer, or surgical incision), probable source of infection, and whether the patient has received antibiotics. Transport immediately to the laboratory.

6. Dress the wound.

PATIENT TEACHING

Explain the purpose of the procedure, that it will take 1 to 2 minutes, and that there may be some discomfort.

GENITOURETHRAL AND RECTAL SPECIMENS

VAGINAL AND CERVICAL EXUDATES

Specimens for vaginal or cervical smears and cultures are obtained during the pelvic examination with the speculum in place. It is essential that only warm water is used for lubricant; any other lubricant will affect laboratory studies. If a Papanicolaou smear is ordered, it should be performed first, followed by vaginal and then cervical specimen collection.

COLLECTION PROCEDURES

1. Assemble this equipment: speculum, gloves, sterile cotton swabs, calcium alginate swab (for *Chlamydia*), glass slides with covers, saline and potassium hydroxide preparations, *Chlamydia* transport media, Thayer-Martin medium, and labels for identification.

2. With gloves on, insert speculum or separate labia.

3. Obtain specimen of vaginal secretions. Roll plain wooden end of sterile swab around in vaginal secretions for about 10 seconds if testing for *Haemophilus*, *Candida*, or *Trichomonas*.

4. Obtain cervical specimen. Insert sterile cotton swab or calcium alginate swab into the opening of the cervical os (Figure 5-3). Move the swab from side to side for 10 to 30 seconds to allow good absorption of the specimen into the swab. If the patient is a child or a woman who has had a hysterectomy, obtain the specimen from the posterior vaginal vault, or if the hymen is intact, the vaginal orifice.

Table 5-4

PREPARATION OF SMEARS FOR MICROSCOPIC EXAMINATION

Type	Suspected organism	Preparation
Dry mount	*Haemophilus vaginalis*	Smear the specimen over a dry glass slide and cover immediately with the coverslip.
Wet mount	*Trichomonas vaginalis*	Smear the specimen over a dry glass slide and add 1 drop of saline. Mix together with wooden end of specimen swab. Cover with coverslip.
KOH (potassium hydroxide)	*Candida albicans*	Smear the specimen over a dry glass slide and add 1 drop of KOH. Mix together with wooden end of specimen swab. Cover with coverslip.

5. Withdraw the swab and prepare the specimen (Table 5-4) for microscopic examination; for gonorrhea see box on p. 86; prepare with transport medium according to laboratory instructions for *Chlamydia.*

URETHRAL SPECIMENS

Urethral secretions are necessary for diagnosing a variety of infections, particularly gonorrhea and nongonococcal urethritis in the male patient. There are two methods for collecting these specimens.

COLLECTION PROCEDURES

For men

1. Assemble this equipment: sterile cotton swab, culture medium for gonococcus, slide and appropriate liquid preparation, as indicated, gloves, and labels for identification.
2. Ask the patient to milk the urethra. This will bring the milky-looking prostatic fluid to the urethral orifice.
3. While wearing gloves, collect the fluid with the cotton tip and prepare the specimen as described in the box on p. 86.

For children, women, or men

1. Assemble this equipment: either a special, thin urogenital alginate swab or wire bacteriologic loop, culture medium for gonococcus, slide and appropriate liquid preparation, as indicated, gloves, sterile gauze, cleansing agent, and labels for identification.
2. Place the patient in a supine position and drape.
3. While wearing gloves, clean the urethral meatus with sterile gauze.
4. Insert the swab or loop about 1 or 2 cm (⅜ or ¾ inch) into the meatus (Figure 5-4). Hold in place for 10 seconds, remove, and inoculate medium.

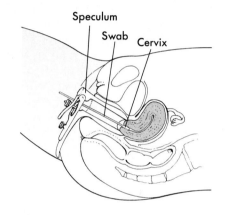
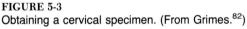

FIGURE 5-3
Obtaining a cervical specimen. (From Grimes.[82])

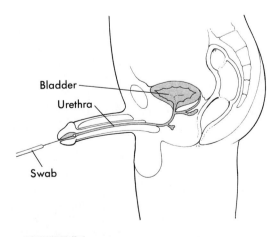

FIGURE 5-4
Obtaining a urethral specimen. (From Grimes.[82])

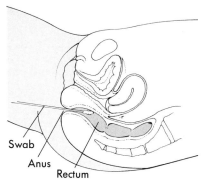

FIGURE 5-5
Obtaining a specimen of exudate from the rectum. (From Grimes.[82])

RECTAL SPECIMENS

The anal canal may be the primary site of gonorrhea infection, or the infection may spread from the genital tract. It is important to note that specimens for gonococcal cultures must not contain fecal material but only secretions from the anal crypts.

COLLECTION PROCEDURES

1. Assemble this equipment: sterile cotton-tipped swab, culture medium (either modified Thayer-Martin medium on a culture plate or Transgrow bottle), gloves, and labels for identification.
2. Position the patient in the left lateral recumbent position and drape.
3. Spread the buttocks and ask the patient to bear down to relax the external anal sphincter.
4. Insert the cotton tip approximately 2.5 cm (1 inch) into the anal canal (Figure 5-5). Move the swab from side to side, allowing 10 to 30 seconds for the swab to absorb organisms.
5. Remove the swab and inoculate culture medium.
6. Dispose of the swab and gloves properly.

GENITAL LESIONS

Cutaneous lesions may appear anywhere on the external genitalia in both women and men and even extend to the buttocks or thighs. Internal lesions may involve the vaginal walls, the cervix, or the anal canal. The appropriate method for collection and culturing depends on the suspected diagnosis.

Regardless of the type of lesion, the specimen must be collected from the exudate—not the surface of the lesion, which will usually yield only flora from the skin surface rather than the pathogen. Although there are minor variations among the procedures, collecting a specimen of a syphilis lesion is presented below.

Treponema pallidum, which causes syphilis, is identified by examination under a darkfield microscope. Because these organisms die quickly when removed from the body, microscopic examination must be done within 15 minutes, while they are still motile.

COLLECTION PROCEDURES

1. Assemble this equipment: sterile cotton swabs, saline, ether, pipette, slide with coverslip, gloves, and labels for identification.
2. While wearing gloves, clean the lesion with a saline-moistened swab to remove extraneous bacteria and debris.
3. Apply an ether-soaked swab to the lesion to release serum exudate.
4. Remove a sample of the exudate with a pipette.
5. Place the specimen on a dry slide and cover with the coverslip.
6. Discard gloves, swabs, and pipette appropriately.
7. Label the slide with the patient's name, time of collection, and location of the lesion.
8. Transport the slide immediately to the laboratory for examination.

FECAL SPECIMENS

Fecal specimens are obtained to culture organisms that are not part of the normal bowel flora. Microscopic examination of the specimen is performed to identify ova and parasites, to detect an increased number of white cells (indicating pathogenic invasion of the intestinal wall), and to detect red blood cells (indicating gastrointestinal bleeding). Some viruses can be identified by either electron microscopy or immunoassay.

Normally, stools contain only normal flora in the expected proportions: over 95% consists of anaerobes (e.g., non-spore-forming bacilli, clostridia, and streptococci) and the remaining consists of gram-negative aerobes (e.g., mostly *Escherichia coli*, other Enterobacteriaceae, and some *Pseudomonas*), gram-positive cocci, and yeasts. The finding of an unusually high population of normal flora is pathogenic, and additional tests may be performed to identify toxin production. Organisms such as *Clostridium difficile* are examples of normal flora that can become pathogenic in immunosuppression.

COLLECTION PROCEDURES

The stool specimen should not contain urine or water from the toilet bowl. The patient may defecate into a clean bedpan or onto a plastic bag or newspaper taped under the toilet seat (Figure 5-6). With proper instructions, ambulatory patients can easily collect their own fecal specimens in the same manner as described below. Fecal specimens may also be obtained directly from the rectum using a sterile swab, if necessary, for unconscious patients or for infants and young children.

Fecal collection

1. If the specimen will be tested for viruses, check with the laboratory for the proper procedure.
2. Assemble this equipment: a waxed or plastic cup with a lid, label for identification, clean gloves, a tongue blade, and either a clean, dry bedpan *or* plastic or newspaper taped securely under the toilet seat.
3. Instruct the patient to defecate without voiding.
4. Wearing gloves, collect the stool specimen with the tongue blade. If the stool is formed, a walnut-sized specimen is sufficient. If the stool is liquid, 15 to 20 ml is collected.
5. Place the specimen in the cup, being careful not to contaminate the outside of the container.
6. Wrap the tongue blade and gloves and discard properly.
7. Place the lid on the container and label it with the patient's name, time of collection, and suspected diagnosis and note if the patient has received antibiotics.
8. Wash your hands.
9. Transport the specimen to the laboratory immediately. (If the fecal specimen will not be tested for parasites, transport may be delayed. However, check with the laboratory for instructions about storing the specimen.)

Rectal swab

1. Assemble this equipment: sterile swab, gloves, and a wax or plastic cup with a tight-fitting lid (label for identification).
2. Place the patient in the left lateral recumbent position, knees bent toward the chest.
3. Separate the buttocks and ask the patient to bear down to relax the external sphincter. Insert the sterile swab into the rectum just inside anal opening (see Figure 5-5).
4. Keeping the buttocks separated, withdraw the swab and deposit the fecal material in the cup. If

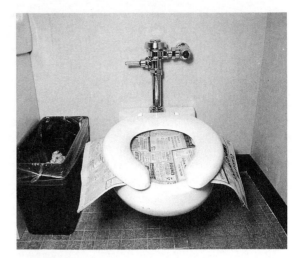

FIGURE 5-6
A stool specimen can be obtained directly from newspaper taped under a toilet seat. (From Grimes.[82])

more material is needed, repeat the procedure with another sterile swab.
5. Discard gloves and swab.
6. See 8 and 9 under Fecal Collection.

PATIENT TEACHING

Explain the procedure and its purpose. If the patient is to collect the specimen without supervision, explain each step in detail, including the importance of not contaminating the fecal material with urine or toilet paper.

CEREBROSPINAL FLUID SPECIMENS

When infection of the central nervous system is suspected, cerebrospinal fluid (CSF) analysis provides the only means of making a definitive diagnosis. CSF is usually obtained by lumbar puncture, which is usually performed between the third and fourth lumbar vertebrae. A cisternal puncture may be necessary if there is an infection or deformity in the lumbar area. Cisternal puncture is done with a short needle inserted below the occipital bone, just above the first cervical vertebra. Both procedures are performed by the physician, usually at bedside.

In rare cases, ventricular puncture must be performed in patients for whom the standard procedures are contraindicated. This is a surgical procedure that requires drilling a hole through the skull and aspirating CSF directly from a lateral ventricle.

A minimum of three tubes of CSF is usually col-

PREPARATION OF GONOCOCCAL CULTURE SPECIMENS

Two methods are used for culturing *Neisseria gonorrhoeae:* modified Thayer-Martin medium and Transgrow bottles. The procedures for inoculation follow.

Modified Thayer-Martin medium

- After collecting the specimen with a sterile cotton swab, remove the plate cover.
- Spread the specimen over the medium in a large **Z** pattern while rotating the swab.
- Cover the plate and label it with the patient's name, age, site from which the specimen was obtained (e.g., cervix, vaginal wall, urethra, or anal canal), and the date and time of collection.
- Transport to the laboratory.

Transgrow bottle

- After collecting the specimen with a sterile cotton swab, remove the bottle cap. Be sure to keep the bottle upright throughout the procedure to prevent the loss of carbon dioxide.
- Insert the cotton swab into the bottle and allow it to absorb excess moisture.
- Roll the swab against the side of the bottle, starting at the bottom of the bottle and working toward the top.
- Replace the cap immediately and label the container with the patient's name, age, site from which the specimen was obtained (e.g., cervix, vaginal wall, urethra, or anal canal), and the time and date of collection.
- Transport to the laboratory.

From Grimes.[82]

lected for laboratory analysis, one of which is for Gram's stains, culturing, and antibiotic sensitivity tests. Additional tests include electrolyte analysis, glucose testing, serologic tests, such as the VDRL for syphilis, and cytologic analysis for protein and unusual cells.

Spinal fluid is normally clear and contains 15 to 45 mg of protein/100 ml, 50 to 80 mg glucose/100 ml, 118 to 130 mEq chloride/L, less than 5 white blood cells (WBCs), and no organisms. Bacterial meningitis, brain abscess, or other infective process of the CNS produces a cloudy CSF containing increased numbers of WBCs, and glucose and chloride levels are often decreased.

CONTRAINDICATIONS

CSF puncture cannot be performed on the uncooperative patient, in patients with severe spine disorders, or if there is an infection at the puncture site. In-creased intracranial pressure is a relative contraindication, requiring that the procedure be performed with extreme caution to avoid cerebellar herniation and compression of the medulla.

COMPLICATIONS

Headache following the procedure is extremely common. Puncture of a nerve root during the procedure may occur.

COLLECTION PROCEDURES

1. Obtain informed consent.
2. Administer sedative as ordered. Be sure the patient urinates immediately before the procedure.
3. Assemble lumbar or cisternal puncture tray, sterile gloves and bandage, local anesthetic, antiseptic solution, and identification labels.

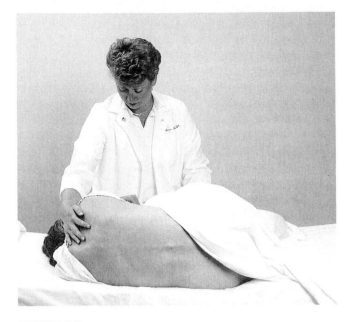

FIGURE 5-7
Positioning patient for lumbar puncture. (From Grimes.[82])

4. Assist the patient into a lateral recumbent position with the spine close to the edge of the bed or table (Figure 5-7). The patient's knees are drawn up against the abdomen and the chin is resting on the chest, curving the spine forward to provide maximum space between the vertebrae. Use pillows as needed to position the spine in a horizontal alignment. You or another nurse must help the patient maintain this position throughout the procedure by placing one arm around the patient's knees and the other arm around his or her neck (or head if a cisternal puncture is performed). (Note: Some physicians prefer performing the procedure with the patient sitting, chest and head bent forward on the thighs.) Quietly reassure the patient throughout the procedure.

5. Medical procedure: The puncture site is scrubbed and draped by the physician, and a local anesthetic is injected to anesthetize the skin. A spinal needle is injected at the midline, usually between L3 and L4 for lumbar puncture, or above C1 for a cisternal puncture. The stylet is removed by the physician, allowing spinal fluid to drip from the needle if it is correctly positioned. The initial CSF pressure is measured with a stopcock and manometer attached to the needle. This initial pressure should be recorded.

CSF samples are then collected and placed into specimen tubes. The CSF pressure is again taken and recorded, and the needle is removed. The puncture site is cleaned with an antiseptic, and a bandage is applied.

6. Fill three or four sterile tubes, following specifications of the laboratory. Label each tube with the words "spinal fluid" and the patient's name, time of collection, and test to be performed. Notify the laboratory that CSF specimens are ready so that the personnel are prepared for immediate analysis, and immediately transport the specimens to the laboratory. Do not refrigerate unless the laboratory requests chilling for viral culture.

7. On the patient's chart, record the color and clarity of the specimen and the patient's reaction to the procedure.

NURSING CARE

During the procedure, observe the patient for any signs of adverse reaction and alert the physician immediately. An elevated pulse rate, pallor, and clammy skin may indicate shock.

After the procedure, maintain the patient in bed as ordered by the physician. Most physicians require that the patient remain flat for 4 to 6 hours, but some allow the head to be elevated 30 degrees. However, the patient may turn from side to side. Monitor the patient's neurologic status (including level of consciousness, mentation, and pupillary reactivity) and vital signs every 15 minutes for 4 hours and then hourly, if the patient remains stable. By 6 hours after the procedure, assess neurologic status every 4 hours or as ordered. Check the puncture site for swelling, erythema, and drainage once an hour for 4 hours and then every 4 hours for the next 24 hours. Encourage the patient to drink fluids. If headache occurs, administer analgesics as ordered.

PATIENT TEACHING

Before the procedure, describe the procedure and explain its purpose. Stress the importance of keeping completely still and breathing normally throughout the procedure. Provide assurance you will help the patient maintain the correct position. Explain that a local anesthetic will be injected first, which will sting, and that the spinal needle will cause some brief pain. Tell the patient to let you know if the pain continues or if any other unusual sensations occur during the procedure, such as pain radiating to either leg. Explain that headache after the procedure is common but staying in bed as ordered by the physician will help minimize this side effect.

Laboratory Tests to Identify Pathogens

As discussed in the introduction to collecting specimens, three general types of laboratory procedures are used for identifying specific organisms involved in infection. These include microscopic examination of a specimen, culture of a specimen, and immunologic tests on a specimen or on serum. All three will be described here.

MICROSCOPIC EXAMINATION

Microscopic examination of a specimen is the only method of identifying parasites and ova, and it distinguishes tissue cells from microorganisms. Because most microorganisms and other cells appear colorless under a microscope, stains are added to highlight their structural characteristics. Microorganisms are classified partly according to their shape, size, and staining characteristics. Thus the type of organism can be identified (e.g., rods versus cocci, gram-positive versus gram-negative bacteria, and viruses versus bacteria) by microscopic examination. The results of microscopy are usually available within hours or even minutes, often permitting a presumptive diagnosis so that treatment can be initiated rapidly.

In addition to the basic brightfield microscope, several other microscopic techniques have been developed to identify specific organisms. They include electron, fluorescent, darkfield, and phase-contrast microscopy.

As soon as a specimen is obtain, it must be prepared immediately to preserve the pathogens and other cells for microscopic examination. Two basic methods are used for microscopy.

- **Wet mounts.** The specimen is smeared on a glass slide, and a liquid is added immediately. (The liquid used depends on the suspected diagnosis.) The specimen is protected with a coverslip for transport. Stains may be added in the laboratory to highlight the characteristics of the organisms. Wet mounts are used when diagnosis requires a live organism (as in *T. pallidum*) and for identifying yeasts, such as *Trichomonas vaginalis*.
- **Smears.** The specimen is smeared on a glass slide, allowed to air dry for a short period, and protected by a coverslip for transport. Stains are added to the smears to highlight cell structures. Smears are used to identify bacteria, viruses, normal tissue cells, and inflammatory cells.

GRAM'S STAIN

Gram's stains are one of the most useful procedures in microbiologic testing. This staining method consists of dropping first methyl violet and then iodine onto the dried smear on a slide. Acetone is then added to wash excess stain away. Organisms that absorb the dye into their cell walls are gram positive and appear violet or blue when examined under the microscope. Gram-negative organisms easily give up the dye and can be counterstained with a red dye, such as fuchsin. Organisms that do not grow in culture, including some anaerobes, can often be identified by Gram's stain. In addition, this technique stains tissue cells, which allows a general evaluation of the patient's inflammatory response.

Finally, the quality of a specimen can be rapidly determined by Gram's staining before culturing. For example, if a "sputum" specimen is found to contain primarily normal flora of the nasopharyngeal tract and large numbers of epithelial cells, the laboratory can notify you that collection should be attempted again. Since cultures require from 24 hours to several weeks for development, microscopic assessment before culturing can save valuable time by excluding poor-quality specimens that might grow little but normal flora.

OTHER STAINS

A multitude of other stains are available. Acid-fast stains can isolate *Mycobacterium*, a genus difficult to culture because of its slow growth, allowing a rapid diagnosis of tuberculosis. Periodic acid–Schiff (PAS) stain is used to identify fungi and *Pneumocystis carinii*. Other commonly used stains include Giemsa stain and Wright's stain, silver stains, and trichrome stain.

QUELLUNG REACTION

A quellung reaction is used to quickly determine the presence of encapsulated bacteria, such as *Streptococcus pneumoniae*, in a sputum specimen. Emulsified sputum is placed on a clear glass slide and mixed with antiserum. When the result is positive, the antibody-antigen reaction causes the capsule of the organism to swell. A positive result is quite specific for encapsulated bacteria. A negative result is inconclusive due to the fact that a particular specimen may not contain the infecting organism.

CULTURES

Bacteria, fungi, and some viruses are positively identified by culturing. Because many microorganisms have very specific requirements for growth, specimens are sent to the laboratory with instructions to culture the suspected pathogen(s). Several types of both liquid and solid culture media are available for supporting different types of organisms. In general, liquid medium is preferred for certain kinds of specimens, such as blood, because fewer microorganisms can be grown, whereas solid medium will grow mixed cultures.

In addition, some organisms have specific temperature, atmosphere, or pH requirements. For example, *N. gonorrhoeae* is sensitive to sudden temperature changes and will not grow when inoculated onto medium just removed from the refrigerator. Mycobacteria grow best when incubated with carbon dioxide. Anaerobic bacteria will not grow in the presence of oxygen.

Accurate results are obtained only when specimens are inoculated into culture media quickly. The bacterial population in room-temperature urine, for example, can quadruple within 60 minutes of voiding. As a result, culture growth will not reflect the actual bacterial level in the urinary tract.

In a few cases, notably when testing for gonorrhea, cultures must be inoculated immediately upon collection. Otherwise, most specimens are placed in a transport medium and sent to the laboratory. Transport media protect the microorganisms from drying, which results in death, and inhibit contaminants. As with culture media, the correct transport medium depends on the suspected pathogen. One method is to obtain the specimen with a polyester culture swab that comes in a plastic tube with an ampule containing the medium. This technique is obviously suitable only for collecting small quantities of exudates (e.g., from mucous membranes, the genitourinary tract, and wounds and lesions).

How quickly the pathogen can be recovered from cultures often depends on the type of microorganism, the type of specimen, and the stage of illness. Culture results are available in 24 to 48 hours on many of the common pathogens, such as streptococci, staphylococci, and enterobacteria. Pneumococcal organisms grow cultures in 3 to 4 days. In contrast, mycobacteria require anywhere from 1 week to 2 months.

Some organisms are detectable in specimens from different sites at varying times. *Salmonella typhosa* is usually detected in blood cultures only during the first 10 days of fever, whereas the organisms appear in stool after 10 days and in urine at 2 or 3 weeks.

Serial cultures are mandatory for positively identifying some organisms. Because *M. tuberculosis* is shed intermittently, negative cultures are common in patients with active tuberculosis. Therefore culture specimens must be collected daily over a 4- to 6-day period.

VIRAL CULTURES

Viral cultures are, in general, difficult to carry out. Most viruses are fragile and die quickly once outside living tissue. They must be kept in a hospitable environment until they are injected into a culture medium. In addition, it is frequently difficult to obtain a specimen that contains enough virus to culture. This is because in many viral syndromes, viral shedding is greatest during the prodromal period before the onset of clinical symptoms. Specimens obtained later in the course of infection may not contain adequate quantities of detectable virus.

Correct handling of the specimen, once obtained, is critical. Because many viruses are heat labile, the sterile container with the specimen requires packing in ice for transport to the laboratory. If some time is likely to pass before the specimen can be cultured, the specimen should be frozen at −70° C. Samples collected on swabs should be placed in a liquid viral transport medium before carrying to the laboratory. Close cooperation between clinicians and the laboratory is essential in order to preserve the highest quality and quantity of the viral specimen. However, even in the best of circumstances, viral cultures are likely to yield a large number of false-negative results.

IMMUNOLOGIC TESTS

Infectious agents cannot always be identified by the direct methods of microscopic examination or culturing. Pathogens that are antigenic stimulate antibodies, which can be detected in patients' serums by adding the specific antigen and observing the antigen-antibody reactions. Similarly, pathogens that release toxins are detected by adding antitoxins to serum. Several immunologic tests are available that measure antibody titers, the most common of which are described below.

It is important to note that the detection of antibodies is not diagnostic of current infection, since previous infection or immunization may account for the presence of antibodies in serum. Therefore antigen-antibody reactions must be evaluated over a period of time before a definite diagnosis can be made. IgM antibody production peaks during active infection and then decreases during the convalescent period. IgG antibodies peak during convalescence and last longer. A blood sample taken during acute infection is compared with a second sample obtained 2 to 3 weeks later. A fourfold rise in antibody titer (the measure of antigen-antibody reactions) during convalescence indicates concurrent infection.

Immunologic tests are less useful for identifying infection with opportunistic organisms in immunosuppressed persons. The reason is that antibody titers are generally high from exposure to these organisms in earlier life. For example, almost every adult in the population has acquired antibodies against herpesviruses. Elevated serum titers for antibodies against herpes simplex virus (HSV), therefore, would not be useful in identifying herpes as a cause of a raging meningitis or encephalitis in an immunosuppressed person.

AGGLUTINATION TESTS

Agglutination tests demonstrate the ability of antibodies and antigens to bind together, a "clumping" reaction that is observed in a test tube, slide, or other specially prepared surface. Several dilutions of the patient's serum are tested against constant amounts of antigen. The highest dilution that still demonstrates agglutination is the agglutination titer. A rise in titer between acute and convalescent serum is more diagnostic than a single high titer.

Two types of agglutination tests are used: direct and indirect. In direct agglutination tests, antibodies attach directly to antigens. In indirect tests, antigens must first be coated with chemicals that attract antibodies. Agglutination tests are used in blood typing and in identifying antibodies against many bacterial, fungal, and parasitic infections and a few viral infections.

Agglutination tests that may be used to identify infections in immunosuppressed persons include the following (with their diagnostic applications):

1. Hemagglutination: amoeba (amebiasis)
2. Hemagglutination inhibition: hepatitis B
3. Heterophil antibody: Epstein-Barr virus
4. Microhemagglutination–*Treponema pallidum: T. pallidum* infection (syphilis)
5. Rapid plasma reagin (RPR): syphilis
6. Venereal Disease Research Laboratory (VDRL): syphilis
7. Widal's reaction: *Salmonella* (salmonellosis)

COMPLEMENT FIXATION

Complement is a group of serum proteins that enter into antigen-antibody reactions, one of which is lysis of antigen cells. One or more of the complement components can be used (or fixed) in an antigen-antibody reaction, rendering complement unavailable for subsequent reactions. Complement fixation (CF) is a multistage test that is based on this principle.

A known amount of complement is added to a patient's serum. Sheep red blood cells (SRBC), which are antigenic in human serum, are then added to the serum. Any unfixed complement will lyse the SRBC. Thus lysis occurs when complement is unfixed, indicating the serum lacks antigen or antibody. No lysis occurs

if all complement is bound. CF test results are given in titers. The CF titer is the dilution of serum that completely fixes complement, with the higher dilutions indicating higher antibody titers.

The CF test detects antigens or antibodies associated with many bacterial, fungal, viral, and parasitic infections. The now obsolete Wassermann test for syphilis was based on complement fixation.

IMMUNODIFFUSION AND COUNTERELECTROPHORESIS

Immunodiffusion, electroimmunodiffusion, electrophoresis, counterimmunoelectrophoresis (CIE), and immunoelectrophoresis are assays that measure precipitation, which is the reaction that occurs when antigen-antibody complexes form and migrate across the test medium. The basic test is immunodiffusion, which uses agar or agarose gel and takes 48 to 96 hours to complete. Precipitin lines form when the concentrations of antigen and antibody are equal, indicating they have formed complexes.

The other four tests are electrophoretic variations on this basic test, in which an electric field is applied to the medium. These tests are much faster, requiring only 1½ to 4 hours to complete.

Precipitation assays detect a variety of viral, bacterial, fungal, and parasitic antigens and antibodies. The Western blot test is an immunoelectrophoresis assay for HIV.

ENZYME-LINKED IMMUNOSORBENT ASSAY

Enzyme-linked immunosorbent assay (ELISA) is a complex and highly sensitive test that measures either antigens or antibodies. Commercial kits, containing specific antigens (or antibodies) that are labeled with an enzyme, provide a testing standard for comparison. The enzyme-labeled antigen (or antibody) is added to serum, where it competes with its unlabeled counterpart to bind to antibody (or antigen) present in the serum. A colorless substrate for the enzyme is added. The bound enzyme acts on the substrate to produce a color change, which can be read visually or with a spectrophotometer. Color increases as the amount of antibody fixed to antigen increases.

ELISA is more sensitive than CIE in detecting antibodies or antigens in certain bacterial, fungal, parasitic, and viral infections. It is particularly useful in diagnosing HIV infection, hepatitis A and B, and rubella.

RADIOIMMUNOASSAY

In radioimmunoassay (RIA), a known amount of a specific antigen (or antibody) that is labeled with radioactive isotopes is added to the specimen, causing antigen-antibody complexes to precipitate. The radioactive count is measured in the precipitate and the result is converted to a titer measurement. RIA is highly sensitive and can detect small amounts of either antibody or antigen. This assay is useful in diagnosing hepatitis B.

IMMUNOFLUORESCENT ANTIBODY ASSAY

With an immunofluorescent antibody (IFA) assay, antigen-antibody binding can be observed under a fluorescent microscope when either antigens or antibodies are tagged with a fluorescent dye. Direct and indirect methods are used. Direct fluorescent antibody uses a specific, labeled antibody to identify viruses from a specimen. Indirect immunofluorescence tests unlabeled patient serum against labeled cell cultures. The highest dilution of patient serum that still shows fluorescence is the IFA titer.

Some commonly used IFA assays are the FTA-ABS (fluorescent treponemal antibody-absorbed test) for syphilis, the IFA for toxoplasmosis, and the Micro-IF (micro-immunofluorescence) for *Chlamydia trachomatis*.

OTHER IMMUNOLOGIC TESTS

The limulus lysate assay detects endotoxins in CSF that are produced by gram-negative bacteria, including *E. coli*, *Neisseria meningitidis*, and *Haemophilus influenzae*. Although the limulus assay is not as specific as CIE and latex agglutination procedures, it is useful for the rapid diagnosis of gram-negative bacterial meningitis.

Three antigen-antibody reactions can be observed microscopically: immobilization, opsonization and phagocytosis, and capsular swelling (quellung reaction). The TPI (*T. pallidum* immobilization) test detects capsular swelling and is used in diagnosing syphilis.

Neutralization tests are sometimes used. A known antigen or toxin is incubated in test serum, which is then inoculated into tissue culture. Neutralizing antibodies or antitoxin, if present, will prevent tissue destruction. Because neutralizing antibodies persist for years, acute and convalescent serums must be compared to identify current infection.

Skin Tests

Skin tests are based on the principle that the immunocompetent person develops a cellular immune response to infection with certain microorganisms. An intradermal injection of these antigens will stimulate this immune response, if present, eliciting inflammation and induration at the site of the injection. A test volume, usually 0.1 ml, of the antigen is injected intradermally (Figure 5-8) into the anterior surface of the forearm. The diameter of the induration at the injection site is measured at a specified time (depending on the test). A positive reaction to the test indicates the presence of T lymphocytes against the antigen, suggesting previous (or present) infection with the organism. A negative test result suggests absence of an immune response, which may or may not indicate absence of infection.

Skin tests are sometimes used to test for an immune response to *Mycobacterium tuberculosis*, *Histoplasma capsulatum* (histoplasmosis), and *Coccidioides immitis* (coccidioidomycosis) in HIV-infected persons. Because these tests are aimed at detecting the cellular immune response to specific organisms, test reactions may be diminished or nonexistent in severely immunocompromised individuals. A positive skin test reaction always indicates previous infection. A negative result may be a false-negative result—that is, it may not indicate absence of infection. A person who is truly infected but is unable to demonstrate a cellular immune response

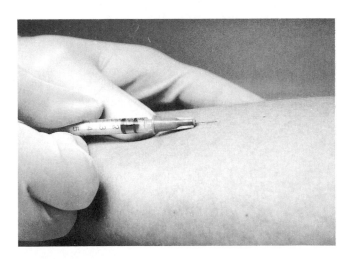

FIGURE 5-8
Administering intradermal injection for skin test. Note that the needle bevel is facing upward and the syringe and needle are parallel to the skin. (From Grimes.[82])

when skin tested is said to be anergic. This state can be confirmed by administering control skin tests against antigens to which the person is known to have been exposed. Antigens commonly administered as controls include *Candida*, mumps, and tetanus. If the control test result is negative (no skin reaction to the antigen), anergy is suspected. A positive reaction to the controls negates the possibility of anergy. This allows one to have more confidence in a negative skin test result with the test antigen, such as *M. tuberculosis*.

Antibiotic Sensitivity Testing

The growing number of pathogens that have developed resistance to antibiotics is a matter of great concern. The widespread, often inappropriate use of antibiotics since World War II has resulted in a varying degree of susceptibility among many species of bacteria. Resistance develops primarily in three ways: genetic mutation of the organism, transmissible genetic particles coding for drug resistance, and the production of beta-lactamase enzymes, which inactivate the drug.

Antibiotic sensitivity testing saves valuable time (and often lives) that might otherwise be wasted waiting for a clinical response. Antimicrobial drugs are added to a culture to determine whether the microorganism is inhibited from growing or is killed. Two methods are used for testing antibiotic sensitivity.

TUBE DILUTION

The tube dilution method uses either broth or agar as the medium, and different concentrations of an antibiotics are added to a known number of organisms to determine the amount of drug that will inhibit visible growth. This dose is termed the *minimum inhibitory concentration (MIC)*.

The MIC is reported as the antibiotic concentration per milliliter of solution and compared with the achiev-able blood level of the antibiotic. An organism is considered sensitive to a drug if the antibiotic blood levels can be attained at two to four times the MIC. Laboratories may also report the *minimum bactericidal concentration (MBC)*, the smallest concentration necessary to kill 99.9% of the organisms. This may or may not be higher than the MIC.

AGAR DIFFUSION

The agar diffusion method is more widely used. This involves exposing a pure culture of the microorganism to a paper disk impregnated with a known amount of antibiotic, which diffuses from the disk into the culture. MIC is measured by the size of the zone around the disk in which growth is inhibited. One advantage of the agar diffusion method is that several antibiotics can be tested on a single culture, allowing a rapid method of identifying the appropriate drug for organisms that are resistant to some antibiotic agents. This multidrug test is the Kirby-Bauer method of agar diffusion.

The results of agar diffusion tests are reported as "resistant" if growth is not altered, "sensitive" if growth is retarded, and "intermediate" if test results are uncertain. Some authorities believe that intermediate sensitivity should be classified as resistant.

CHAPTER 6

Dermatologic Manifestations

The skin is a marvelous organ, capable of carrying out multiple functions to allow the body to interface safely with a sometimes hostile environment. HIV infection alters and impairs the skin and one or more of its functions at some time during the long course of infection.

One important function is to act as an armor against constant bombardment by billions of environmental microorganisms. An intact skin can be an impenetrable barrier against most invaders, thus functioning as the most important defense against these pathogens. Unfortunately, microorganisms can enter the body through breaks in the skin or through other portals of entry, such as mucous membranes, causing pathologic manifestations in the skin. Impairment of skin integrity, from whatever mechanism, opens the body to further invasion by microorganisms. Therefore, the frequent infections and skin lesions associated with HIV not only cause pain and embarrassment, but also increase vulnerability to environmental pathogens.

The skin not only is a passive barrier against infection but actively fights potential invaders as well. One of its armaments is the secretion of bactericidal substances. Another defense mechanism is the presence of a normal flora of organisms. The skin's normal flora competes with environmental organisms for nutrients on the skin, thus preventing colonization by potential pathogens. The marvelous checks and balances provided by normal flora can be disrupted by antibiotic therapy. Antibiotics may kill many of the organisms that have previously acted to check the growth of potential pathogens, resulting in an overgrowth of these pathogens. HIV-infected persons frequently take multiple antibiotics to control serious systemic infections. They take these antibiotics for long periods of time, causing nonstop interference with normal flora.

The skin also functions to regulate body temperature through a number of interacting mechanisms. One is by providing a large surface area to conduct heat away from the body into the atmosphere. The amount of heat dispersed in this fashion is regulated by blood vessels in the skin that dilate or constrict to allow less or more blood to be cooled. In addition, sweat produced when the body overheats hastens cooling as it evaporates. The immunocompromised person experiences a great amount of diaphoresis due to chronic and recurrent fevers associated with HIV itself and/or opportunistic infections. Constant diaphoresis not only leads to fluid and electrolyte imbalance but also impairs the skin's integrity further by leading to maceration, excoriation, and overgrowth of fungi.

Skin also is a major sensory organ. Free nerve endings and special receptors in the skin assist the body to recognize and interpret environmental stimuli by producing pain, itching, heat, cold, pressure, and kinesthesia. Such sensations are critical to protecting the body from injury. Progressive neuropathy, which is as-

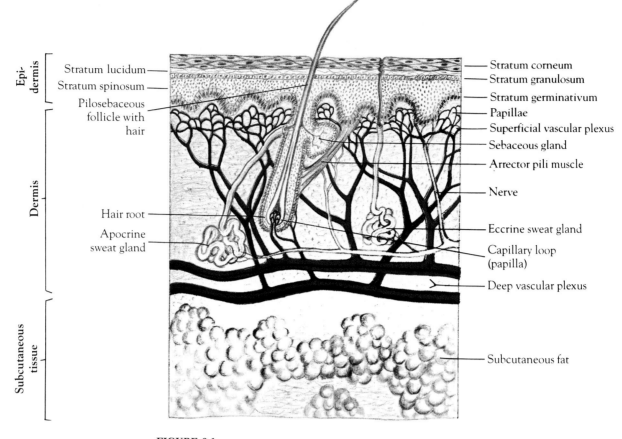

Epi-dermis

Stratum lucidum

Stratum spinosum

Pilosebaceous follicle with hair

Dermis

Hair root

Apocrine sweat gland

Subcutaneous tissue

Stratum corneum

Stratum granulosum

Stratum germinativum

Papillae

Superficial vascular plexus

Sebaceous gland

Arrector pili muscle

Nerve

Eccrine sweat gland

Capillary loop (papilla)

Deep vascular plexus

Subcutaneous fat

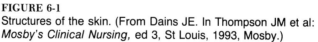

FIGURE 6-1
Structures of the skin. (From Dains JE. In Thompson JM et al: *Mosby's Clinical Nursing,* ed 3, St Louis, 1993, Mosby.)

sociated with HIV infection (see Chapter 8), interferes with sensory ability. This predisposes the person to further injury from heat, pressure, trauma, etc., and to further impairment in skin integrity.

The skin has been described as a window to the internal functioning of the body. Many systemic infections, such as measles and hepatitis, manifest themselves with characteristic skin changes or eruptions. These manifestations are often used as important diagnostic clues to the presence of underlying infection. For example, herpes zoster infections are diagnosed based on the characteristic grouping of vesicular lesions along a nerve pathway. Some systemic infections, such as tuberculosis, may produce exudative skin lesions. This permits the clinician to identify the causative pathogen from a specimen of the exudate. In addition, skin rashes, swelling, or itching reflects systemic allergic reactions, which would otherwise go unnoticed.

Thus, the HIV-infected person may have many dif-

ferent pathologies that are reflected by the skin. These can be uncovered by a careful history of skin changes and a physical examination of the skin.

Figure 6-1 shows the basic structures of the skin. It will assist the reader to interpret Table 6-1, which presents the principal dermatologic problems associated with HIV infection. Color plates 42-57 in the front of the book illustrate the most commonly used terms to describe types of skin lesions (e.g., papules, vesicles). These illustrations can be used in conjunction with Table 6-1 to interpret findings from physical assessment of a patient.

The skin can become infected and/or diseased in more than one manner. First, pathogens may invade the skin and cause either localized pathology or localized and systemic pathology. Second, an infectious or pathologic process may occur elsewhere in the body and manifest with skin lesions.

Table 6-1 _____

OVERVIEW OF DERMATOLOGIC MANIFESTATIONS

Condition	Description	Signs and symptoms
Folliculitis	Bacterial infection and irritation of the hair follicle, usually caused by *Staphylococcus aureus;* occasionally caused by other organisms, particularly after antibiotic therapy.	Infection usually begins as a small 1-2 mm pustule surrounded by erythema, which often has a hair in its center; most likely to appear on the central trunk, face, and groin in the HIV-infected person.
Impetigo/ecthyma (Color Plate 4)	Impetigo is a superficial vesiculopustular infection; ecthyma is the ulcerative form of impetigo; may be caused by *S. aureus,* by beta-hemolytic streptococci, or by both. Autoinoculation is common, with satellite lesions developing.	Initial lesion is an erythematous macule that changes into a bulla with a thin roof. In streptococcal impetigo, the bulla becomes pustular within hours of forming; it ruptures and becomes covered with a thin, honey-colored crust. In staphylococcal impetigo, a thin, clear crust forms from the exudate.
Cellulitis	A diffuse, acute infection of the skin and subcutaneous tissue caused by streptococci or staphylococci; enzyme byproducts of the invading organism break down cellular components that would normally contain and localize the inflammation; lymphangitis and septicemia are potential complications.	Diffuse erythema with ill-defined borders; skin is red, hot, indurated, and tender; may have an infiltrated surface resembling the skin of an orange, purulent discharge and/or abscesses, and/or red striae radiating from the central inflammatory area.
Tinea	Generalized term used to describe a group of superficial fungal infections that are common and difficult to treat in HIV-infected persons; they include:	
	Tinea capitis (ringworm)	Scaling, itchy scalp, friable hair, and balding
	Tinea cruris (jock itch)	Small areas of erythema, scaling, and vesicular patches in groin
	Tinea pedis (athlete's foot)	Erythema, scaling, maceration, fissures, and burning pain, primarily between the toes
	Tinea versicolor	Pale, tan patches in Caucasians; depigmented patches in dark-skinned persons; appears primarily on the trunk and upper arms
Insect bites	Hypersensitive reactions to insect bites are common in HIV-infected persons.	Mosquito bites appear as pruritic, erythematous, urticarial papules on exposed parts of the body. Flea bites appear as hemorrhagic punctures in the center of small wheals, usually appearing at wrists, ankles, and waist. Scratching results in secondary infections.
Scabies	Transmissible parasitic infestation of the skin whereby a mite burrows into the skin to lay its eggs, creating inflammation, intense pruritus, and potential for secondary infections from scratching.	Papules, vesicles, or lines of burrows, often obscured because of excoriation due to scratching; may appear as a generalized dermatitis; usually found in webs of fingers, flexor surfaces of wrists and elbows, belt line, axillary folds, and thighs.
Molluscum contagiosum (Color Plate 17)	Chronic, cutaneous viral infection; transmitted by direct contact or through fomites; new lesions form from autoinoculation; condition may persist for years.	Smooth-surfaced, firm, spherical papules 2-5 mm to 1 cm in diameter; lesions may be flesh colored, white, translucent, or yellow; common on the face, groin, and genitalia but may appear anywhere.
Human papillomavirus (HPV) (condylomata acuminata) (Color Plates 13-16)	A viral infection manifested by a variety of skin and mucous membrane lesions (warts); generally sexually transmitted. HPV types 16 and 18 have been associated with cervical neoplasia (see Chapter 10).	Soft, moist, pink or red papules that grow rapidly and become pedunculated; usually found in clusters (cauliflower-form) on the genitalia, around the anus, and within the anal canal.

Continued.

Table 6-1

OVERVIEW OF DERMATOLOGIC MANIFESTATIONS—cont'd

Condition	Description	Signs and symptoms
Candidiasis (Color Plate 18)	Fungal infection, in which *C. albicans*, a normal flora organism of the skin and mucous membranes, becomes pathogenic; occurs in the absence of inhibiting organisms or because of decline in cell-mediated immunity.	Initial lesion is a thin-walled pustule, with an inflammatory base, that extends under the stratum corneum; produces an exudate that is a whitish-yellow, curdlike substance. Lesion typically is found in moist areas, such as the mouth and skin folds, around fingernails, and in the vulvovaginal areas; enlarges until it reaches dry skin; may burn or itch.
Bacillary angiomatosis	New skin disorder seen exclusively in HIV infection; apparently caused by a rickettsia called *Rochalimaea henselae*.	Friable, vascular papules or cellulitic plaques; lesions may become pedunculated; may spread to liver, bone, spleen, and lymph nodes. Lesions have an appearance similar to those of Kaposi's sarcoma.
Syphilis (Color Plates 19 and 20)	Chronic, systemic, sexually transmitted infection of the blood vessels caused by *Treponema pallidum*, a spirochete; characterized by three stages: primary, secondary, and tertiary syphilis. Dermatologic signs appear in primary and secondary syphilis; the latent stage is a quiescent, asymptomatic stage; systemic manifestations, including neurosyphilis, appear in the tertiary stage. Infection progresses very rapidly in HIV-infected persons.	Primary syphilis: single painless papule at site of invasion of the spirochete (generally found on the head of the penis, vulva, or anus); papule becomes a hard, indurated chancre without exudate and resolves spontaneously. Secondary syphilis: generalized or localized macular, papular, pustular, or papulosquamous rash; appears bilaterally and symmetrically, first on the trunk and proximal extremities, extending to the palms of the hands and the soles of the feet. Latency is an asymptomatic stage. Tertiary syphilis is characterized primarily by neurologic signs.
Herpes zoster (Color Plates 7 and 8)	Acute cutaneous eruption of the herpes zoster virus, which has been dormant since a previous infection with the virus (chickenpox). Eruption is accompanied by inflammation of the cutaneous nerve.	Clusters of vesicles on an erythematous base, localized along one or more posterior root ganglia; accompanied by intense pain and skin sensitivity to touch.
Herpes simplex (Color Plates 11, 12, 21-26)	Recurrent, cutaneous, viral infection; generally resolves in 1-2 weeks in immunocompetent persons, becoming chronic in immunosuppressed persons.	Clusters of vesicles, filled with clear fluid, on an erythematous base; appear on lips, mouth (see Chapter 7), genitalia, anus, and, occasionally, on the conjunctiva and cornea. Vesicles may coalesce and form large, erosive ulcers.
Seborrheic dermatitis	Chronic, recurrent, erythematous scaling eruption that is localized in areas where sebaceous glands are concentrated; cause is unknown; may be complicated with yeast infections; common in HIV infection.	Lesions appear as scaly, white or yellow inflammatory plaques; usually found on the face or behind the ears, although may appear on the chest and axillae; accompanied by mild pruritus. Scalp lesions are associated with dandruff.
Psoriasis (Color Plate 6)	Chronic relapsing skin disorder associated with systemic processes of unknown origin; lesions result from cellular proliferation and inflammation leading to excess production of epithelial cells. Condition can arise spontaneously after infection with HIV or can worsen in HIV-infected persons with a history of psoriasis.	Circumscribed red patches covered by thick, dry, silvery, adherent scales. Lesions may appear on back, buttocks, scalp, and extensor surfaces of extremities such as the knees and elbows.
Eosinophilic folliculitis	Condition is specific to HIV infection; characterized by inflammatory infiltration with eosinophils clustered around hair follicles; cause is unknown.	Pruritic, papular/vesicular rash on an erythematous base; usually appears on the face, neck, upper trunk, arms, and back.

Table 6-1

OVERVIEW OF DERMATOLOGIC MANIFESTATIONS—cont'd

Condition	Description	Signs and symptoms
Photodermatitis	Cutaneous eruptions that are believed to be related either to HIV infection or to sensitivity to sulfa and/or nonsteroidal antiinflammatory drugs.	Pruritic, scaly patches or manifestations of an intense sunburn; may become excoriated, thickened, and hypopigmented. Appears first on areas exposed to the sun, progressing to nonexposed areas.
Erythema multiforme (Color Plates 9 and 10)	Acute inflammatory eruption; cause is unknown but condition seems to be due to allergic hypersensitivity to certain drugs, particularly sulfa and penicillin. May progress to a potentially fatal condition called Stevens-Johnson syndrome, where lesions occur in internal organs.	Symmetric, erythematous, edematous or bullous lesions; typically appear as dark plaques with raised, circular borders and a depressed inner ring. After a few days the central area of erythema becomes dusky purple and may become bullous. In mild cases the lesions appear symmetrically on hands, feet, and face. In severe cases, lesions cover the trunk or entire body.
Pressure ulcers (decubiti)	Localized necrosis of skin and deeper tissues, which results from interruption of capillary blood supply to the area; generally due to prolonged pressure, immobility, malnutrition, etc. Ulcers are generally categorized as to their severity from stages 1-4. The first signs of a stage 1 ulcer indicate that irreversible impairment has already occurred. Progression of the necrosis and ulceration can result in septicemia and death.	Stage 1 ulcer: small area of skin, at pressure points (sacrum, heels, iliac crest, inner knees, elbows, shoulder blades), becomes "dusky" in coloration; blister may be present; stage 2: erosion of epidermis; stage 3: ulceration into dermal layers and subcutaneous tissue; stage 4: ulcer exposes muscle and bone.
Xerosis (dry skin)	Extremely common in HIV-infected persons throughout their infection; cause is unknown; may be the result of HIV itself or reaction to medications.	Generalized itching and scaling of skin; scratch marks.

Skin Manifestations That Result from Direct Invasion of Organisms

Once external pathogens survive the skin's defenses and invade dermal tissue, they meet the body's second line of defense against invaders, the inflammatory response. Neutrophils migrate to the junctional zones between the vascular endothelial cells. If the neutrophils do not neutralize the invader, lymphocytes will accumulate in the area and will attempt to create a cellular barrier against spread of the organism. As part of the process of neutralizing the invader, neutrophils, lymphocytes, and monocytes signal the body to produce granulation tissue around the lesion to contain the invader. If the inflammatory response fails to halt infec-

tion, other immune mechanisms generally take over. Because these other immune mechanisms are not fully functional in the HIV-infected person, successful pathogen invasion can result in uncontrolled local and disseminated infection.

The conditions caused by direct invasion are often preventable. A person can avoid anything that breaks the skin's integrity, such as trauma, scratching, and insect bites; can avoid direct contact with organisms transmitted sexually, such as molluscum and human papillomavirus; and can reduce colonization of organisms on the skin by aseptically cleaning wounds and by regularly bathing and shampooing. However, when organisms are already in the body in a latent form, progression of the immunosuppression is responsible for manifestation of dermatologic conditions.

The conditions listed in Table 6-1 that are caused by invading organisms that create only localized pathology in the skin include folliculitis, impetigo/ecthyma, cellulitis, tinea, insect bites, scabies, molluscum contagiosum, the human papillomavirus (HPV) that causes warts, and candidal inflammations. Another listed disorder, bacillary angiomatosis, has been so recently described that its pathophysiology is still vague. Conditions that present with skin and systemic pathologies include syphilis, herpes zoster, and herpes simplex.

Folliculitis is the term generally used to describe a bacterial infection around hair follicles. There are, however, other types of folliculitis. The lesions seen in the bacterial form are the result of the inflammatory response to chemotactic factors and enzymes that occur when bacteria proliferate rapidly. While relatively easily treated, the condition is also relatively easily prevented through good skin hygiene and avoidance of trauma that may result from scratching or shaving. HIV-infected men who experience recurrent facial folliculitis often are helped by growing a beard, which prevents both the lesions associated with ingrown hairs and trauma associated with shaving.

Impetigo/ecthyma (Color Plate 4) is a superficial, vesiculopustular infection caused by coagulase-positive staphylococci or beta-hemolytic streptococci, with both organisms sometimes present. The condition is called ecthyma if ulceration occurs. In streptococcal impetigo the infection localizes beneath the stratum corneum and produces macules, which develop into vesicles and bullae. Staphylococcal lesions tend to produce an exudate that hardens to form a honey-colored crust. The ulceration of ecthyma results when the infecting organism invades the dermal layers, which sometimes results from scratching the more superficial lesions. Ecthyma is characterized by thick, adherent, crusted plaques with underlying ulceration, purulent exudate, and subsequent scarring. Both impetigo and ecthyma are easily spread by autoinoculation and to others. Scratching should be avoided, and itching should be treated with antipruritics. One should take care in handling materials, such as clothing, that have been in contact with the lesions, since they may be highly infectious.

Cellulitis is the term used to describe a diffuse, inflamed area of skin, which is caused by bacterial overgrowth. The area is diffuse because enzymes produced by the organism break down some of the cellular components that would usually localize the infection. The organism is then able to infiltrate all layers of the skin and subcutaneous tissue. The lesion is characteristically red, hot, indurated, and tender and is often accompanied by irregular lymphangitic streaks (red streaks) leading away from the infection site. The condition may progress to skin breakdown with purulent discharge and/or bacteremia and septicemia. Timely treatment with systemic antiinfectives is important to prevent progression of the infection.

Tinea refers to a group of superficial fungal infections that invade the stratum corneum, nails, and hair. These infections are caused by a group of fungi called dermatophytes, which are very prevalent in the environment. They thrive in warm, moist areas of the skin. Specific tinea infections are named according to the body site where the lesion occurs (see Table 6-1). These conditions range in severity from mild inflammation to acute vesicular eruptions. They are difficult to treat in HIV-infected persons, particularly when the nails are involved. Even when successfully treated, tinea infections frequently recur.

Insect bites and **scabies** are as common in HIV-infected persons as they are in the immunocompetent. Bites may cause more severe reactions in the immunocompromised and may precipitate scratching and breaks in the skin. Therefore, they should be prevented if possible. Scabies must be treated in all household members and sexual partners to avoid reinfestation.

Molluscum contagiosum (Color Plate 17) appears as a flat, spherical, smooth papule. The lesions result from invasion of the molluscipoxvirus into epithelial cells, causing them to divide. The papule has a central core containing extremely infectious exudative material. The lesions are seldom painful, and usually are only mildly disfiguring. They tend to resolve without treatment within a few months. New lesions, however, may appear in different places as old lesions resolve. Individual lesions may be treated with topical drugs, curettage, cryotherapy, or electrosurgery.

Human papillomavirus (**HPV**) infection (Color Plates 13-16) (also called condylomata acuminata) of the anal-genital area is relatively common in HIV-infected individuals. HPV invades epithelial cells, causing the cells to divide rapidly, forming bulky lesions. These lesions, commonly called warts, vary in size and shape. The warts are not only unsightly, but they can grow large enough to interfere with urination, defecation, or childbirth. HPV infections have also been implicated as precursors to cervical and rectal cancer.

Candidal inflammations (Color Plate 18) can manifest on moist areas of the skin such as in skin folds, at sites where central lines have been installed, and around the fingernails. The most common dermatologic site for *C. albicans* overgrowth, however, is in the vulvovaginal area. This normal flora organism grows unchecked because of immunosuppression, antibiotic therapy, hormone changes, use of birth control pills, or some combination of these factors. Vulvovaginitis due to *C. albicans* does occur in immunocompetent women, but it is generally self-limiting or rapidly clears when the cause of the overgrowth is removed. In HIV-infected women, vulvovaginal candidiasis is much more severe and persistent, even with treatment. While topical treatments are sometimes effective, systemic antifungals are frequently required. This infection tends to recur frequently in HIV-positive women. Recurrent vulvovaginal candidiasis is so characteristic of HIV infection that some clinicians use it as a marker to suggest HIV testing for women at risk whose serostatus is unknown.

Syphilis is a systemic infection of the vascular system with four distinct stages: primary, secondary, latency, and tertiary syphilis. Both the primary and secondary stages have dermatologic manifestations. Primary syphilis is characterized by a red papule that appears at the site where the treponemal organism penetrated the skin or mucous membrane. The papule soon erodes to form an indurated, painless ulcer (chancre) with a serous exudate that contains *Treponema* (see Color Plate 19). The ulcer will heal spontaneously in 4 to 6 weeks. About the time that the ulcer resolves, the secondary stage is heralded, for 80% of people infected with syphilis, by the appearance of a characteristic generalized rash. This maculopapular rash is pinkish or pale red in Caucasians and is pigmented or copper colored in people of color. It appears bilaterally on the body but is particularly evident on the soles of the feet and palms of the hands (see Color Plate 20). During secondary syphilis, lesions sometimes appear on the mucous membranes (mouth, pharynx, glans penis, vulva, anus, and/or rectum). These lesions begin as erosions that form mucous patches that are circular and grayish-white with a red areola. Papules that develop at mucocutaneous junctions or in moist areas of the skin (e.g., the groin) become hypertrophic, flattened, and dull pink or gray. These lesions are called condylomata lata. They are highly infectious. Any of the lesions associated with secondary syphilis usually resolve spontaneously, even without treatment, within a few months, although sometimes they persist for a year. It is important that health care providers recognize signs of primary and secondary syphilis in the HIV-infected person so that treatment can be initiated. Latency, a prolonged asymptomatic period in the immunocompetent, is extremely abbreviated in HIV-infected individuals. If syphilis is allowed to progress untreated, the HIV-infected person may rapidly progress to tertiary syphilis. The manifestations of tertiary syphilis vary depending on the body system most compromised by the pathology.

Herpes zoster (shingles) is the reactivation of a latent infection with varicella-zoster virus, the virus that causes chickenpox. Almost all adults have been infected since childhood with this virus. Following initial infection, the virus remains dormant in dorsal root ganglia until some stimulus in later life causes its reactivation. Under conditions of immunosuppression, the virus multiplies and travels along nerve pathways, inflaming them and often causing severe, intractable pain. The skin area supplied by these nerve pathways manifests with the characteristic skin lesions of shingles (Color Plates 7 and 8). These are large patches of vesicles on an erythematous base, the arrangement of which corresponds to the cutaneous distribution of one or more posterior root ganglia. Shingles can usually be diagnosed by observing these lesions and by noting the patient's description of the pain.

Herpes simplex is a viral infection that is characterized by localized primary vesicular lesions, latency, and a tendency for localized recurrence. Two types of herpes simplex virus (HSV), type 1 and type 2, each with distinct clinical characteristics, have been implicated in herpes infections. Herpes simplex 1 is usually associated with oral lesions (cold sores), and herpes simplex 2 is associated with anal-genital lesions. Either virus may infect either area of the body, depending on the portal of entry. Differentiation of the two types is not clinically important, because treatment is the same.

The pathologic mechanisms also are the same for both viruses. During primary infection, the virus invades epithelium of broken skin or mucous membranes, where it causes inflammation, intracellular and extracellular edema, and cell lysis. Vesicular lesions form on a base of inflamed epithelium at the site of viral invasion. The superficial epithelium of the lesions eventually collapses and sloughs, leaving single shallow ulcers or coalesced, large, painful ulcers (see Color Plates 11, 12, 21-26). The lesions usually resolve spontaneously in 10 to 12 days in immunocompetent persons. The HSV then travels along sensory nerve pathways to a sensory nerve ganglion, where it remains in a latent stage. Latent infections are widespread in the population, with 90% of adults infected with HSV type 1 and 60% of sexually promiscuous adults infected with HSV type 2.

The exact mechanism for reactivation of the virus is not known but is believed to be associated with immune status. Immunocompromised persons experience not only severe primary infections but also severe recurrence of lesions. The presence of lesions also may signal the development of herpes-related syndromes in the lungs, nervous system, or viscera. These can be life-threatening events requiring aggressive medical treatment. HIV-infected patients with herpes frequently require IV therapy with acyclovir followed by prolonged oral therapy for suppression of the virus. As acyclovir-resistant strains of HSV are appearing, other antiviral drugs may be required to treat this virus.

Skin Manifestations Associated with Systemic Pathology

Some of the skin manifestations of HIV disease seem to be related to systemic, rather than local, pathology. These conditions are thought to be an inflammatory response of the skin to some systemic disease, the cause of which is frequently unknown. These inflammatory skin conditions include seborrheic dermatitis, psoriasis, eosinophilic pustular folliculitis, photodermatitis, erythema multiforme, decubiti, and xerosis.

Seborrheic dermatitis is quite common, with 80% of HIV-infected persons experiencing this condition at some time during HIV infection. The cause is not known. The syndrome is characterized by vasodilation and discharge of inflammatory cells into the epidermis from the capillary roots. Scales are produced as a result of an increased mitotic rate and accumulation of cells of the stratum corneum. In HIV-infected persons, seborrhea-prone areas include the central face, eyebrows, behind the ears, the scalp, chest, upper back, axillae, and groin. These lesions also may contain an overgrowth of fungi. As a result, therapy may include antifungal creams to treat the fungi and topical corticosteroids to treat the inflammation. Treatment is difficult, eradication is almost impossible, and recurrence is expected.

Psoriasis (Color Plate 6) is another common condition in HIV-infected persons, particularly those who had a previous history of psoriasis before becoming HIV infected. Even persons with no previous history can develop severe, recalcitrant psoriasis. Some experts suggest that clinicians offer HIV testing to their patients whose serostatus is unknown and who suddenly develop severe psoriasis.[46]

The exact cause of psoriasis is unknown. The pathology is characterized by an increased rate of cell mitosis, resulting in rapid turnover of cells and shortening of the time for cells to travel from the basal layer to the epidermis. The usual transit time of 1 month is shortened to 1 week or less. This process is accompanied by faulty keratinization of the horny layer, resulting in its loss. This in turn leads to dilation of upper dermal vessels and discharge of polymorphonuclear leukocytes into the dermis. Psoriasis occasionally is related to a condition called Reiter's syndrome, which includes conjunctivitis, nonbacterial urethritis, and arthritis.

Eosinophilic pustular folliculitis is characterized by an inflammatory infiltrate with eosinophils clustered around the hair follicle. This condition is seen only in HIV-infected persons. Its cause is unknown but sometimes is attributed to an inflammatory response to HIV. Its pathophysiology is not well described. Severe itching (and scratching) leads to superficial infections.

Photodermatitis is another poorly understood condition, which seems to be related to interactions between exposure to sunlight and certain medications, such as sulfonamides and nonsteroidal antiinflammatory drugs, and, perhaps, HIV itself. Manifestations first appear in skin areas exposed to sunlight. The condition is successfully treated by avoiding exposure to the sun, eliminating the offending drugs, and administering topical steroids. If these preventive measures are not taken, the condition may spread to other areas and become refractory to treatment.

Erythema multiforme (Color Plates 9 and 10) is frequently found in HIV-infected persons, particularly those who are taking sulfonamides. Reports estimate that 50% of patients taking TMP/SMX to prevent *Pneumocystis carinii* pneumonia develop erythema multiforme. This condition is characterized by dilation of peripheral blood vessels, which become surrounded by lymphohistiocytic infiltrate. There is substantial edema of the papillary dermis. Edema of the outer dermis leads to formation of bullae, which become necrotic in the center. Treatment usually consists of withdrawal of medication that might be causing the reaction and provision of antiinflammatory drugs such as corticosteroids and antihistamines. Untreated, the condition can progress and create lesions in other body tissues, including the kidneys, bladder, pharynx, larynx, esophagus, trachea, and bronchi, a condition called Stevens-Johnson syndrome.

Pressure ulcers (decubiti) result from disruption of circulation to the skin. Any condition or situation that impairs the capillary circulation of oxygen and nutrients to dermal cells causes the cells to die, necrose, and slough. Persons at greatest risk for developing decubiti are those with impairment in mobility, those with generalized changes in vascular structure or function (such as diabetics and the aged), and those with any condition that alters circulation of blood and nutrients to tissue (such as those who are malnourished). Many persons with HIV- and AIDS-related conditions, particularly at later stages of AIDS, experience all of the factors contributing to developing decubiti. They are malnourished and have lost weight, including subcutaneous fat pads. They are weak and debilitated, leading to inactivity and sitting or lying in bed in one position for long periods of time. They may also have generalized changes in their blood vessels and skin due to multiple diseases and drug therapies. Early decubiti provide a large opening for invading organisms. Infection easily leads to bacteremia and septicemia. Stage 1 ulcers can progress rapidly to stage 4, with destruction of fascia, connective tissue, muscle, and bone.

Treatment of decubiti in HIV-infected patients is as difficult and futile as it is in any other patient. For this reason, decubiti should be prevented whenever possible. Caregivers and patients must learn methods for preventing skin pressure and for intervening early if an ulcer begins.

Xerosis (dry skin) is an extremely common manifestation in HIV, and the cause is unknown. Some authorities attribute the condition to action of the virus.

DIAGNOSTIC STUDIES AND FINDINGS FOR DERMATOLOGIC MANIFESTATIONS

Diagnostic Test	Finding
Culture and/or microscopic examination of biopsied tissue or exudate from skin lesion	Presence/absence of suspected organism or dermal cells characteristic of suspected pathology
Tests specific for herpes:	
Microscopic examination of stained smear from base of vesicles (Tzanck test)	Direct identification of multinucleated giant cells with intranuclear inclusions
Virus tissue culture of specimen from base of vesicles using fluorescent antibody or neutralization techniques	Identification of type 1 or type 2 viral cytopathogenic effect in tissue culture in 24-48 h
Complement fixation or neutralization tests	Fourfold increase in antibody titer in convalescent serum; difficult to differentiate type 1 from type 2
Indirect immunofluorescence and radioimmunoassay	IgM antibodies detected in primary and recurrent infections

Persons with a new infection with herpes should also be examined for syphilis, gonorrhea, and chlamydia.

Tests specific for syphilis:	
Darkfield or phase-contrast microscopic examination of exudate or cells from lesions or regional lymph nodes	Positive for *T. pallidum* in primary and secondary stages; not useful for latent or tertiary stages
Nontreponemal serologic tests:	Useful for screening; many false-positive results.
Venereal Disease Research Laboratory (VDRL)	Increase in nonspecific antibodies 1-3 weeks after appearance
Rapid plasma reagin (RPR)	of the chancre or 4-6 weeks after infection. Become negative
Automated reagin test (ART)	in 6-12 months after treatment of primary syphilis; 12-18
Reagin screen test (RST)	months after treatment of secondary syphilis. Serologic tests may not revert to negative if treatment is delayed beyond 2 years; results should be reported quantitatively (e.g., >1:512)
Treponemal serologic tests:	Useful for confirmation of positive screening tests. Reported
Fluorescent *Treponema* antibody absorption (FTA-ABS)	as nonreactive, borderline, or reactive. These tests become
Microhemagglutination assay (MHA-TP)	reactive earlier in the primary stage and remain reactive
***T. pallidum* hemagglutination assay (TPHA-TP)**	longer in latent and late syphilis; remain reactive, even after treatment; results do not vary with disease activity.

MEDICAL MANAGEMENT

DRUG THERAPY FOR DERMATOLOGIC MANIFESTATIONS

Bacterial folliculitis: Dicloxacillin, 250-500 mg PO qid. For recurrent or refractory folliculitis and to reduce nasal carriage: add rifampin, 300-600 mg PO qd for 10 days. Chlorhexidine gluconate (Hibiclens) cleanser used for bathing qd for 1 week, then used in bath q 1-2 wk for 2-3 months. If patient is a nasal carrier of *S. aureus,* apply topical antibiotic ointment such as polymyxin B sulfate/zinc bacitracin (Polysporin), Bactroban, or bacitracin (Baciquent) into nares with a cotton-tipped applicator bid for 10-14 days.

Impetigo/ecthyma: Penicillin V, erythromycin, or cephalexin, 250-500 mg PO q 6 h for 7-10 days. Antibacterial washes with chlorhexidine or povidone-iodine (Betadine) qd for 1-2 weeks followed by periodic washes. In mild cases, antibiotic ointments, such as mupirocin (Bactroban), may help.

Cellulitis: Penicillin V, 250 mg PO qid for mild cases. If severe, aqueous penicillin G, IV q 6 h; alternative for mild cases: erythromycin, 250 mg PO qid; alternative for severe cases and for patients allergic to penicillin: clindamycin, 150 mg IV q 6 h.

Tinea: Ketoconazole, 200 mg/day PO for 3-5 days only; selenium sulfide (Exsel, Selsun) lotion, 2.5% qd left on for 15-20 min. Also: Lotrimin cream or ketoconazole ointment can be tried.

Insect bites: Antipruritics and antihistamines.

Scabies: Lindane, 1% lotion; apply twice, 1 week apart; keep application on skin for 12 hours.

Molluscum contagiosum: Retinoic acid (Retin A) applied to skin; cannot be used on eyelids or genitalia; *or* liquid nitrogen applied for 5-15 sec per lesion.

Human papillomavirus warts: 25% podophyllum resin (Pod-Ben-25) in tincture of benzoin, apply weekly; leave chemical in contact with skin for no more than 4-6 hours, then wash off.

Vulvovaginal candidiasis: Topical applications of miconazole (Monistat-Derm), clotrimazole (Lotrimin, Mycelex), econazole nitrate (Spectazole), or ciclopirox olamine (Loprox) 1-2 times/day for at least 2 weeks after clinical resolution.

Bacillary angiomatosis: Erythromycin ethylsuccinate, 250-500 mg PO q 6 h for 4 weeks; *or* dicloxacillin sodium (Dycill, Dynapen, Pathocil), 250-500 mg PO q 6 h with local excision.

Syphilis: If primary stage, benzathine penicillin G, 2.4 million U IM/wk for 3 weeks. If secondary stage, penicillin G procaine, 2.4 million U IM/wk for 3 weeks. Because syphilis in HIV infected may recur, some clinicians advocate more aggressive regimens.

Herpes zoster: Acyclovir (Zovirax), 10-12 mg/kg IV, infused over 1 h, q 8 h for 7-14 days; *or* acyclovir, 800-1000 mg PO q 4 h.

Herpes simplex: Acyclovir (Zovirax), 5.0 mg/kg IV, infused over 1 h, q 8 h for 7 days; *or* 200-600 mg PO q 4 h. Suppressive therapy is acyclovir, 400 mg PO bid or 200 mg PO tid indefinitely.

Seborrheic dermatitis: Hydrocortisone, 2.5% cream, and ketoconazole, 2% cream, applied bid until lesions resolve. If severe: ketoconazole, 200-400 mg PO qd for 3-4 weeks. Alternative: Lotrisone cream. Maintenance therapy: 1% hydrocortisone cream and 2% ketoconazole cream bid.

Psoriasis: Triamcinolone acetonide, 0.1% cream tid indefinitely.

Esoinophilic folliculitis: Oral antihistamines and topical steroids or ultraviolet light.

Photodermatitis: Topical steroids; discontinue photosensitizing medications.

Erythema multiforme: Analgesics for pain; antihistamines and corticosteroids; discontinue drugs, particularly sulfa, which might be precipitating the reaction.

Xerosis: Emollients after bath and twice daily and/or weak topical steroids (e.g., 1% hydrocortisone in ointment base); teach patient to avoid soap if possible and to use a mild soap in groin area and axillae.

MEDICAL MANAGEMENT—cont'd

OTHER MEDICAL MANAGEMENT

For lesions caused by molluscum contagiosum and HPV*:

Cryotherapy:　Liquid nitrogen or dry ice is applied briefly to a lesion to kill cells. Following treatment, a blister forms with subsequent necrosis.

Electrocautery:　Application of a needle heated by electric current to cause necrosis of lesions.

Electrodesiccation:　Application of an electric spark to burn tissue; often used in conjunction with curettage.

Curettage:　Application of a blunt or sharp instrument or suction to remove tissue from a cavity or lesion; often used with other measures discussed here to kill cells.

*Recent research suggests that removal of warts may increase the risk of malignancy at the site of removal.

See Chapter 11 for nursing management of persons with dermatologic manifestations.

CHAPTER 7

Oral and Gastrointestinal Manifestations

Oral and gastrointestinal manifestations are being discussed together for two reasons. First, it is often difficult to determine whether a given disease is oral or gastrointestinal. For example, it may not be clear whether oral candidiasis is extending to the esophagus or whether esophageal candidiasis has spread to the mouth. What is clear is that the patient suffers from a disease process that is painful, debilitating, and treatable. The second reason for discussing these manifestations together is that they often work synergistically to produce the severe weight loss, poor nutritional status, and energy depletion that are seen in HIV-infected people. Individuals who have tender oral lesions or have lost teeth often drastically reduce their intake of solid foods and liquids. It is simply too painful to eat or drink. This dramatically reduced caloric intake, combined with the decreased absorption associated with the gastrointestinal manifestations of HIV disease, contributes to the rapid weight loss seen in the HIV wasting syndrome. The problems are compounded by loss of energy and weakness—making simple activities like grocery shopping and food preparation beyond the capability of the person. To further complicate matters, caloric needs are greater because of increases in metabolism from fevers and infections. Consequently, oral and GI diseases work against the overall health and well-being of the immunocompromised person.

Oral Manifestations

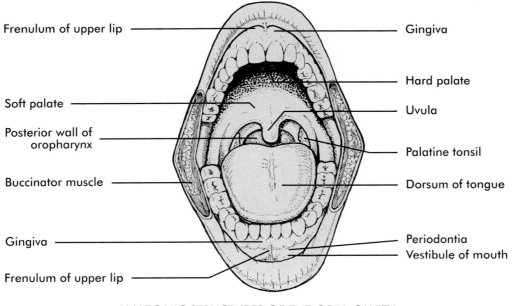

Frenulum of upper lip

Soft palate

Posterior wall of
oropharynx

Buccinator muscle

Gingiva

Frenulum of upper lip

Gingiva

Hard palate

Uvula

Palatine tonsil

Dorsum of tongue

Periodontia
Vestibule of mouth

ANATOMIC STRUCTURES OF THE ORAL CAVITY

Virtually all HIV-infected people will experience one or more HIV-related oral diseases. These range in severity from the relatively benign but cosmetically displeasing, to severely painful, to life threatening. The disfiguring aspects of visible lesions or tooth loss should not be ignored, as they compound the HIV-infected person's self-image problems. Poor appearance may also reduce the person's social interaction at a time when support from others, distraction from symptoms, and intellectual stimulation are crucial to the person's well-being. Insertion of bridges, plates, and other dental replacement devices should always be considered. No one should have his or her appearance or ability to eat compromised simply because he or she is HIV infected. Dental pain can be excruciating and debilitating, and obtaining relief from such pain is critical in enabling a person to carry out activities of daily living. Oral manifestations of HIV can also create life-threatening conditions related to nutritional deficiency, dehydration, and septicemia. For all of the above reasons, nurses must attend to the oral manifestations of their HIV-infected patients.

Unfortunately, oral assessment and intervention are often neglected in education programs for nondental professionals. Therefore, comprehensive oral assessment is reviewed in Chapter 5.

Table 7-1 presents an overview of the most common oral lesions associated with HIV infection. Readers unfamiliar with the appearance of these conditions may wish to refer to the color plates that are identified in the table and presented at the beginning of this book.

While oral lesions are often disfiguring, painful, or life threatening, most are susceptible to treatment. The lesions can be eliminated or reduced in scope through preventive hygiene, dental treatment, or systemic drug therapy. A review of these conditions and their treatment follows.

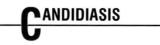

CANDIDIASIS

This infection is an overgrowth of a usually nonpathogenic, normal flora fungus. The organism, which thrives on moist mucosal surfaces, becomes pathogenic in situations of immunosuppression or steroid therapy, or following antibiotic therapy. Lesions first appear as thin-walled vesicles under the stratum corneum. They have an inflammatory base that may burn or itch. The accumulation of inflammatory cells may produce a whitish-yellow, curdlike exudate on the mucosa. This characteristic white-yellow appearance will not be found in

Table 7-1 _____

OVERVIEW OF ORAL MANIFESTATIONS ASSOCIATED WITH HIV INFECTION

Condition	Description	Signs and symptoms
Candidiasis: pseudomembranous form (white candidiasis): see Color Plates 29-31	Very common opportunistic fungal growth causing characteristic lesions of the oral cavity; occurs in over 50% of people with AIDS.	Characterized by white, raised lesions that can be wiped off with gauze, exposing an erythematous, sometimes bleeding, mucosa; often painless in the oral cavity, becoming extremely painful if lesions spread to the esophagus.
Candidiasis: erythematous form (red candidiasis):	An uncommon (<5% of people with AIDS) fungal overgrowth with characteristic lesions.	Characterized by smooth, red patches on the dorsal surface of the tongue, on the buccal mucosa, or on the hard or soft palate; sometimes accompanied by mucosal bleeding. Lesions are often painless in the oral cavity, becoming extremely painful if they spread to the esophagus.
Candidiasis: hyperkeratotic form (candidal leukoplakia)	A very rare (<1% of people with AIDS) fungal overgrowth causing a characteristic lesion; differentiated from other leukoplakia by microscopic exam or by response to antifungal therapy.	Characterized by adherent white lesions that cannot be wiped off.
Candidiasis: angular cheilosis form	Uncommon (<5% of people with AIDS) fungal overgrowth in the corners of the mouth.	Characterized by uncomfortable, often painful, erythematous cracks and fissures in the corners of the mouth.
Human papillomavirus (oral warts, HPV)	Rare (<2%) viral infection appearing as single or multiple lesions; appears to be related to activation of latent infection, not to recent sexual transmission.	Characterized by painless lesions, which may appear as white, spikelike projections or as pink, cauliflower-like masses or as a flat plaque that resembles focal epithelial hyperplasia.
Oral hairy leukoplakia (OHL): see Color Plate 28	Common (up to 30% of people with AIDS—rare in immunocompetent) oral lesion, probably caused by the Epstein-Barr virus (EBV). The lesions are benign.	OHL lesions are painless and characterized by white thickening of the oral mucosa and/or the lateral portion of the tongue, often with vertical folds or corrugations; lesions may have fingerlike extensions (hairs) leading away from the main mass of the lesion.
HIV-associated gingivitis: see Color Plate 32	Relatively common (20% of people with AIDS) inflammation of the gums near the tooth line. It is caused by a wide variety of bacteria that are found in plaque and that infiltrate gum tissue. While gingivitis is common in non-HIV-infected people, HIV-associated gingivitis is very aggressive and may result in acute necrosis of gingival tissue. The condition is exacerbated by poor dental hygiene, which can be difficult to maintain due to pain associated with the inflammation.	The inflammation generally appears as a thin red line at the portion of the gums touching the teeth. Gingivitis can be extremely painful and can be accompanied by spontaneous bleeding and severe halitosis.

Table 7-1

OVERVIEW OF ORAL MANIFESTATIONS ASSOCIATED WITH HIV INFECTION—cont'd

Condition	Description	Signs and Symptoms
HIV-associated periodontitis: see Color Plate 33	A common manifestation affecting one third of people in late stages of HIV infection; more common in smokers; caused by a variety of bacteria and generally follows gingivitis; characterized by inflammation and degeneration of the dental periosteum, alveolar bone, cementum, and adjacent gingiva; results in suppuration, resorption of supporting bone, recession of gingiva, and loss of teeth. Severe infection can spread beyond teeth and create an osteomyelitis.	Characteristic appearance is massive erosion of the gums, which gives teeth the appearance of being longer. Condition is painful and often accompanied by spontaneous bleeding. Tooth loss severely affects nutrition.
Herpes simplex virus (cold sores, HSV): see Color Plates 21-26	Common manifestation (up to 25% of people with AIDS) with characteristic lesions on the lips, hard palate, dorsal surface of the tongue, or gingiva; may extend to esophagus; condition can be so painful as to interfere with nutrition and hydration.	Painful lesions, which begin as small vesicles on an erythematous base; vesicles erupt and ulcerate; ulcers may coalesce, creating large areas of ulceration.
Aphthous ulcers (canker sores): see Color Plate 27	Idiopathic ulceration, which is relatively common (up to 10%) in people with AIDS; while also common in the non-HIV infected, ulcers are more severe and prolonged in the HIV infected. Can become severe enough to interfere with speech, hydration, and nutrition.	Acute onset, characterized by painful ulcers that are usually found on the buccal mucosa, oropharynx, soft palate, or ventral surface of the tongue; may subside spontaneously but are likely to recur.
Kaposi's sarcoma (KS): see Chapter 10.	Relatively common progressive neoplastic disease in males with AIDS (up to 10%); very rare in women. Produces characteristic lesions, which regress when patients receive chemotherapy.	Vascular lesions appearing as red or purple macules, papules, or nodules on any area of the oral cavity; occasionally are the same color as the adjoining normal mucosa. Generally painless, unless lesions are associated with traumatic ulceration, inflammation, and/or infection.
Other oral conditions	Many other rare lesions are found in the oral cavity of persons with AIDS. They can be caused by fungi (i.e., histoplasmosis, geotrichosis, cryptococcosis), viruses (CMV), or cancers (lymphomas, squamous cell).	Conditions can result in severe pain and/or painful lesions.
Drug reactions	Painful oral lesions are often the result of drug therapies.	Variable

the less common red candidiasis, even though the pathogenic process is similar. In immunocompromised people, the infection may rapidly extend to the esophagus. Both oral and esophageal forms can become extremely painful, interfering with nutrition and hydration.

Candidiasis following antibiotic therapy generally subsides when the antibiotic is discontinued. Because of the potential for the infection to extend and to develop into more serious disease, oral candidiasis is generally treated with antifungal troches or mouth rinses. Esophageal candidiasis must be treated with systemic antifungal drugs. Although *Candida* strains that are resistant to some antifungal drugs have developed, a variety of highly effective antifungal drugs are available. Some experts recommend the use of rinses and troches as the first approach to treatment, reserving the systemic antifungal drugs for disseminated infections or more serious disease in later HIV infection. They advocate this approach in order to discourage development of drug-resistant organisms.

Angular cheilosis is another fungal overgrowth of *Candida albicans*. The characteristic lesions are found in the corners of the mouth, causing breakdown of tissue. The macerated tissue and lesions are disfiguring and painful, causing difficulty with speaking, eating, smiling, and so forth. Treatment with topical antifungal creams or systemic antifungal medications improves this condition.

In summary, oral candidiasis is a treatable and controllable opportunistic infection. Cure is often dramatic and is greatly appreciated by the patient.

ORAL HAIRY LEUKOPLAKIA

This essentially is a benign, painless condition that produces mildly disfiguring lesions on the tongue. Its appearance is almost diagnostic of HIV infection in the absence of any other indication of immunosuppression. The cause of this condition is not known, but is thought to be related to an overgrowth of the Epstein-Barr virus (EBV). Treatment with acyclovir is successful in resolving these lesions; however, they tend to recur when drug therapy is stopped. Many clinicians advocate not treating leukoplakia because the lesions are painless and seldom noticeable and do not interfere with ingestion. These clinicians are concerned that unnecessary use of acyclovir may produce an acyclovir-resistant strain of herpes, which can cause severe oral, GI, and skin disease. In addition, it probably is best to limit the number of drugs in the patient's regimen to those that are absolutely essential, in order to reduce the risk for drug interactions.

In general, oral hairy leukoplakia should be considered a benign condition for which treatment is available but not generally necessary. The condition should be monitored, however, to ensure that it is not masking other treatable diseases such as candidiasis.

HIV-ASSOCIATED GINGIVITIS

Gingivitis is a frequently painful inflammation of the margin of the gums (gingiva) that seems to be due to an overgrowth of a variety of organisms in gum tissue. It is usually visible as a thin, very bright red line on the gums along the tooth line. The causative organisms are generally found to be gram-negative bacteria. However, a recent study has implicated a previously unidentified spirochete as being instrumental in this condition and in HIV-associated periodontitis.[136] Unchecked gingivitis can lead to separation of the gum from the teeth, creating pockets that collect food debris and organisms. Such a situation stimulates further inflammation, leading to exacerbated gingivitis and, eventually, periodontitis. Gingivitis can be retarded in its development by a combination of meticulous oral hygiene with a soft toothbrush and plaque removal by a dentist or hygienist every 2 to 3 months. The disease can also be slowed by the regular use of oral rinses with antiseptics such as Betadine or chlorhexidine gluconate (Peridex), a simple but extremely valuable treatment. Some report success with administration of systemic antibiotics. Once established, gingivitis is very difficult to eliminate; it can, however, generally be controlled by the methods described above. This condition can often be prevented or delayed by regular brushing and flossing after eating. Nurses can have an impact on prevention by instructing patients in oral hygiene (see Chapter 11). Nurses can also prevent deterioration by arranging for the patient with signs of gingivitis to be treated by a dentist.

HIV-ASSOCIATED PERIODONTITIS

Periodontitis is characterized by necrosis of bone and other underlying support structures of teeth. It is a common, very slowly developing condition in non-HIV-infected people that progresses more rapidly in those who practice poor oral hygiene. In the HIV infected, periodontitis is an aggressive, rapidly developing condition that can go from absent to severe with attendant tooth loss in a matter of months. It is associated with overgrowth of a number of different gram-negative bacteria in the affected tissues. A history of severe pain is a distinguishing feature. The condition can so severely compromise the support structures of teeth as to cause the teeth to become loose. These teeth either fall out or can be removed easily by what one dentist called "fingertip extraction." Treatment, as with gingivitis, requires a combination of approaches, including meticulous oral hygiene with a soft toothbrush, plaque removal by a dentist or hygienist every 2 to 3 months, regular use of oral rinses with antiseptics such as Betadine or chlorhexidine gluconate (Peridex), and administration of systemic antibiotics. As with gingivitis, oral rinses are considered to be invaluable in the treatment of this condition. In addition, surgical debridement of the affected tissues by a dentist may be necessary. Periodontitis is very difficult to cure and usually can only be arrested. This condition, like gingivitis, is easier to prevent through good oral hygiene than to treat once it is progressing. The nurse can educate the patient about oral hygiene and can arrange for dental referral when the condition is observed.

HERPES SIMPLEX VIRUS

This is a commonly occurring infection in immunocompetent persons. As much as 70% to 90% of the population has serum antibodies against herpes simplex 1, the virus associated with most oral herpes lesions. In addition, at least 20% of adults have antibodies to herpes simplex 2, which also causes oral lesions. Following an initial infection with these viruses and healing of the lesions, the virus remains dormant along the peripheral nerves innervating the area of initial infection. Immunocompetent people may experience an occasional exacerbation of lesions (i.e., cold sores), which generally resolves spontaneously without treatment within 1 or 2 weeks. In the immunocompromised, these eruptions can become extensive and persistent.

Oral herpes lesions are characterized by epidermal vesicles, which show extensive intracellular and extracellular edema upon microscopic examination. Cells lose their intercellular bridges, undergo ballooning degeneration with eosinophilic intranuclear inclusion bodies, and become multinucleated. Widespread tissue destruction with poor healing is common in the HIV infected who are not treated for this condition.

Acyclovir is the primary treatment for both cure and suppression. Widespread and continuous use of this drug has resulted in acyclovir-resistant strains of HSV.

Patients who have a poor response to acyclovir or who develop disease while on suppressive therapy are usually treated with foscarnet. Response to these drugs is generally quite good, with resolution of the oral lesions and prevention of extension of the disease to the esophagus.

HSV can be transmitted by direct person-to-person contact and by indirect contact through hands or equipment contaminated with lesion exudates. The latter is a particular risk within health care settings, and can be avoided by strict adherence to universal precautions. The virus can also be transmitted from one part of the body to another by autoinoculation. Patients should, therefore, be instructed to wash their hands after touching the lesions.

APHTHOUS ULCERS

The pathophysiology of these lesions, commonly called "canker sores," is poorly understood. The ulcers are generally described as being idiopathic in origin, although at times they are clearly associated with administration of certain drugs. Most of the time they resolve spontaneously in a short period of time. When they persist, the patient's medication should be reviewed and altered if aphthous ulcers are a known side effect. Treatment consists of topical medications or mouth rinses that reduce pain and inflammation.

HUMAN PAPILLOMAVIRUS

At least 50 human papillomavirus (HPV) types have been identified.[11] Each is probably specific to different conditions. While many of these types rarely cause clinical disease, some cause skin warts; others are sexually transmitted, causing warts at the site of contact. Unusual HPV types have been implicated in oral and laryngeal warts in the HIV infected. These opportunistic HPVs are not of the types that are sexually transmitted. Their presence in the HIV infected is attributed to reactivation of a latent HPV skin infection or autoinfection from skin or face lesions. Treatment usually consists of surgical or laser excision of the wart. This treatment does not eliminate the virus, which maintains its viability in tissue even when the wart is removed. These lesions often recur at the same site or elsewhere in the mouth.

DIAGNOSTIC STUDIES AND FINDINGS FOR ORAL MANIFESTATIONS

Diagnostic Test	Finding
Microscopic examination of KOH-prepared slide	Visualization of characteristic fungus cells
Culture	Visualization of organism (seldom helpful in HIV-associated periodontitis or gingivitis)
Biopsy	Visualization of organism or tumor cells
Visual inspection	Characteristic clinical appearance of oral lesions

DENTAL/MEDICAL MANAGEMENT OF ORAL MANIFESTATIONS

DRUG THERAPY

Candidiasis: Clotrimazole oral troche (Mycelex), 10 mg tablet dissolved slowly in the mouth five times/day (topical treatment is not used if there is esophageal involvement). Ketoconazole (Nizoral), 200 mg/day or bid PO until condition resolves; or fluconazole (Diflucan), 200 mg PO first day and then 100 mg PO once/day until improvement. Suppressive therapy: either ketoconazole or fluconazole is administered in acute dose once/week.

Oral hairy leukoplakia: Usually not treated except for cosmetic purposes. Acyclovir, 10 mg/kg IV q 8 h for 7 days (not yet approved by FDA); lesions reappear when therapy is discontinued.

HIV-associated gingivitis and periodontitis: Topical Betadine and chlorhexidine gluconate (Peridex) mouthwash, used to retard these conditions. Systemic treatment to eliminate gram-negative pathogens: Metronidazole (Flagyl), 500 mg PO q 12 h. Drug treatment must be accompanied by debridement of diseased tissue.

Herpes simplex virus: For persistent lesions: acyclovir (Zovirax), 200-400 mg PO five times/day for 7-14 days. Suppressive therapy: acyclovir, 400 mg PO bid indefinitely. Acyclovir-resistant HSV: foscarnet (Foscavir), 40 mg/kg IV (infused over 2 h) q 8 h for 21 days; followed by 40 mg/kg IV daily indefinitely for suppressive therapy.

Oral Kaposi's sarcoma and lymphoma: See Chapter 10.

Aphthous ulcers: Fluocinonide (Lidex), 0.05% ointment mixed with equal quantities of Orabase applied to the lesion 6 times daily. Decadron elixir, 0.5 mg/ml as a rinse (and spit) several times daily; useful when lesion is located in a hard-to-reach area. Corticosteroids injected into the affected area.

Oral pain from any type of lesion: Topical anesthetics; anesthetic mouth rinses; systemic analgesics and narcotics, if indicated.

SURGICAL AND OTHER DENTAL/MEDICAL MANAGEMENT

Radiation therapy and surgical removal of lesions of Kaposi's sarcoma and lymphomas (see Chapter 10).

Dental care, including cleaning and scaling of teeth every 2 to 3 months; debridement of decayed tissue, performed with local anesthetic. CO_2 laser surgery for removal of warts.

GENERAL MANAGEMENT

IV therapy and nutrition supplementation to relieve dehydration, electrolyte imbalance, and malnutrition.

Patient education on oral hygiene.

Refer to Chapter 11 for nursing management.

Gastrointestinal Manifestations

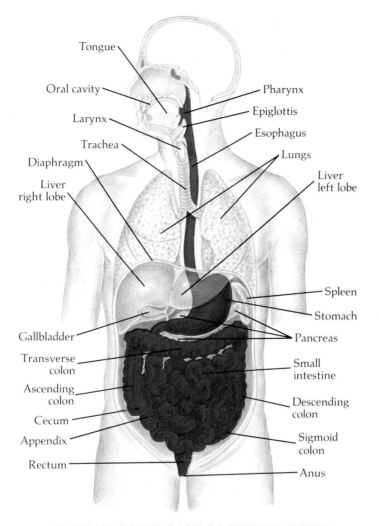

Tongue
Oral cavity
Larynx
Trachea
Diaphragm
Liver right lobe
Pharynx
Epiglottis
Esophagus
Lungs
Liver left lobe
Spleen
Stomach
Pancreas
Small intestine
Descending colon
Sigmoid colon
Anus
Gallbladder
Transverse colon
Ascending colon
Cecum
Appendix
Rectum

ANATOMY OF THE GASTROINTESTINAL SYSTEM

Almost all HIV-infected people experience at least one gastrointestinal disease during the course of HIV infection. The likelihood and frequency of this occurring increase as the CD4+ lymphocyte count declines. Up to 70% of those with a count below 100 cells/mm^3 will develop chronic GI disease. The problem is often complicated by iatrogenic GI manifestations resulting from drug side effects and/or disruption of normal flora from antibiotic therapy.

The human immunodeficiency virus itself, as well as a large number of opportunistic organisms and neo-plasms, can affect the GI tract anywhere from the esophagus to the colon. The cause of any particular set of symptoms can be very difficult to diagnose and treat. Often the pathogen is part of the body's normal flora. Thus, its presence in a body specimen may or may not indicate that the organism is causing the pathology and symptoms. Additionally, many of the techniques used to identify organisms (e.g., microscopy of tissue or stool specimens) elicit a large number of false-negative results. So, failure to identify a suspected organism does not necessarily rule out its being the cause of an episode of illness. Diagnostic procedures, such as endoscopy, can be useful for visualizing pathologic tissue. However, the lesions that are characteristic of certain organisms sometimes become so ulcerated as to make them indistinguishable from one another. In addition, more than one organism can be the cause of a GI problem, making it necessary to identify and successfully eradicate two or three pathogens before a patient's symptoms are relieved.

Throughout this whole diagnostic and treatment process, the patient will require supportive care ranging from symptomatic relief to life-sustaining measures. With respect to the latter, people with certain HIV-related opportunistic infections may excrete 15 to 20 liters of fluid per day. Such fluid and electrolyte loss, if untreated, can precipitate circulatory collapse. Symptomatic treatment (e.g., antidiarrheal medication) will be employed during the diagnostic process. Often, antimicrobial therapy will be started on a "best guess" basis while a more definitive diagnosis is being sought. Sometimes the diagnosis is made by treatment failure. In this situation the "best guess" treatment failed; therefore a different organism must be responsible for the disease. Another "best guess" treatment is then initiated, and the process continues until diagnostic and treatment success is achieved or until the patient can no longer tolerate changing drug regimens.

Treatment options for GI manifestations of HIV disease range from drugs that have been safely administered for years to recently developed medications with dangerous and/or unknown side effects and interactions. Depending on the organism, the medications can be highly effective, orally administered, and require short-term therapy; or they can be partially effective, intravenously administered, and require therapy for the remainder of the patient's life. No drugs have demonstrated effectiveness against some organisms. In these cases, clinicians may use experimental drugs, high doses of potentially effective drugs, or combination therapies.

Thus, the GI manifestations present the patient with pain, debilitation, and life-threatening events. They present the clinician with diagnostic puzzles; demands for effective, rapid, supportive care; and difficult choices for therapy. Management and control of the GI aspects of HIV/AIDS is, perhaps, the most difficult and challenging area in the care of the HIV-infected person. Table 7-2 presents an overview of gastrointestinal manifestations commonly associated with HIV/AIDS.

The major gastrointestinal manifestations are discussed here according to the area of the tract where symptoms present (i.e., esophagus, stomach, or intestinal tract) and the diseases related to those areas (esophagitis, gastritis, and enteritis/diarrhea).

ESOPHAGITIS

Esophagitis is an inflammation of the esophagus, which is usually caused by reflux of gastric contents into the esophagus or by ingestion of irritants in immunocompetent people. Rarely, esophagitis is caused by infection. Immunocompromised people are subject to both gastroesophageal reflux and irritation of the esophagus, but their esophagitis is more often due to pathogens. The organism most often causing esophagitis in immunosuppressed people is *Candida albicans*. This is a yeastlike fungus that can be found on the mucous membranes and skin, in the gastrointestinal tract, and in the vagina. It is seldom pathogenic, because cell-mediated immunity prevents the organism from replicating. However, *Candida* is likely to overgrow and cause tissue destruction in the immunosuppressed. Primary sites for overgrowth are the mouth and esophagus. Estimates are that over one half of HIV-infected people will get oral candidiasis and one third will acquire esophageal candidiasis. Candidal infections at these two sites are so linked together that many experts suggest that esophageal symptoms (pain and difficulty in swallowing) together with visible presence of candidal infection in the mouth constitute sufficient evidence to treat with antifungal drugs. No further diagnostic testing is required unless the esophageal symptoms fail to clear up on antifungal therapy.

Candida typically affects only the outer layers of mucous membranes. The initial lesion is a thin-walled vesicle that extends under the epithelial layer with an inflammatory base. The accumulation of inflammatory cells and exudate produces a whitish-yellow, curdlike substance covering the lesion. This resembles a membrane and is termed pseudomembranous candidiasis. As the infection progresses, the lesions become extremely painful, frequently interfering with eating and drinking.

Treatment of esophagitis due to *C. albicans* is usually successful in removing the organism from the esophagus. However, healing of the lesions may take up to several months. Thus, treatment usually keeps things from becoming worse but is slow in making things better. Patients are treated with an antifungal drug suspended in liquid, which is administered as a "swish and swallow," or with systemic oral or IV antifungal drugs.

A second microbiological cause of esophagitis in immunocompromised persons is herpes simplex virus. This organism produces lesions, which begin as multiple, small, distinct vesicles. The vesicles eventually rupture and form deep ulcers with overhanging tissue. Their characteristic appearance has led to their being

Table 7-2

OVERVIEW OF GASTROINTESTINAL MANIFESTATIONS

Condition	Description	Signs and symptoms
Esophageal candidiasis	Common fungal infection, which is an AIDS-defining condition in 13% of HIV patients; affects 20% to 30% of persons during the course of HIV infection; frequently associated with concurrent oral candidiasis; lesions persist for a while after treatment.	Pain (odynophagia) and difficulty (dysphagia) in swallowing. Patients report, "Food sticks in my throat."
HSV esophagitis	Relatively uncommon (<5%) viral infection of the esophagus, which can progress rapidly from small vesicles to large ulcers; lesions persist for a while after treatment.	Mild pain and difficulty in swallowing.
HIV esophagitis	Uncommon (<1%), self-limiting cause of esophageal lesions.	Mild pain and difficulty in swallowing; suspected in absence of other causes.
CMV esophagitis	Relatively uncommon (<2%) viral infection characterized by large, shallow ulcers that may reach 10 cm in length.	Mild pain and difficulty in swallowing.
Gastritis due to: Kaposi's sarcoma and lymphoma	See Chapter 10.	All of these forms of gastritis may manifest with nausea, vomiting, feeling of fullness, hematemesis, and black, tarry stools (melena).
CMV	Viral infection of the stomach that causes large (up to 10 cm) lesions.	
Drug side effects	Antiinfective drugs and steroids may cause gastritis/duodenitis and gastric and duodenal ulcers.	
Diarrhea due to: *Cryptosporidium* spp (cryptosporidiosis)	Protozoan infection of the jejunum affecting 10% of HIV-infected persons; AIDS-defining condition for 2% of HIV infected.	Persistent and severe watery diarrhea with excretion of up to 15-20 liters/day; severe dehydration; wasting, malabsorption, intestinal cramping, and abdominal pain; may have fever, malaise, anorexia, nausea, vomiting.
Isospora belli (isosporiasis)	Protozoan infection of the mucosa of the small intestine; affects 3% of HIV-infected persons.	Similar to cryptosporidiosis; may be accompanied by lactose intolerance.
Enterocytozoon bienensi (microsporidiosis)	Protozoan infection that may be found throughout the intestinal tract; commonly found in the small intestine; causes diarrhea in 5% of HIV-infected persons.	Similar to cryptosporidiosis.
Entamoeba histolytica (amebiasis, amebic dysentery)	Protozoan infection of the colon; may cause liver abscesses. Subclinical and occasional symptomatic infections are common in male homosexuals. Becomes virulent in immunosuppression, causing diarrhea in 8% of HIV infected.	Flatulence, diarrhea, cramping, abdominal pain; mucus and blood in stool; malabsorption, weight loss, liver tenderness.
Giardia lamblia (giardiasis)	Protozoan infection of the duodenum, jejunum, and small intestine; causes diarrhea in 5% of HIV-infected persons.	Intermittent nausea, flatulence, epigastric pain, abdominal cramps, diarrhea; weight loss.
Mycobacterium avium complex (MAC, MAI)	Mycobacterial infection of the mucosa of the small intestine and, less frequently, of the colon; AIDS-defining condition in 4% of HIV-infected persons and affects 30% to 40% of persons during the course of HIV infection.	Diarrhea, abdominal pain; weight loss, malabsorption, anemia, thrombocytopenia; fever and night sweats.

Continued.

Table 7-2

OVERVIEW OF GASTROINTESTINAL MANIFESTATIONS—cont'd

Condition	Description	Signs and symptoms
Salmonella spp. (salmonellosis)	Acute bacterial infection causing enterocolitis in 5% to 10% of HIV-infected persons; may cause recurrent bacteremia.	Abdominal pain, diarrhea, nausea and vomiting; dehydration and headache.
Shigella spp. (shigellosis, bacillary dysentery)	Acute bacterial infection of the mucosa of the large and distal small intestine, causing 5% of diarrhea in HIV-infected persons.	Gripping abdominal pain, urgency to defecate, diarrhea containing mucus, pus, and blood; tenesmus; dehydration.
Campylobacter jejuni (campylobacteriosis)	Bacterial infection of the colon causing 4% to 20% of HIV-related diarrhea; rarely bacteremia occurs.	Watery, occasionally bloody diarrhea with abdominal pain; fever up to 104° F, hepatosplenomegaly; symptoms may mimic acute appendicitis.
Clostridium difficile (pseudomembranous colitis, antibiotic-associated colitis)	Overgrowth of a normal flora bacteria during antibiotic therapy; accounts for 3% of diarrheas in HIV infected.	Intermittent, watery diarrhea, abdominal pain, weight loss; sometimes fever.
Cytomegalovirus (CMV)	Frequent viral infection in HIV infected, occurring anywhere in the intestinal tract.	Diarrhea, nausea, vomiting, abdominal pain and cramping, fever; occasional colonic perforation with acute bleeding.
Herpes simplex virus (HSV)	Viral infection occurring anywhere in the intestinal tract; causes about 5% of diarrheas in HIV infected; may cause proctitis.	Cramping, large-volume diarrheas; weight loss.

called volcano ulcers. Untreated, or sometimes even with treatment, the ulcers coalesce to form giant ulcers covering most of the esophagus.

Treatment of HSV esophagitis with acyclovir or foscarnet (for acyclovir-resistant strains) is reasonably successful. Progression of ulceration may suggest acyclovir resistance. Some clinicians recommend a trial of vidarabine before trying foscarnet, because of the cost of foscarnet.

Cytomegalovirus also causes esophagitis. This virus invades and destroys epithelial and endothelial cells and fibroblasts, creating large, generally shallow ulcers. These ulcers often reach 10 cm in diameter and can cause extreme pain. Treatment of CMV esophagitis is controversial, as anti-CMV drugs have not been shown to improve this condition. However, both ganciclovir and foscarnet have demonstrated an effect on CMV retinitis. As a result, many clinicians utilize these drugs in treating CMV esophagitis.

Esophagitis may be caused by other organisms, including HIV. There have been case reports of isolating HIV from esophageal lesions from which no other organism could be cultured. There is no treatment for these lesions. Esophagitis has also been reported as a side effect of zidovudine therapy. HIV-infected persons also acquire non-HIV-related esophagitis from gastroesophageal reflux or by ingestion of irritants. On occasion, medications such as Bactrim will lodge and dissolve in the esophagus, causing ulcers. This can be minimized by swallowing pills with adequate fluid.

GASTRITIS

Gastritis, with or without nausea and vomiting, is common in HIV-infected people. However, it is almost always secondary to another condition, particularly diarrhea. If an opportunistic infection is more than transitory, the organism is far more likely to colonize in the intestinal tract than in the stomach. These opportunistic infections will be discussed with diarrheas. Nausea and vomiting in HIV-infected people are also frequently a side effect of medications, including antimicrobial drugs. For example, 46% of patients on high-dose zidovudine (1200 mg/day) experience nausea, and 20% report GI pain. As many as 80% of patients taking foscarnet report nausea. Persistent nausea and vomiting should alert the health care provider to review the patient's prescribed and over-the-counter medications.

ENTERITIS, COLITIS, AND DIARRHEA

Persistent and intractable diarrhea is the most frequent complication of enteritis (inflammation of the small intestine) and/or colitis (inflammation of the large intestine). While oral and esophageal lesions are associated with dehydration and weight loss, persistent diarrhea is the principal cause of severe wasting and dehydration in HIV-infected people. A dozen major organisms have been implicated in these diarrheal conditions, particularly *Mycobacterium avium* complex and *Cryptosporidium* spp. Many of these organisms are normal inhabitants of the intestinal tract but overgrow as a result of immunodeficiency, antibiotic use, or other HIV-related inflammatory processes. Environmental organisms, which usually are not pathogenic in immunocompetent persons, also cause severe diarrhea in immunosuppressed persons.

These various organisms cause pathology in either the small intestine or the colon and precipitate either increased secretion into the tract lumen or interference with nutrient and fluid absorption, or both. Typically, the small intestine absorbs about 6 liters of fluid per day. It is able to absorb this much because it has several million fingerlike projections, called villi. These villi are covered with large numbers of microvilli, which together form a large mucosal surface for absorption, called the brush border. Some HIV-related pathogens directly attack this brush border, reducing its absorption ability. Extra unabsorbed fluid is then passed to the colon. Diarrhea results when the amount of fluid exceeds the colon's capacity to absorb it. Other organisms produce toxins, which attack the intestinal mucosa, causing inflammation and secretion of fluid into the lumen. In all cases, the amount of fluid can quickly overwhelm the absorbing capacity of both the small and large intestines and can destroy the body's fluid and electrolyte balance.

Destruction of mucosal villi and microvilli and rapid passage of material through the colon mean that fewer nutrients are absorbed. Often this occurs at the same time that the person is exhausted from coping with severe diarrhea and no longer has the energy to shop, to prepare food, and to eat. Very rapid loss of body mass

and weight (wasting syndrome) occurs (see Color Plate 34). Many clinicians advocate use of total parenteral nutrition as a means of forestalling the wasting syndrome, although studies in cancer patients have shown this to be detrimental to the patient.

Treatment of the organisms that cause HIV-related diarrhea is not an easy process. Some organisms respond rapidly to treatment. However, there is no effective treatment for others, particularly cytomegalovirus, *Cryptosporidium* spp., *Microsporidium*, and *Mycobacterium avium* complex. Symptoms sometimes resolve spontaneously or become episodic rather than persistent. Supportive care, which enables the patient to cope with periodic crises, is essential.

Three organisms have been implicated as the principal causes of colitis in HIV-infected people. These are herpes simplex virus, cytomegalovirus, and *Clostridium difficile*. Other organisms that occasionally have been implicated are *Mycobacterium avium* complex, *Microsporidium* spp., and *Entamoeba histolytica*. Both HSV and CMV can cause large ulcers in the colon, which can lead to perforation. *Clostridium difficile* is an opportunistic organism that multiplies when the normal flora, which normally inhibits the growth of *C. difficile*, is eradicated by antimicrobial therapy. Under these circumstances, the organism produces two toxins that attack colonic mucosa. Usual treatment is to eliminate currently administered antibiotics and to treat with vancomycin or metronidazole.

Persistent diarrhea, like persistent nausea and vomiting, also suggests drug reactions. HIV-infected individuals often take multiple medications, many of which have diarrheas as a side effect. For example, Sande and Volberding listed 49 drugs commonly administered in HIV disease, 19 of which have diarrhea as a side effect. Drugs commonly causing diarrhea are didanosine (ddI, Videx), interferon, recombinant erythropoietin, granulocyte colony stimulating factor (G-CSF), granulocyte-monocyte colony stimulating factor (GM-CSF), flucytosine, clarithromycin, and azithromycin. Persistent diarrhea should always prompt a review of the patient's currently prescribed drugs, particularly those that have been prescribed recently.

DIAGNOSTIC STUDIES AND FINDINGS FOR GASTROINTESTINAL MANIFESTATIONS

Diagnostic Test	Finding
Endoscopy in esophagus for lesions due to:	Visualization of:
Candida albicans	Yellow-white plaque overlying ulcers
Herpes simplex virus	Multiple, small, deep ulcers that may coalesce into large ulcerated lesions; overhanging erythematous, edematous mucosa ("volcano ulcers")
HIV	Small ulceration (2-15 mm in size) is diagnostic when all other causes have been excluded
Cytomegalovirus (may also be extended to stomach)	Shallow, large (up to 10 cm) ulcers
Endoscopy in intestinal tract for:	Visualization of:
Cryptosporidium spp.	Mild villus atrophy, crypt enlargement
Isospora belli	No characteristic findings
Enterocytozoon bienusi (microsporidia)	Diffuse erythema overlain by a thin mucoid coating
Entamoeba histolytica	Ragged undermined ulcers that are focal and discrete in mild cases, which may coalesce with hemorrhage; edema and sloughing of large areas of mucosa of colon only
Giardia lamblia	No characteristic findings
Clostridium difficile	Erythematous, friable mucosa with yellow-white pseudomembranous plaques in colon only
Mycobacterium avium complex	Erythema, edema, and friability of mucosa; small erosions and fine white nodules possible
Salmonella spp. (nontyphoidal)	No characteristic findings
Shigella spp.	Hyperemia, edema, superficial mucosal ulcers in lower colon; mucosa covered with mucus
Campylobacter jejuni	No characteristic findings
Cytomegalovirus	Localized hyperemia progressing to deep ulceration
Herpes simplex virus	Small discrete vesicles progressing to erosions and large coalesced ulcers
Examination of biopsied tissue from esophagus for signs of:	Visualization of:
Candida albicans	Tissue invasion by pseudomycelia, hyphae, pseudohyphae, and yeast forms
Herpes simplex virus	Presence of intranuclear inclusion bodies
Cytomegalovirus (tissue also may be taken from stomach)	Large intranuclear inclusion cells with surrounding inflammation; may be surrounded by a space called the "owl's eye halo"
Examination of biopsied tissue from the colon for signs of:	Visualization of:
Cryptosporidium spp.	Characteristic organisms found in brush border of epithelial cells
Isospora belli	Localized inflammation and atrophy of mucosa; organisms found within the lumen or within cytoplasmic vacuoles in enterocytes
Enterocytozoon bienusi	Degenerative necrosis and sloughing of infected enterocytes
Entamoeba histolytica	Characteristic organism
Mycobacterium avium complex	Characteristic acid-fast organisms
Salmonella spp. (nontyphoidal)	Characteristic organism
Shigella spp.	Characteristic organism in epithelial cells
Campylobacter jejuni	No characteristic finding
Cytomegalovirus	Large mononuclear, epithelial, endothelial, or smooth muscle cells containing intranuclear or cytoplasmic inclusion bodies
Herpes simplex virus	Intranuclear inclusions in multinucleated cells
Culture of stool specimen or biopsied tissue	Can seldom be considered definitive because GI tract contains multiple organisms that may not be causing pathology or multiple organisms may be responsible for the pathology; findings are diagnostic for organisms that don't ordinarily inhabit the GI tract, e.g., *Shigella*.

DIAGNOSTIC STUDIES AND FINDINGS FOR GASTROINTESTINAL MANIFESTATIONS—cont'd

Diagnostic Test	Finding
Microscopic examination of stool specimen	May be positive for ova and parasites; same cautions as for culture of stool specimen apply
Modified acid-fast bacilli stain	Confirmatory but not diagnostic of *M. avium* complex, cryptosporidia, and *I. belli*
Stool assay for *C. difficile* toxin	Positive result indicates organism is present; other organisms may be coinfecting; may be false-negative results
Fecal white blood count	Positive result suggests infection with salmonella, *Shigella, C. jejuni,* or *C. difficile;* distinguishes between inflammatory and secretory diarrhea
Serum ferritin	Anemia associated with blood loss in bowel
Serum electrolytes	Alterations in sodium, potassium, bicarbonate, and chloride associated with diarrhea
X-ray	May confirm presence of a bowel perforation

MEDICAL MANAGEMENT OF GASTROINTESTINAL MANIFESTATIONS

DRUG THERAPY

Esophagitis due to *Candida albicans:* Fluconazole (Diflucan), 200 mg PO first day, then 100-200 mg qd until improvement; or ketoconazole (Nizoral), 200-400 mg PO qd until improvement; or clotrimazole troches, one 10 mg troche 5 times/day; or nystatin solution, 500,000-1 million units "swish and swallow" 3-5 times/day for 14 days. If no response in 1 week: amphotericin B (0.3 mg/kg IV qd for 7 days). Suppressive therapy: fluconazole, 100 mg PO q week, *or* nystatin *or* clotrimazole *or* ketoconazole.

Esophagitis due to herpes simplex virus: Acyclovir (Zovirax), 5.0 mg/kg IV (infused over 1 h) q 8 h; or acyclovir, 200 mg PO 5 times/day for 10 days; or foscarnet (Foscavir), 40 mg/kg IV (infuse over 2 hours) q 8 h for 21 days in well-hydrated patient. Suppressive therapy: Acyclovir, 400 mg PO bid indefinitely; or foscarnet, 40 mg/kg IV qd indefinitely.

Esophagitis due to cytomegalovirus: Ganciclovir, 5 mg/kg IV bid for 14-21 days; or foscarnet, 60 mg/kg IV q 8 h for 14-21 days (efficacy of this treatment is not established).

Diarrhea due to *Cryptosporidium spp:* Paromomycin, 500 mg PO bid for 7-10 days (efficacy not established).

Diarrhea due to *Isospora belli:* TMP/SMX, 1 double-strength tablet PO qid for 10 days, then bid for 3 weeks, then 1 double-strength tablet of TMP/SMX 3 times/wk indefinitely. (Double-strength trimethoprim is 160 mg and sulfamethoxazole is 800 mg.)

Diarrhea due to *Entamoeba histolytica:* Metronidazole (Flagyl), 750 mg PO tid for 10 days, followed by either iodoquinol, 650 mg PO tid for 20 days, or paromomycin, 500 mg PO tid for 7 days.

Diarrhea due to *Giardia lamblia:* Metronidazole (Flagyl), 250 mg PO tid for 5 days; or quinacrine, 100 mg PO tid after meals for 5 days.

Diarrhea due to *Mycobacterium avium complex:* No antimicrobial therapy has been demonstrated to reduce MAC-related diarrhea.

MAC bacteremia: Clarithromycin, 500-1000 mg PO bid. Azithromycin, 600-1200 mg PO qd, may be added to regimen. Prophylaxis for MAC bacteremia in patients with CD4+ counts <100: rifabutin, 300 mg qd.

Diarrhea due to *Salmonella* spp: Ampicillin, 8-12 g IV/day for 1-4 wk, then amoxicillin, 500 mg PO tid to complete a 2-4 week course. Alternative therapy: ciprofloxacin, 500-750 mg PO bid for 2-4 wk.

Continued.

MEDICAL MANAGEMENT OF GASTROINTESTINAL MANIFESTATIONS—cont'd

DRUG THERAPY—cont'd

Diarrhea due to *Shigella* spp: Ciprofloxacin, 500 mg PO bid for 5-7 days. If recurrent, a maintenance dose of 500 mg PO bid is administered indefinitely.

Diarrhea due to *Campylobacter jejuni:* Ciprofloxacin, 500 mg PO bid for 7-10 days; or erythromycin, 500 mg PO qid for 7-10 days.

Diarrhea due to *Clostridium difficile:* Metronidazole, 250 mg tid for 10 days, *or* vancomycin, 125 mg PO q 6 h for 7-10 days. Because diarrhea caused by *C. difficile* is related to antibiotic use, previously ordered antibiotics should be discontinued or modified.

Diarrhea due to cytomegalovirus: Ganciclovir, 5 mg/kg IV bid for 14-21 days; or foscarnet, 60 mg/kg IV q 8 h for 14-21 days. Efficacy is not proven.

Diarrhea due to herpes simplex virus: Acyclovir, 30 mg/kg/day IV for at least 10 days; or vidarabine, 15 mg/kg IV for at least 10 days.

Antiemetics: Dimenhydrinate, 50 mg IM q 4 h; or chlorpromazine, 25 mg/day IM.

Antidiarrheal drugs: Any one of the following may be ordered: diphenoxylate (Lomotil), 2.5-5 mg PO qid; or codeine phosphate, 15-30 mg bid or tid; or paregoric (camphorated), 15 ml q 4 h; or opium tincture (DTO) (paregoric), 0.6 ml PO qid (maximum dose 6 ml qd); loperamide hydrochloride (Imodium), 2-4 mg tid; bismuth subsalicylate (Pepto-Bismol), 30 ml or 2 tabs PO tid, may be increased up to 8 doses per day for 2 days. Psyllium (Metamucil), 1-2 tsp PO tid in fluid. (While usually administered for constipation, in severe diarrhea it absorbs water and expands to increase bulk.)
Kaolin and pectin compounds, 30-60 ml PO q 6 h act to decrease water content of stools but do not reduce the total amount of fluid lost.
Octreotide (Sandostatin), 50 mg subcutaneous q 8 h for 48 hr; if no response, increase stepwise to 500 mg q 8 h for 48 hr. Less than 50% of patients respond.

SUPPORTIVE THERAPY

Fluid and electrolyte replacement: Based on amount of fluid and electrolytes lost and may equal 15-20 liters per day. Oral fluids, except those that cause GI distress (fluids with caffeine and milk), are recommended and should be encouraged, if tolerated. Oral rehydration fluid containing 1 tsp table salt, 1 tsp baking soda, and 4 tsp table sugar dissolved in 1 quart water (flavoring can be added) may be administered up to 75 ml/kg over 4 hours.

Refer to Chapter 11 for nursing management.

CHAPTER 8

Central Nervous System and Neurosensory Manifestations

Approximately 60% of HIV-infected people will suffer at least one neurologic manifestation during the course of disease, with 10% to 20% having neurologic signs as the first symptom of their infection. Many of the neurologic conditions are progressive and have subtle early manifestations, such as forgetfulness, change in speech patterns, or a decrease in sensation of the hands and feet (peripheral neuropathy). The actual occurrence of these conditions may not be noticed initially and may only be recognized in retrospect. Therefore, as stressed in Chapter 5, health care providers must have a well-documented baseline neurologic and cognitive assessment, against which comparisons can be made as the client's disease progresses. To complicate matters, HIV-infected persons are also subject to a wide range of acute infections, such as meningitis and encephalitis, that also produce acute neurologic symptoms. These conditions can progress very rapidly and become life threatening if the person does not receive timely antiinfective treatment and supportive care. Acute neurologic infections are not limited to the central nervous system. CMV retinitis, for example, can lead to blindness within days if untreated. In addition, medication given to HIV-infected persons can produce neurologic symptoms as side effects. This chapter will provide an overview of both acute and chronic HIV-related manifestations associated with the central and peripheral nervous systems and the sensory system.

Central Nervous System Manifestations

People infected with HIV experience a variety of conditions affecting the central nervous system (CNS). These include both chronic and acute infections causing encephalitis, meningitis, or myelopathy. An overview of CNS manifestations with definitions and signs and symptoms is provided in Table 8-1.

HIV ENCEPHALOPATHY (AIDS DEMENTIA COMPLEX)

The most common chronic infection is caused by the human immunodeficiency virus itself. The exact mechanisms of destruction of brain tissue is not clear. The virus has been found in brain macrophages and, presumably, causes their eventual destruction. HIV also infects glial cells, causing localized edema and occasional demyelination within the brain. In addition, early brain atrophy can be detected through diagnostic procedures such as CT scans and magnetic resonance imaging (MRI). No one seems to know how all these factors combine to cause the progressive cognitive and motor losses found in HIV-infected people. It is clear, however, that many, if not most, HIV-infected people will experience a noticeable decline in both their cognitive and motor abilities. This deterioration is collectively referred to as AIDS dementia complex, or ADC. ADC is attributed to this subacute infection with HIV and might even be more correctly referred to as cognitive and motor deficits due to chronic, subacute HIV infection of the cerebrospinal fluid (CSF) and brain tissue. Because the condition is caused by HIV infection itself, there is no curative therapy. Some clinicians believe that the condition can be slowed by increased doses of antiretroviral drugs so that higher levels of the drugs cross the blood-brain barrier. However, there are neurotoxic adverse reactions to ddI and ddC, and there are hematopoietic side effects to AZT. The side effects of high-dose therapies with these drugs present difficult choices for the clinician.

MENINGITIS

Atypical aseptic meningitis, a chronic infection with periodic acute exacerbations, is found in up to 10% of HIV-infected people. It appears that this condition also is caused by HIV itself and, therefore, has no specific drug therapy. Aseptic meningitides associated with her-

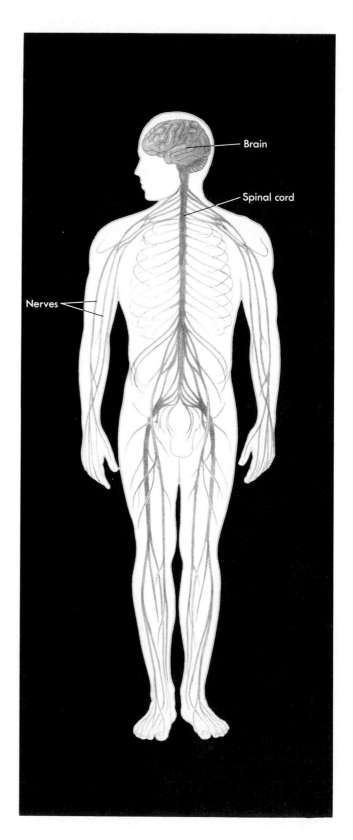

Table 8-1 _____

OVERVIEW OF CENTRAL NERVOUS SYSTEM MANIFESTATIONS

Condition	Description	Signs and symptoms
Primary viral syndromes due to HIV		
HIV encephalopathy (AIDS dementia complex [ADC], subacute encephalitis)	Chronic, subacute encephalitis in which there is progressive deterioration of cognitive, motor, and behavioral functions; it is unique to HIV infection and produces clinical symptoms in up to 40% of people with HIV; 75% of HIV infected show signs of CNS effects on autopsy	Poor concentration, forgetfulness, general slowness indicating global dementia, disturbances in balance and hand-eye coordination, dysarthria progressing to mutism, apathy, social withdrawal, inattention, psychomotor slowing, inability to do complex mental processes, ataxia, tremor, hypertonia, paraparesis, incontinence, spasm
Aseptic meningitis	Chronic or recurring meningitis, which may be occasionally acute; it is characterized by elevated intracranial pressure and excess lymphocytes in CSF, meningeal irritation, and cranial neuropathy; occurs to 5% to 10% of HIV-infected persons	Fever, headache, meningeal signs, cranial nerve V, VII, and VIII involvement
Spinal vacuolar myelopathy	Diffuse degeneration of the spinal cord that is most severe in the lateral and posterior areas of the thoracic cord; may be related to direct effect of HIV or to malnutrition; found at autopsy in 25% of HIV-infected persons	Leg weakness, incontinence, paraparesis, spasticity, ataxia
Non-HIV viral syndromes		
Progressive multifocal leukoencephalopathy (PML, papovavirus JC infection)	Chronic, progressive CNS demyelinating disease; affects up to 3% of HIV-infected persons	Dementia, blindness, aphasia, alteration in level of consciousness or cognition, hemiparesis, unsteadiness, ataxia, headache
Herpes meningitis, encephalitis, or myelitis (herpes simplex or herpes zoster)	Acute or chronic infection presenting as meningitis, encephalitis, or myelitis; occurs to 1% of HIV-infected persons	Headache, fever, seizures, focal neurologic deficits, altered mental status
Cytomegalovirus (CMV) encephalitis	Acute, severe, afebrile inflammation of the brain that may involve the cortex, white matter, and/or meninges; occurs to 1% to 3% of HIV-infected persons	Headache, nuchal rigidity, fever, positive Babinski reflex, tremors, irritability, lethargy, nausea, vomiting; may progress to delirium and loss of consciousness, motor weakness, seizures, and aphasia
Nonviral infections		
Toxoplasma encephalitis (*T. gondii*, toxoplasmosis)	Acute encephalitis with focal or diffuse inflammation of the brain; occurs in up to 15% of HIV-infected persons	Seizures, bifrontal headache unrelieved by analgesics, fever, altered mentation and cognition, lethargy, psychosis, nausea, vomiting, hemiparesis, ataxia, unsteady gait, cranial nerve palsies, aphasia, visual disturbances
Cryptococcal meningitis (*Cryptococcus neoformans*, cryptococcosis)	Acute, chronic, or recurring meningitis; occurs in up to 12% of HIV-infected persons	Headache, fever, night sweats, impaired consciousness and cognition, cranial nerve abnormalities, photophobia, seizures

Continued.

Table 8-1

OVERVIEW OF CENTRAL NERVOUS SYSTEM MANIFESTATIONS—cont'd

Condition	Description	Signs and symptoms
Neurosyphilis (*Treponema pallidum*)	Acute or chronic inflammation of cerebrovascular system and meninges; prevalence in HIV infected is unknown; it is a risk factor for sexually active people and may confuse diagnosis of other neurologic conditions	Progressive dementia, alterations in speech, weakness with hyperreflexia, irritability, grandiose delusion and hallucinations, ataxia, paresthesia, trophic joint disease and granulomatous lesions (gummas)
Coccidioidomycosis (valley fever, San Joaquin fever, *Coccidioides immitis*)	Acute, rapidly progressive, and fulminating meningitis that becomes chronic after initial manifestation; occurs rarely outside desert areas of Southwest; occurs to 1% of HIV infected from that area	Fever, night sweats, headache, meningeal signs, altered mentation, progressive lethargy
Neoplasms (see also Chapter 10), primary CNS lymphoma	Neoplasm of lymphoid tissue in the brain with a subacute onset; occurs in 2% of HIV infected	Altered mental status, headache, seizures, focal weakness, aphasia, incontinence

pes simplex virus (HSV) and cytomegalovirus (CMV) occur in both acute and chronic forms during HIV infection. Specific therapies do exist for infections with these organisms.

SPINAL VACUOLAR MYELOPATHY

Another disorder, which is believed to be related to the direct effect of HIV, is vacuolar myelopathy in the spinal cord. Autopsy studies show that about 25% of HIV-infected people exhibit diffuse degeneration of the spinal cord, particularly of the white matter of the lateral and posterior columns. Degeneration can also be observed in the white matter of the brain. As in HIV encephalopathy, the mechanism of destruction is not understood. Research has demonstrated that HIV infects macrophages in the spinal cord, and edema can be observed in the myelin sheath. Because this degeneration closely resembles the destruction caused by vitamin B_{12}, some investigators have suggested that there may be a nutritional cause to this condition. This hypothesis has some logic, given the nutritional deprivation found in people with AIDS. However, attempts to link serum vitamin B_{12} levels to this condition have not been successful. Nonetheless, concern about maximizing nutrition in HIV-infected persons may be warranted and certainly will do no harm. There is no specific drug therapy for this condition, which progresses until death.

PROGRESSIVE MULTIFOCAL LEUKOENCEPHALOPATHY (PML)

Progressive multifocal leukoencephalopathy (PML), another viral syndrome, is caused by the papovavirus JC, an opportunistic organism, which is present in most adults. The virus causes clinical disease in about 3% of people infected with HIV. PML is characterized by focal loss of myelin without destruction of axons. The areas of demyelination are surrounded by damaged delicate neuroglial cells, particularly oligodendrocytes and astrocytes. PML is a progressive disease affecting nerves associated with motor, sensory, or cognitive function. No specific drug therapy against papovavirus JC is available.

HERPESVIRUS INFECTIONS

Infections of the CNS with herpes simplex or herpes zoster occur in 1% of HIV-infected people. Herpesviruses are generally acquired earlier in life and manifest as self-limiting skin or mucous membrane lesions. Both viruses remain in a latent state along nerve pathways in the body, resurfacing to cause disseminated serious disease in the immunosuppressed. These infections may manifest as meningitis, encephalitis, or myelitis. Antiviral treatment is available; however, the therapy is suppressive rather than curative. Patients may have to be maintained on therapy for the remainder of their lives. In addition, therapy may not always be successful, as drug-resistant strains of herpesviruses are continually being observed. Another opportunistic herpesvirus, cytomegalovirus (CMV), can cause acute encephalitis as well as pathology in the lungs, retina, and gastrointestinal tract. Antiviral therapy is available to suppress this organism, but not eliminate it.

TOXOPLASMA ENCEPHALITIS

Toxoplasma gondii, a protozoan, causes encephalitis in 15% of HIV-infected people. This organism is opportunistic, infecting anywhere from 25% to 80% of the population, depending on the area of the United States. The organism rarely causes symptomatic clinical disease except in the immunosuppressed. A variety of antibiotics are effective against *Toxoplasma* encephalitis. However, the disease recurs in 50% of the cases, necessitating lifelong suppressive therapy. Therapies that suppress *Toxoplasma* have a side benefit of being effective at preventing *Pneumocystis carinii* pneumonia, which is also caused by a protozoan.

CRYPTOCOCCAL MENINGITIS

Cryptococcal meningitis occurs in up to 12% of people with HIV. The organism causing this infection is widespread in the environment. It rarely causes disease in immunocompetent people, suggesting natural resistance to the organism. Cryptococcus is an aggressive pathogen in the immunosuppressed. Pathology includes granulomatous lesions in the meninges and granulomas and cysts in the cortex of the brain. Antibiotic therapy is now available to fight this potentially fatal infection. Therapy must be maintained for life in order to prevent recurrence.

NEUROSYPHILIS

Treponema pallidum is not a true opportunistic organism in HIV infection in that it may be acquired after infection with HIV or may be present as a latent infection acquired earlier in life. Infection with *T. pallidum* appears to be much more aggressive in the HIV infected, progressing to neurosyphilis in just a few years. The organism attacks small arteries and arterioles anywhere in the body, causing inflammation, endothelial swelling, and fibrosis. Fibrotic thickening of the vessels impairs arterial circulation, resulting in necrosis and tissue death. When this pathologic process occurs in the brain, any number of neurologic changes may occur, affecting cognitive, motor, or sensory functions. Because the risks associated with acquiring HIV infection are the same as those associated with syphilis, syphilis is to be suspected in persons with HIV. Some clinicians recommend that anytime CSF is obtained from an HIV-infected patient, it should be examined for indicators of neurosyphilis. The treatment for neurosyphilis involves high-dose antibiotic therapy with penicillin or third-generation cephalosporin, which may require hospitalization. Such therapy is generally successful.

COCCIDIOIDOMYCOSIS

The fungus *Coccidioides immitis* can cause meningitis in 1% of people exposed to it. This is both an acquired and an opportunistic organism, commonly found in soil and dust in the southwestern United States (generally from central Texas to southern California) or certain areas of Mexico and Central America. A travel or residence history may reveal a person's risk for this infection. Most infections are subclinical and do not cause problems in an immunocompetent host. However, when a person harboring the fungus becomes immunosuppressed, the pathogen may become aggressive, causing caseation and calcification of brain tissue. Symptoms vary depending on the location and size of the lesions. Long-term administration of antifungal drugs, generally through a central line, is required.

NEOPLASMS

About 2% of HIV-infected persons develop a primary lymphoma in the central nervous system. A smaller percent develop metastatic lymphomas in the CNS. Kaposi's sarcoma may also disseminate to the central nervous system, causing CNS symptoms. All of these conditions are described in Chapter 10.

Peripheral Nervous System Manifestations

Chronic distal peripheral neuropathy and *demyelinating polyneuropathy* are two major types of peripheral neuropathies associated with HIV infection (Table 8-2). Experts believe that both are caused by direct attack of HIV on the myelin covering axons or on myelin covering nerve sheaths. The exact pathologic mechanism is not clear. Demyelinization of nerve sheaths seems to predominate in chronic distal peripheral neuropathy. Treatment consists of efforts to obtain symptomatic relief with analgesics and tricyclic antidepressants. When axonal demyelination predominates, the result is inflammatory demyelinating polyneuropathy. Plasmapheresis and steroids seem to alleviate this condition.

Steroids must be used with caution because of their immunosuppressive effects. Analgesics are also used for symptomatic relief. No specific drug treatment is available.

VARICELLA ZOSTER VIRUS AND HERPES SIMPLEX VIRUS

Both varicella zoster virus (VZV) and herpes simplex virus (HSV) are associated with acute and recurring dermatologic infections and painful neuropathies in immunocompromised people. These are discussed in Chapter 6.

Sensory Manifestations

Two pathologies cause vision defects in persons with HIV infection (Table 8-3). HIV can directly attack retinal tissue and does so in at least 50% of HIV-infected people. This is noted by observation of small, white, fluffy lesions ("cotton-wool spots") in the retina. These lesions have regular borders and are seldom larger than one disk diameter. They are benign and generally resolve within weeks. In contrast, 10% to 20% of HIV-infected persons will have retinitis, with irreversible reti-

nal damage, caused by cytomegalovirus. CMV retinitis, if left untreated, will cause blindness in the involved eye. With time, both eyes will become infected. Unlike the lesions in HIV retinopathy, CMV retinitis lesions have diffuse borders and will expand rapidly. Treatment is intravenous administration of antiviral drugs. This is another condition where treatment merely suppresses the organism rather than eliminates it. Lifelong maintenance therapy is required.

Table 8-2

OVERVIEW OF PERIPHERAL NERVOUS SYSTEM MANIFESTATIONS

Condition	Description	Signs and symptoms
Chronic distal symmetric peripheral neuropathy	Chronic disorder of the peripheral nerves characterized by loss of sensory function as opposed to motor function; usually affects hands and feet; occurs in 50% of HIV infected	Numbness, tingling, hyperesthesia, sensory ataxia, weakness, hypoactive deep tendon reflexes
Inflammatory demyelinating polyneuropathy	Acute, subacute, or chronic neuropathy affecting motor functions as opposed to sensory functions; almost all HIV-infected people experience demyelination, but few are actually symptomatic	Weakness, hypoactive tendon reflexes, or areflexia
Varicella zoster virus (VZV) and herpes simplex virus (HSV) infection	See Chapter 6	

Table 8-3

OVERVIEW OF SENSORY MANIFESTATIONS

Condition	Description	Signs and symptoms
HIV retinopathy	Chronic, benign, self-limiting inflammation of the retina caused by HIV; occurs in over 50% of HIV infected	"Cotton-wool" spots with regular borders on retina; occasional small retinal hemorrhages
Cytomegalovirus (CMV) retinitis (Color Plate 35)	Aggressive, acute infection of the eye resulting in destruction of retinal tissue, leading to loss of vision and/or blindness; occurs in 10% to 20% of HIV infected in late-stage disease	Initially small, white "cotton-wool" spots with irregular borders on the retina, which progressively enlarge to fluffy, white exudates with associated hemorrhages; vision loss progressing to blindness

DIAGNOSTIC STUDIES AND FINDINGS

Diagnostic Test	Finding
CSF determinations:	
Pressure	Elevated
Pleocytosis	Present
Culture	Positive for organisms
Gram's stain	Positive for organisms
Antigen titers	Increased
Protein	Elevated
Glucose	Elevated
Serology for antibodies	Elevated; fails to decline following therapy
CT scan and MRI	Observations of diffuse or focal lesions, atrophy, presence and location of white matter abnormalities; presence of hydrocephalus or space-occupying lesions
Brain biopsy	Identification of type of organism or tumor; may not be recommended due to frequency of complications following procedure (10%)
Electroencephalography (EEG)	Identification of focal or diffuse slowing
Electromyography	Disruption in nerve conduction
Mental status exam	Determination of capacity of client to perform cognitive tasks (see Chapter 5)
Retinal photographs	Presence of lesions, their size and shape; growth or resolution of lesions

---

MEDICAL MANAGEMENT

DRUG THERAPY FOR CNS MANIFESTATIONS

HIV encephalopathy: AZT dosage raised to 1000-1200 mg/day PO; controversial (see text).

Atypical aseptic meningitis: Antipyretics and analgesics.

Spinal vacuolar myelopathy: No drug treatment available.

Progressive multifocal leukoencephalopathy (PML): No drug treatment available.

Herpes simplex virus encephalitis: Acyclovir, 10 mg/kg IV q 8 h for 10-14 days; or foscarnet if virus is resistant to acyclovir; sedatives for seizures, antipyretics, analgesics.

Continued.

MEDICAL MANAGEMENT—cont'd

Herpes zoster encephalitis: Acyclovir, 10-12 mg/kg IV q 8 h for 7 days; or foscarnet if virus is resistant to acyclovir; sedatives for seizures, antipyretics, analgesics.

CMV encephalitis: Ganciclovir, 5 mg/kg IV bid for 14-21 days, or foscarnet, 60 mg/kg IV q 8 h for 14-21 days; sedatives for seizures, antipyretics, analgesics.

***Toxoplasma* meningitis/encephalitis:** Pyrimethamine, 50-100 mg PO qd following one loading dose of 200 mg PO; plus sulfadiazine, 4-6 g/day PO in 4 divided doses; plus folinic acid, 5 mg/day for 4-6 weeks; alternative in case of sulfadiazine sensitivity: clindamycin, 450-600 mg PO qid or 600-900 mg IV q 6 h; corticosteroids for cerebral edema.

Suppressive therapy for *Toxoplasma*: Pyrimethamine, 25-50 mg PO qd, plus folinic acid, 5 mg/day, plus sulfadiazine, 2-4 g/day PO in 4 divided doses; clindamycin 300-450 mg PO q 6-8h may be substituted for sulfadiazine in case of sulfadiazine sensitivity; lifelong therapy is required.

Cryptococcal meningitis: Amphotericin B, 0.5-0.8 mg/kg/day IV infused over 2-4 hours, plus flucytosine, 25 mg/kg PO q 6 h if WBC is normal; therapy is maintained for 10-14 days; analgesics and antipyretics.

Suppressive therapy for *Cryptococcus* (begin when CSF is negative for organism): Fluconazole, 200 mg PO qd; lifelong therapy is required.

Neurosyphilis with CSF positive for *T. pallidum*: Aqueous penicillin G, 2-4 million units IV q 4 h for 10 days, or procaine penicillin, 2-4 million units IM qd, plus probenecid, 500 mg PO qd for 10 days. Either regimen should be followed by benzathine penicillin, 2.4 million units IM every week for 3 weeks.

Coccidioidomycosis meningitis: Amphotericin B, 0.5-1.0 mg/kg/day IV for 8 weeks; intrathecal amphotericin B is usually added.

Suppressive therapy for coccidioidomycosis: Amphotericin B, 1.0 mg/kg/wk, or fluconazole, 400 mg PO qd.

Neoplasms: Multiple drug regimens or radiation therapy (see Chapter 10).

GENERAL MANAGEMENT FOR CNS MANIFESTATIONS

HIV encephalopathy: Psychiatric counseling; referral to support groups and case managers; instructions on simplifying one's life and tasks.

Atypical aseptic meningitis: Intratracheal intubation, ventilatory assistance, IV fluids (restrict fluids if intracranial pressure is elevated), control of intracranial pressure, supportive care.

Spinal vacuolar myelopathy: Supportive care and nutrition therapy; obtain assistance with activities of daily living (ADLs); provide assistive devices (canes, walkers, etc.).

PML: Supportive care with attention to safety needs; obtain assistance with ADLs.

Meningitis and encephalitis (due to herpesviruses, CMV, *T. gondii,* and *Cryptococcus* and *Coccidioides*): Intratracheal intubation, ventilatory assistance, IV fluids and electrolytes (restrict fluids if intracranial pressure is elevated), control of intracranial pressure, supportive care; maintain a safe environment to minimize harm from seizures; refer client with residual disabilities for rehabilitation and assistance with ADLs.

Neurosyphilis: Refer patient for case management and assistance with ADLs.

MEDICAL MANAGEMENT—cont'd

DRUG THERAPY FOR PERIPHERAL NERVOUS SYSTEM MANIFESTATIONS

Chronic distal peripheral neuropathy: Analgesics for pain; capsaicin-containing topical ointments such as Zostrix or lidocaine ointment (10%-30%); tricyclic antidepressants such as nortriptyline, 10-75 mg hs.

Inflammatory demyelinating polyneuropathy: Analgesics for pain; steroids are sometimes used, although they decrease cellular immune function; plasmapheresis may be helpful.

Herpes zoster virus (HZV) and herpes simplex virus (HSV) infections: See Chapter 6.

GENERAL MANAGEMENT FOR PERIPHERAL NERVOUS SYSTEM MANIFESTATIONS

Refer for assistance, as necessary, with ADLs; provide assistive devices (walkers, canes, etc.) and safety equipment for the home.

DRUG THERAPY FOR SENSORY MANIFESTATIONS

HIV retinopathy: No drug treatment.

CMV retinitis: Foscarnet, 60 mg/kg IV q 8 h for 14-21 days; as an alternative, ganciclovir, 5 mg/kg IV bid for 14-21 days; dosages may have to be reduced based on creatine clearance tests.

Suppressive therapy for CMV: Foscarnet, 90 mg/kg/day IV; or ganciclovir, 5 mg/kg/day IV.

GENERAL MANAGEMENT FOR SENSORY MANIFESTATIONS

HIV retinopathy: Reassure client that condition is benign and self-limiting.

CMV retinitis: Refer for assistance with ADLs.

Refer to Chapter 11 for nursing management.

CHAPTER 9

Respiratory Manifestations

The most vital element in the maintenance of life is oxygen. If a person is deprived of it for even a few minutes, cerebral infarction and irreversible brain damage occur. Death rapidly follows. HIV-infected individuals are subject to a variety of infections and conditions that compromise oxygen exchange. As a result, pulmonary diseases are the major cause of HIV-related deaths. The majority of HIV-related pulmonary diseases are pneumonias, followed by a significant number of mycobacterial respiratory infections. In addition, as many as 60% of HIV-infected people will also have recurrent or persistent sinus infection. Manifestations of these sinus infections can range from mild, but embarrassing, halitosis to painful sinus headache to life-threatening sinocerebral mucormycosis. The important point is that almost all HIV-infected individuals will experience at least one life-threatening episode of pulmonary disease.

Pneumonias

Pneumonia is the inflammatory response of the lungs to a foreign invader. When pathogens infect the tissue of the lungs, the body responds by flooding the area with alveolar fluid and leukocytes specific to the type of invader. Instead of being protective, these inflammatory reactions sometimes create a favorable medium for replication of the organism. The net result of vascular engorgement, the accumulation of debris, and scarring of the alveolar capillary lining is interference with oxygen exchange in the alveoli. In the normal host, immunologic destruction of the pathogen and reabsorption of the alveolar debris usually occur more rapidly than pathogen replication and debris production; eventually, the inflammation subsides. Antimicrobial therapy greatly speeds this process. In the immunocompromised host, pathogens are destroyed very slowly, if at all, and the lungs become overwhelmed. Oxygen exchange becomes so compromised that death can result unless appropriate and rapid antiinfective therapy is instituted. Therefore, any lung infection in an HIV-infected person must be promptly and vigorously treated. Even then, the pathogen may not be eliminated but merely suppressed, necessitating lifelong antiinfective drug therapy.

Almost all HIV-infected people will experience an opportunistic pneumonia at some time during the course of HIV disease. Because most of these conditions result in progressive deterioration in oxygen exchange, they can quickly become life threatening. The goal of management of these conditions is to provide supportive care (e.g., oxygen therapy) while seeking the exact causative organism. Once the organism is known, appropriate antibiotic therapy is employed. Because these conditions can become so rapidly life threatening, antibiotic therapy often is started on a "best-guess" basis while waiting for the results of laboratory cultures and drug sensitivity tests. In such circumstances, close monitoring of the patient's condition is required. Any positive or negative change in the patient's condition should immediately be brought to the attention of the prescribing clinician.

Pneumonia in the HIV infected can be bacterial, viral, or fungal in origin. The most common of these pneumonias are described in Table 9-1.

Table 9-1

OVERVIEW OF PNEUMONIAS ASSOCIATED WITH HIV INFECTION

Condition	Description	Signs and symptoms
Pneumonia (general)	An acute inflammation of the lung involving the bronchioles and alveoli; due to an infectious organism	Severe chills, fever, diaphoresis, cough, chest pain, painful breathing, purulent (sometimes rust-colored) sputum, shortness of breath, rapid respirations, characteristic breath sounds, and lack of energy
Pneumococcal pneumonia due to *S. pneumoniae*	Infection can be acquired or opportunistic and is common in all stages of HIV infection. Immunization is available and recommended at first knowledge of HIV infection.	Usually sudden onset; may present with referred pain suggestive of appendicitis; may have only a single episode of chills
Pneumonia due to *H. influenzae*	Infection can be acquired or opportunistic and is common in all stages of HIV infection. Organism commonly colonizes in the upper respiratory tract of healthy adults. Immunization is available. Although effectiveness of vaccine in immunocompromised is unclear, experts recommend immunization at first knowledge of HIV infection.	Not distinguishable from other bacterial pneumonias
Cytomegalovirus (CMV) pneumonia	CMV is very commonly found in the respiratory tract. It is seldom pathogenic, accounting for less than 5% of pneumonias in HIV infected, and generally occurs only in the later stages of HIV infection.	Generally has gradual onset, resembling an interstitial pneumonia; differentiated from other pneumonias through laboratory studies to rule out other organisms

Continued.

Table 9-1

OVERVIEW OF PNEUMONIAS ASSOCIATED WITH HIV INFECTION — cont'd

Condition	Description	Signs and symptoms
Herpes simplex pneumonia	A rare form of viral pneumonia in HIV-infected persons	Not distinguishable from other pneumonias except through laboratory studies to rule out other organisms
Pneumocystis carinii pneumonia (PCP)	The most common form of pneumonia in the HIV infected, occurring in 80% of people with AIDS; prophylaxis is effective and is recommended after the first episode of PCP or when CD4+ cells fall below 200/mm³	Generally has a subacute course characterized by fever, dyspnea, and nonproductive cough; decreased tolerance for activity and dyspnea are generally the presenting symptoms
Cryptococcal pneumonia	Moderately common asymptomatic pulmonary infection in the immunocompetent; occurs in about 5% of people with AIDS and is usually (80% of the time) accompanied by cryptococcal meningitis	Presenting symptoms are usually neurologic (see Chapter 8); not distinguishable from other pneumonias if not accompanied by meningitis
Histoplasmosis	Common (500,000 cases/year in U.S.) pulmonary infection in areas where the fungus (*H. capsulatum*) is found in the soil, particularly central and northeastern U.S. along the Canadian border. The infection occurs in 5% to 20% of persons with AIDS, particularly those who live in or have traveled to the areas where the organism is endemic. The infection is benign in the immunocompetent, but can be an aggressive disseminated disease in people with AIDS.	Not distinguishable from other pneumonias
Coccidioidomycosis (coccidioidal pneumonia)	Generally (95% of the time) benign, asymptomatic, and self-limiting pulmonary infection in the immunocompetent. The fungus is endemic in southwestern U.S., Mexico, and Central America and is opportunistic in 1% to 2% of persons with AIDS who live in or travel to these areas.	Not distinguishable from other pneumonias except by laboratory studies to rule out other causes

BACTERIAL PNEUMONIA: PNEUMOCOCCAL PNEUMONIA

Pneumococcal pneumonia, caused by *Streptococcus pneumoniae*, is the most common type of bacterial pneumonia in the HIV infected and in the general population. The organism first invades and replicates in the bronchioles, stimulating an inflammatory response and release of large quantities of serous fluid. The fluid serves as a culture medium and as a mechanism for transporting the organism to nearby alveoli. Inflammation and accumulation of fibrin and leukocytes in the alveoli continue until the alveoli become consolidated into solid tissue, losing their ability to hold air. The pathologic process resolves with the disintegration of the fibrin and neutrophils and digestion of the bacteria by macrophages.

Pneumococcal pneumonia can occur at any stage of HIV infection. Therefore, its appearance in a previously healthy individual may raise suspicion about an undiagnosed HIV infection. Clients will present with complaints of sudden-onset fever, coughing, purulent sputum, and pleural pain associated with coughing. The person may report single or multiple episodes of chills. Some clients report abdominal pain that mimics appendicitis, although there is no abdominal pathology.

Treatment of *S. pneumoniae* is straightforward and is usually successful. Penicillin is administered orally, or parenterally in severe cases. Other antiinfectives are employed in cases of penicillin allergies or penicillin resistance. Most patients show marked improvement in a few days. All patients should have follow-up chest x-rays to ensure that resolution has occurred and to rule out other causes of lung pathology, such as tuberculosis.

Pneumococcal pneumonia vaccine, which protects against most strains of *S. pneumoniae,* is available. This vaccine should be given to any person diagnosed HIV positive in order to prevent any occurrence of this pneumonia.

BACTERIAL PNEUMONIA: HAEMOPHILUS INFLUENZAE

Haemophilus influenzae is the second major cause of bacterial pneumonia in HIV-infected persons. The pathophysiology of this pneumonia is less well understood than that of pneumococcal pneumonia. One similarity is the occurrence of an inflammatory response with serous exudate, consolidation, and alveolar macrophage assistance in elimination of the invader. This pneumonia also can occur in all stages of HIV infection, and its occurrence in the previously healthy may be a clue to undiagnosed HIV infection. This condition is also successfully treated with antibiotics. The drug of choice has been ampicillin/amoxicillin, but resistant strains have been identified. These are treated with a second- or third-generation cephalosporin, such as cefuroxime or cefotaxime. Trimethoprim-sulfamethoxazole (TMP/SMX) is preferred by many clinicians because of its effect on other pneumonia-causing organisms (e.g., *Pneumocystis*) in HIV-infected patients. However, TMP/SMX has dose-limiting side effects, including severe rash, fever, and abdominal pain, and is contraindicated for anyone with an allergy to sulfa.

Haemophilus influenzae b (HIb) vaccine is available. Clinicians recommend administration of the vaccine early in HIV infection. Although it is effective in preventing pneumonia in the general population, the effectiveness of the vaccine in HIV-infected persons has not been determined.

VIRAL PNEUMONIA: CYTOMEGALOVIRUS AND HERPES SIMPLEX VIRUS

Viruses cause pathology in the respiratory system by destroying ciliated epithelial cells, goblet cells, and bronchial mucous glands. The bronchial epithelium sloughs, preventing mucociliary clearance and thus interfering with a major defense against invasion by other pneumonia-causing pathogens. Bronchial walls become edematous and infiltrated with leukocytes. Fibrin, monocytes, neutrophils, and serous fluid clog alveoli, as in bacterial pneumonias.

The two most common viral pneumonias seen in the immunocompromised are cytomegalovirus (CMV) and herpes simplex virus (HSV), occurring in 5% of HIV-infected people. Both of these organisms can frequently be isolated in specimens taken from the lungs of HIV-infected persons, even those without respiratory symptoms. Because these viruses are rarely pathogenic, they are only considered to be causative if no other pathogen can be isolated in a person with respiratory symptoms. Diagnosis is assisted by x-ray findings of interstitial involvement and by a dominance of monocytes in sputum specimens.

CMV is treated with intravenous ganciclovir or foscarnet. No acceptable treatment regimen has been established against pneumonia caused by herpes simplex virus, the rarest of these pneumonias. Some clinicians advocate treatment with intravenous acyclovir in doses similar to those used for treatment of gastrointestinal herpes simplex infections.

FUNGAL PNEUMONIA: PNEUMOCYSTIS CARINII PNEUMONIA

Pneumocystis carinii pneumonia (PCP) is the most common opportunistic infection experienced by people with HIV infection. PCP is the AIDS-defining condition in over one half of people with AIDS. Of those who have other AIDS-defining conditions, about one half will experience PCP at some point in their HIV infection. *Pneumocystis carinii,* once classified as a protozoan, is now considered to be a fungus because it cannot grow on an artificial medium. The organism is ubiquitous in the environment, can be transmitted from person to person via the respiratory passages, and remains in a dormant state in lungs of immunocompetent hosts.

Pneumocystis carinii multiplies aggressively in the alveoli of immunocompromised persons, causing interstitial irritation and inflammation. The alveoli become infiltrated with a proteinaceous material containing fluid, inflammatory cellular debris, and numerous *Pneumocystis* organisms at all stages of development (e.g., cysts, sporozoites, and trophozoites). Eventually, the alveoli become so choked with organisms that oxygen exchange is impaired. Symptoms develop slowly over 2 to 8 weeks. Early manifestations are often nonspecific and include fatigue, fever, shortness of breath on exertion, nonproductive cough, and weight loss. Once established, PCP can progress rapidly, leading to respiratory failure if untreated.

PCP is treated relatively successfully with trimethoprim-sulfamethoxazole (TMP/SMX, Bactrim, Septra) if therapy is begun before fulminating infection is present. Because of its insidious onset, PCP is often well developed before infected people seek medical care. While best treated in early stages, advanced PCP has been successfully treated with corticosteroids in addition to antiinfective therapy.

One of the biggest advances in the care of people with AIDS has been the use of prophylactic drugs for

PCP. Lifelong suppressive therapy with TMP/SMX or dapsone (or aerosolized pentamidine, if other drugs are not tolerated) is now recommended for any HIV-infected individual who has had an episode of PCP or whose CD4+ T lymphocyte count falls below 200/mm^3. The success of this therapy can be demonstrated by the fact that at one time PCP was the AIDS-defining condition for 70% of HIV-infected people. Now, PCP defines 50% of new AIDS diagnoses. At one time, 50% of those treated for PCP experienced a relapse within 1 year of treatment. The annual relapse rate is now down to 3% to 5% in those taking prophylactic TMP/SMX and 15% to 20% for those using aerosolized pentamidine.

FUNGAL PNEUMONIA: HISTOPLASMOSIS, CRYPTOCOCCAL PNEUMONIA, AND COCCIDIOIDOMYCOSIS

Pathologic processes in the lungs associated with other fungi, such as *Histoplasma capsulatum*, *Cryptococcus neoformans*, and *Coccidioides immitis*, cause disease either by primary pulmonary infection or by reactivation of previous infections (histoplasmosis, coccidioidomycosis).

All of the fungal diseases are considered to be opportunistic for two reasons. First, most of the population in areas where the fungi are endemic will show immune evidence that in the past they have experienced subclinical pulmonary infections with these organisms. Second, treatment never eradicates, but merely suppresses, these organisms in the immunosuppressed, because a competent immune system is required for a cure. Consequently, suppressive therapy for these fungi must be maintained for the life of immunosuppressed people.

All of these fungi are diagnosed by microscopic examinations of specimens obtained from sputum, bronchoalveolar lavage, or tissue biopsy or from cultures grown from the specimens. Presence of a specific fungus is generally considered diagnostic. One exception to this is *Candida albicans*, a common normal flora fungus, which is often found in respiratory specimens. *Candida* is usually not pathogenic. The presence of *Candida* is considered to be diagnostic for pneumonia when there are symptoms of pneumonia and no other organism is found in the respiratory specimen. Histoplasmosis and cryptococcosis can be diagnosed by a positive antigen test. Any patient with pulmonary cryptococcal infection should have a lumbar puncture to rule out cryptococcal meningitis.

Drug treatment for cryptococcosis, coccidioidomycosis, and histoplasmosis is intravenous amphotericin B. This drug is usually used for suppression therapy also, although fluconazole increasingly is used for suppression of cryptococcosis and coccidioidomycosis because it can be administered orally. Itraconazole is used to suppress histoplasmosis and to treat patients with isolated cryptococcosis who are not seriously ill. The treatment of choice for candidal pneumonia has not been established, although both ketoconazole and fluconazole are used for other systemic candidal infections.

Other organisms occasionally cause pneumonia in the HIV infected. These include *Legionella*, *Nocardia*, *Aspergillus*, and gram-negative bacilli. The latter are often associated with hospital-acquired (nosocomial) infections. They should be suspected in patients admitted to the hospital for nonpulmonary problems who develop sudden-onset, fulminant pneumonias, particularly if the patient is neutropenic.

Mycobacterial Diseases

HIV-infected people have up to a 10% probability of contracting a mycobacterial pulmonary infection. Usually the offending organism is *Mycobacterium tuberculosis*, but occasionally *M. kansasii* and *M. avium* complex are involved. Most of the *M. tuberculosis*–related conditions will result from activation of latent (inactive) infections acquired earlier in life. In the immunocompetent, 95% of new infections with *M. tuberculosis* are successfully suppressed by a cellular immune (T lymphocyte) response. These infections become dormant, and 90% remain in a latent state for the remainder of the person's

life. If the immune system becomes impaired due to age, chronic disease, immunosuppressive therapy, malnutrition, or HIV infection, latent *M. tuberculosis* reactivates and becomes an aggressive pathogen in the lungs and elsewhere in the body. In addition, HIV-infected people may spend time in the company of other HIV-infected people, particularly during medical visits, who may have active and communicable *M. tuberculosis*. This increases their risk for exposure to new *M. tuberculosis* infections. Up to 50% of new tuberculosis (TB) infections in HIV-infected people become active within 60

Table 9-2

OVERVIEW OF MYCOBACTERIAL RESPIRATORY MANIFESTATIONS

Condition	Description	Signs and symptoms
M. tuberculosis	A chronic, recurrent infection of the lungs and any other body organ. Most (90%) of infections in immunocompetent do not result in active, symptomatic disease. Progression to active disease is most common during the first 2 years after infection or later in life when a person becomes immunocompromised due to aging, chronic disease, or HIV infection. Once active, TB disease usually progresses slowly, except in HIV infected, in whom the organism rapidly destroys tissue. *Health care workers are at risk for infection from patients with active TB.*	Low-grade fever, night sweats, chills, weight loss; dry, nonproductive cough progressing to mucopurulent; dyspnea, hypoxemia, anorexia; painful skin lesions, meningitis, or lymphadenitis in severely immunosuppressed
M. kansasii	A rare cause of tuberculosis-like disease in the AIDS patient	Productive cough; rarely accompanied by systemic signs and symptoms
M. avium	A moderately common pulmonary infection in the late stages of AIDS	Productive cough; rarely accompanied by systemic signs and symptoms

days of exposure. If an HIV-infected individual develops active tuberculosis with a strain of *M. tuberculosis* that is resistant to available drugs, he or she has a 50% chance of death within 60 days.

In order to discuss the course of tuberculosis, it helps to differentiate tuberculosis infection from tuberculosis disease (Table 9-2). *M. tuberculosis* is transmitted in aerosolized mucous droplets through the cough of a person with active disease. Infection begins if inhaled bacilli invade the tissue of the alveoli of the middle or lower lobes of the lung, replicate, and create an inflammatory lesion. Replicating bacilli proceed to infiltrate the lymphatic system, causing further inflammation, hematogenous dissemination of the bacilli, and establishment of inflammatory lesions throughout the body. In 95% of TB-infected people who are immunocompetent, a cellular and humoral immune response is initiated. This immune response produces a fibroblastic response in the inflammatory lesions. Dense connective tissue surrounds the bacilli and inflamed tissue and forms a granuloma. This heralds the onset of the period of inactive infection called latency. This immune response is detectable with an intradermal skin test using purified protein derivative (PPD) in 4 weeks after infection (see Diagnostic Studies). During latency, mycobacteria continue to be viable in the granuloma, although they are not replicating or being shed. As long as the bacilli are viable, there is a potential for reactivation and active disease at a later time.

Initial active disease or reactivation of a latent infection is possible if the integrity of the immune system is compromised for any reason, such as aging, disease, or certain immunosuppressive drug therapies. Activation of the mycobacteria and progression to tuberculosis disease, either early in the infection or after a period of latency, results in replication and spread of mycobacteria in the sputum. Active disease is definitively diagnosed by detection of the mycobacteria in a sputum specimen (see Diagnostic Studies). Active mycobacteria cause a caseating necrosis and cavitation in the tubercular lesions. The lesions may rupture, spreading necrotic debris and bacilli throughout the body. These circulating bacilli form new lesions, which progress through stages of inflammation and caseating necrosis. Untreated tuberculosis can slowly or, as in the immunocompromised, rapidly destroy the lungs. Extrapulmonary lesions can appear in almost any organ or organ system. Even the skin and meninges can become sites for tubercular lesions.

Treatment of active *M. tuberculosis* is as successful in persons with AIDS as it is in the immunocompetent. Standard three- or four-drug therapies are employed and maintained for 9 months or longer, depending on the severity of the disease when treatment is begun. Treatment is also recommended for HIV-infected persons and other recently infected individuals who have a latent (inactive) *M. tuberculosis* infection. Recommended treatments for both latent infections and active tuberculosis are listed under Medical Management. Patients receiving therapy for tuberculosis should be monitored carefully for adherence to the medication regimen, as drug-resistant strains of *M. tuberculosis* are being found increasingly in the HIV infected. Infection with such strains has resulted in rapid death. The Centers for Disease Control now recommends that drug sensitivity testing be performed whenever a specimen is cultured for mycobacteria. This is to ensure that drug therapy is specific to the strain of mycobacteria from the onset of treatment.

It should be noted that persons caring for HIV-infected people have a risk for exposure to *M. tuberculosis*. Preventive measures, such as protective masks, negative-pressure ventilation rooms, or use of ultraviolet lights, are necessary (see Chapter 14). Vigilance for preventing transmission of *M. tuberculosis* is particularly important in places where aerosolized pentamidine is administered.

M. kansasii and *M. avium* very rarely cause pulmonary disease in HIV-infected people. Treated *M. kansasii* infections have a prognosis as favorable as treated *M.*

tuberculosis. The organism is susceptible to the same drug regimens that are employed for *M. tuberculosis*. *M. avium* infections in the lungs have a poor prognosis, as this organism is not susceptible to most of the anti-TB drugs. Fortunately this organism is a rare cause of pulmonary disease. While four- and five-drug regimens have been employed, there is little evidence that they have any effect on the outcome of the disease. However, continuing regimens of clarithromycin and azithromycin are considered by some clinicians to be the most effective. Recent studies have shown that administration of rifabutin prophylactically reduces the risk for *M. avium* bacteremia. Many clinicians use rifabutin also as a preventative for gastrointestinal infections caused by *M. avium* in persons with CD4+ counts less than 100 cells/mm^3. Perhaps the widespread use of this drug will further reduce the low incidence of pulmonary *M. avium* infections.

Sinus Disease

HIV-infected individuals are quite likely to report symptoms associated with sinusitis, such as fever, nasal congestion, and severe headache. Sinusitis is an uncomfortable phenomenon that, while typically self-limiting in the immunocompetent, can be severe and chronic in the immunosuppressed. In addition, the pain can mask other symptoms, such as those associated with early central nervous system infections (see Chapter 8).

Sinusitis is generally bilateral and may be localized in any of the paranasal sinuses, including the maxillary, frontal, ethmoid, and/or sphenoid sinuses. The infections are characterized by significant, mucoperiosteal thickening that is sometimes accompanied by erosion of the bones of the sinus cavities (Table 9-3).

Determining the cause of the infection can be difficult. While sinus aspiration can yield material for examination, specimens are frequently contaminated with multiple normal flora organisms. Determining which organism is causing the infection and choosing the appropriate antibiotic may be problematic. The general approach to treatment is to use broad-spectrum antibiotics together with decongestants and analgesics. Some studies have reported the use of steroidal nasal sprays. In general, treatment is not very successful. In one study 50% of patients reported improvement while only one third reported remission of symptoms.

MUCORMYCOSIS

Mucormycosis (also called phycomycosis or zygomycosis) is a group of fungal infections usually caused by fungi of the family Mucoraceae of the class Zygomycetes. These fungi localize in blood vessels, causing thrombosis, infarction, gangrene, and perforation of all infected tissues. Infection begins in the mucous membranes of the nose and paranasal sinuses and progressively spreads to the palates, eyes, and lower respiratory tract. Infection may penetrate to the internal carotid artery and disseminate to the brain, or it may extend directly to the brain. These organisms are extremely virulent and destructive once established in the tissue of immunocompromised persons. Fortunately, this is a relatively rare condition in HIV-infected persons.

Diagnosis cannot be made by culture of the fungi in a secretion specimen, because the organisms are ubiquitous in the environment. The diagnosis can be confirmed by microscopic examination and observation of broad, nonseptate hyphae in biopsied tissue. Surgical debridement slows the progression of the disease. Amphotericin B is administered systemically and topically. However, the disease usually progresses to death from cerebral infarction and hemorrhage.

Table 9-3

OVERVIEW OF SINUS DISEASES ASSOCIATED WITH HIV INFECTION

Condition	Description	Signs and symptoms
Nonspecific sinusitis	A chronic, nonspecific syndrome that affects 60% of HIV-infected people and seems to increase in frequency as the CD4+ count falls below 200/mm^3; may clear up as a result of antibiotic treatment of other infections	Fever, nasal congestion, headache
Mucormycosis (phycomycosis, zygomycosis)	A relatively rare rhinocerebral complication of a fungal infection that can penetrate the sinus structures into the brain, becoming more common as severely immunocompromised people live longer	Facial, orbital pain, fever, orbital cellulitis, proptosis, necrotic nasal passages, purulent nasal drainage; spread to the brain can cause convulsion, aphasia, and hemiplegia

DIAGNOSTIC STUDIES AND FINDINGS FOR PULMONARY MANIFESTATIONS

Diagnostic Test	Finding
Culture of blood specimen	Positive results are confirmatory for *H. influenzae* and *S. pneumoniae*
Culture of biopsied tissue	Presence of *Cryptococcus neoformans, Coccidioides immitis, M. tuberculosis, M. kansasii,* or *M. avium* complex (MAC) is diagnostic; presence of other organisms, which may be part of normal flora, is not diagnostic unless other organisms are ruled out
Culture of specimen from bronchoalveolar washing	Presence of *Coccidioides immitis, Histoplasma capsulatum, Cryptococcus, M. tuberculosis, M. kansasii,* or MAC is diagnostic
Culture of sputum specimen	Many organisms, particularly *H. influenzae,* CMV, HSV, and *Candida,* are frequently part of the normal flora; presence of these organisms in a specimen is, therefore, not diagnostic for these organisms. Presence may be confirmatory if no other organism can be found. Presence of *Coccidioides immitis, Histoplasma capsulatum, M. tuberculosis, M. kansasii,* or *M. avium* is diagnostic for these organisms. May take as long as 6 weeks to obtain growth of mycobacteria
Microscopic examination of biopsied tissue	Presence of cells with intranuclear inclusion bodies is confirmatory for CMV and HSV; confirmatory for characteristic cells of PCP, *Histoplasma capsulatum, Cryptococcus neoformans, Coccidioides immitis, Candida,* and *Mycobacterium*
Microscopic examination of specimen from bronchoalveolar washing, percutaneous transbrachial aspiration, or sputum	Presence of gram-positive diplococci and a positive quellung reaction suggest *S. pneumoniae;* visualization of budding forms is confirmatory for PCP; diagnostic for *Coccidioides immitis, H. capsulatum, Cryptococcus neoformans, M. tuberculosis*
Acid-fast with Ziehl-Neelsen stain smear of sputum (blood or CSF in extrapulmonary disease)	Positive for acid-fast mycobacteria
Antigen-antibody tests	Not performed for organisms that frequently are found in normal flora, such as *H. influenzae, S. pneumoniae,* CMV, HSV, PCP, and *Candida albicans*
Complement fixation	Antibodies develop within 10-21 days; titers of above 1:16 are suggestive of *Histoplasma capsulatum*

Continued.

Diagnostic Test	Finding
Precipitation	Precipitating antibodies against *Coccidioides immitis* develop within 4 weeks and last for 4-6 weeks; presence is diagnostic of recent infection
Antigen test of alveolar lavage fluid	Positive antigen results are interpreted as probable for histoplasmosis. Presence of cryptococcal antigen is diagnostic; absence does not rule out disease.
Drug sensitivity testing (essential when mycobacteria are suspected, because of growing concern for drug-resistant *M. tuberculosis*)	Listing of antimicrobials to which the organism is susceptible and the degree of susceptibility; sometimes reported as sensitive, resistant, or intermediate
X-ray	For tuberculosis, findings may show calcification at original site of infection, enlargement of hilar lymph nodes, parenchymal infiltrate representing extension of original site of infection, or the appearance of pleural effusion or cavitation. A multinodular infiltrate above or behind the clavicle suggests recrudescence of an old infection. With *M. kansasii* or *M. avium*, cavitation is thin walled and pleural effusion is rare. See Table 9-4 for summary of common findings in all pulmonary infections
Gallium scan	Reading of 3 or more suggests microscopic examination for PCP
Diffusing capacity of the lung for carbon monoxide (DLCO)	Results less than 75% of expected suggest microscopic examination for PCP. If chest x-ray, gallium scan, and DLCO are negative, the patient is most likely negative for PCP.
Pulmonary function tests, arterial blood gases, and acid-base imbalances	Although not diagnostic of infection, these tests are used to monitor the patient's condition and response to therapy. For further discussion, see Wilson and Thompson, 1990.[169]
Lactic dehydrogenase (LDH)	Elevated in PCP and histoplasmosis
Skin testing	(See Chapter 5 for general discussion of skin testing)
Histoplasma capsulatum	Used in epidemiologic investigations; not routinely performed for diagnostic purposes; test interferes with results of serologic tests
Coccidioides immitis	Useful for showing conversion if a previous test was negative; skin test is not positive until 4 weeks after infection; skin test interferes with results of serologic tests for histoplasmosis; false negative results are common in HIV-infected persons
M. tuberculosis	The Mantoux test is administered by intradermal injection of 0.1 ml of PPD tuberculin containing 5 tuberculin units (TU) into the volar or dorsal surface of the forearm. The test is read in 48-72 hours by measuring induration, not erythema. A positive reaction indicates past infection and presence of cellular antibodies; does not indicate active disease; nonspecific reactions during first 48 hours can be overlooked. If reaction is questionable or negative (when infection is suspected), a second test should be done 1 week later. A reaction of 5 mm or greater is considered positive for persons with HIV infection, for those with close personal contact with a person with infectious tuberculosis, and for persons who have chest radiographs with fibrotic lesions likely to represent old healed tuberculosis. A reaction of 10 mm or greater is positive for persons with other medical risk factors, foreign-born persons, low-income and high-risk minority populations, intravenous drug users, residents of long-term care facilities and correctional institutions, and health care workers. A reaction of 15 mm or greater is positive for all other persons. A negative reaction may mean absence of infection or absence of cellular immunity, as in the case of HIV-infected people with decreased CD4+ cells. HIV-infected persons should be tested for anergy at the same time that they receive the Mantoux test

Table 9-4 _____

COMMON X-RAY FINDINGS IN PULMONARY DISEASE

Organism or condition	Diffuse interstitial or alveolar infiltrate	Pleural effusion	Nodular infiltrates	Focal infiltrates	Cavity	Intrathoracic adenopathy
Haemophilus influenzae	X			X		
Streptococcus pneumoniae		X		X		
CMV/HSV	Rare/0					
Pneumocystis carinii	X		X	X	X (rare)	
Cryptococcus neoformans	X	X	X	X	X	X
Candida albicans						
Histoplasma capsulatum	X		X			X
Coccidioides immitis	X				X	X
Lymphoma		X	X			X
Kaposi's sarcoma	X	X	X	X		X
Mycobacterium tuberculosis disseminated (d) or late in HIV	X	X(d)	X(late)		X	X(late)
Mycobacterium tuberculosis avium			X			

Adapted from Peiperl.[176]

DIAGNOSTIC STUDIES AND FINDINGS FOR SINUS DISEASE

Diagnostic Test	Finding
Culture or microscopic examination of specimen obtained by direct sinus aspiration or biopsy	Positive for growth of organism or characteristic nonseptate hyphae associated with mucormycosis. Nasal discharge is considered to be poor culture material because it contains so many normal flora organisms. Inform the laboratory of the organism that is expected, particularly if it is *Mucor.*
Transillumination of maxillary and frontal sinuses	Normal findings rule out sinusitis. Dull transillumination suggests sinusitis.
Sinus x-rays	Air-fluid level implies infection; complete opacity of the cavity is consistent with acute infection; mucosal thickening of over 5 mm suggests acute sinusitis; spotty, diffuse craniofacial bone destruction indicates mucormycosis.
CT scan or MRI	Positive for characteristic swelling and blockage; particularly useful for diagnosing posterior sinus involvement, which is frequently missed by radiography.

MEDICAL MANAGEMENT

DRUG THERAPY FOR PULMONARY MANIFESTATIONS (BASED ON ORGANISM)

S. pneumoniae: Penicillin G or V, 250 to 500 mg PO q 6 h.

H. influenzae: Cefuroxime or ampicillin; alternative: trimethoprim, 15 mg/kg/day, with sulfamethoxazole, 75 mg/kg/day, in divided doses.

Cytomegalovirus: Ganciclovir, 5 mg/kg IV bid for 14-21 days, or foscarnet, 60 mg/kg IV q 8 h for 14-21 days.

Continued.

MEDICAL MANAGEMENT—cont'd

Herpes simplex virus: Acyclovir (dosage and route of administration not established).

Pneumocystis carinii: Mild disease: trimethoprim-sulfamethoxazole, 2 double-strength tablets each containing 160 mg TMP/800 mg SMX PO tid to qid. Severe disease: trimethoprim, 15 mg/kg/day, plus sulfamethoxazole, 75 mg/kg/day, IV in 3 to 4 divided doses for 21 days; or trimethoprim, 15 mg/kg/day PO, plus dapsone, 100 mg/day PO, for 21 days. Corticosteroids are also administered to patients with Po_2 <70 mm Hg. Alternative: atovaquone, trimethoprin, dapsone, or pentamidine IV.

PCP prophylaxis: Given to any HIV-infected person who has had a bout of PCP or who has a CD4+ count of <200/mm^3. Trimethoprim-sulfamethoxazole, 1 double-strength tablet PO qd or 3 days per week (optimum dosing and schedule have not been determined). Alternatives include dapsone, 50 mg/day PO or 100 mg 2 times per week, or aerosolized pentamidine, 300 mg/q mo or 60 mg q 2 wk

Candida albicans: Systemic antifungals (dosage depends on the drug utilized).

Histoplasma capsulatum: Amphotericin B, 0.5 to 1.0 mg/kg/day IV for 4 to 8 weeks. Maintenance therapy is amphotericin B, 1.0 mg/kg/wk IV, or itraconazole, 200-400 mg PO daily.

Cryptococcus neoformans: Amphotericin B, 0.5 to 0.8 mg/kg/day IV for 10-14 days, with or without 5-flucytosine, 100-150 mg/kg/day in 4 doses PO. Alternative for patients without meningitis: fluconazole. Maintenance therapy is fluconazole, 200-400 mg/day PO; usually started after 15 mg/kg of amphotericin B has been administered.

Mycobacterium tuberculosis: Drug therapy for tuberculosis in all persons, including HIV infected, has been complicated by emergence of drug-resistant organisms. Effective regimens must contain multiple drugs to which the organisms are susceptible. CDC now recommends a four-drug regimen, with INH, RIF, pyrazinamide (PZA), and SM or EMB, for the initial treatment of TB. Recent recommendations are reproduced in Tables 9-5 and 9-6.

Mycobacterium kansasii: Treated like *M. tuberculosis.*

Mycobacterium avium complex: This organism is refractory to antibiotic treatments; regimens containing three to five drugs (rifampin, EMB, clarithromycin, azithromycin, ciprofloxacin, and amikacin) have been utilized. Prophylactic use of rifabutin and clarithromycin has been shown to prevent *M. avium* bacteremia.

GENERAL MANAGEMENT FOR PULMONARY MANIFESTATIONS

Humidification, if secretions are thick and copious.

Oxygen administration if Po_2 <60 mm Hg.

Fluid administration.

Isolation of patients who are sputum positive for mycobacteria is essential (see AFB isolation in Chapter 14).

DRUG THERAPY FOR SINUS DISEASE

Nonspecific sinusitis: Decongestants, analgesics, and broad-spectrum antibiotics.

Mucormycosis: Amphotericin B, 0.75 mg/kg/day IV, increasing to 1.0 mg/kg/day; irrigation with amphotericin B may be used.

GENERAL MANAGEMENT FOR SINUS DISEASE

Nonspecific sinusitis: Sinus drainage procedures are sometimes utilized.

Mucormycosis: Regular surgical debridement of abscessed tissue.

Refer to Chapter 11 for nursing management of clients with respiratory manifestations of AIDS and HIV.

Table 9-5

REGIMEN OPTIONS FOR THE INITIAL TREATMENT OF TB AMONG CHILDREN AND ADULTS

TB without HIV infection			TB with HIV infection
Option 1	Option 2	Option 3	
Administer daily INH, RIF, and PZA for 8 weeks followed by 16 weeks of INH and RIF daily or 2-3 times/ week* in areas where the INH resistance rate is not documented to be <4%. EMB or SM should be added to the initial regimen until susceptibility to INH and RIF is demonstrated. Continue treatment for at least 6 months and 3 months beyond culture conversion. Consult a TB medical expert if the patient is symptomatic or smear or culture positive after 3 months.	Administer daily INH, RIF, PZA, and SM or EMB for 2 weeks followed by 2 times/ week* administration of the same drugs for 6 weeks (by DOT‡), and subsequently, with 2 times/week administration of INH and RIF for 16 weeks (by DOT). Consult a TB medical expert if the patient is symptomatic or smear or culture positive after 3 months.	Treat by DOT, 3 times/ week* with INH, RIF, PZA, and EMB or SM for 6 months.† Consult a TB medical expert if the patient is symptomatic or smear or culture positive after 3 months.	Options 1, 2, or 3 can be used, but treatment regimens should continue for a total of 9 months and at least 6 months beyond culture conversion.

*All regimens administered 2 times/week or 3 times/week should be monitored by DOT for the duration of therapy.
†The strongest evidence from clinical trials is the effectiveness of all four drugs administered for the full 6 months. There is weaker evidence that SM can be discontinued after 4 months if the isolate is susceptible to all drugs. The evidence for stopping PZA before the end of 6 months is equivocal for the 3 times/week regimen, and there is no evidence on the effectiveness of this regimen with EMB for less than the full 6 months.
‡*DOT*, Directly observed therapy.

Table 9-6

DOSAGE RECOMMENDATION FOR THE INITIAL TREATMENT OF TB AMONG ADULTS

	Dosage		
	Daily	2 times/week	3 times/week
Drugs	Adults	Adults	Adults
Isoniazid (INH)	5 mg/kg Max. 300 mg	15 mg/kg Max. 900 mg	15 mg/kg Max. 900 mg
Rifampin (RIF)	10 mg/kg Max. 600 mg	10 mg/kg Max. 600 mg	10 mg/kg Max. 600 mg
Pyrazinamide (PZA)	15-30 mg/kg Max. 2 g	50-70 mg/kg Max. 4 g	50-70 mg/kg Max. 3 g
Ethambutol (EMB)	5-25 mg/kg Max. 2.5 g	50 mg/kg Max. 2.5 g	25-30 mg/kg Max. 2.5 g
Streptomycin (SM)	15 mg/kg Max. 1 g	25-30 mg/kg Max. 1.5 g	25-30 mg/kg Max. 1 g

From CDC.[26]

CHAPTER 10

HIV-Related Malignancies

James Halloran

PATHOPHYSIOLOGY OF CANCER

The term "cancer" refers to a group of diseases characterized by changes in cellular structure (the arrangement of cellular components), differentiation (maturity or ability to function normally), and proliferation. Growth and development of normal cells are regulated by mechanisms that restrict the number and location of specific types of cells. Cells that are malignantly transformed reproduce unrestricted by these mechanisms. The unchecked reproduction of malignant cells results in *neoplasia* (new growth), which may appear as a tumor in solid cancers. Malignant cells can be invasive, extending into local tissues, and are capable of *metastasis* (spread to other parts of the body), replacing normal cells and disturbing metabolic and/or mechanical function.

Current theories postulate that malignant disease arises through a multistep process. Initiation involves damage to cellular DNA, such as might be caused by oncogenic viruses or other organisms, chemical exposure, or other means. Left unrepaired, these genetic changes may lead to promotion of malignant disease. Progression of malignant disease involves development of local invasiveness and metastasis. While potentially malignant changes routinely occur in cells, the normal immune system maintains surveillance to identify and remove damaged cells that display cancerous characteristics. When, for whatever reason, this immune surveillance system fails, malignantly transformed cells may proliferate and produce clinical disease.

Cancers are named according to the type of cell involved, the degree of disturbance in organization or differentiation of cellular components (*grade*), and the extent of disease in the body (*stage*). Higher grade correlates with increased disorganization of cellular components and function. Staging systems use parameters specific to the type of cancer and its natural history to establish the degree to which disease has progressed. Different staging systems may exist for some types of cancers. In general, the higher the stage and grade, the more extensive the disease, and the poorer the prognosis.

HIV AND CANCER

The specific physiology of cancer development in HIV-infected persons is not well understood. Immunosuppression is associated with increased risk of malignant disease regardless of the etiology of the immune suppression. The risk of specific cancers increases in persons with congenital immune deficiencies and in those receiving immunosuppressive drugs following organ transplantation. Degradation of the immune system caused by HIV infection is also associated with increased risk of specific cancers.

A type of malignant disease (cancer) known as Kaposi's sarcoma (KS), observed in the early 1980s among young, previously healthy men, was one of the

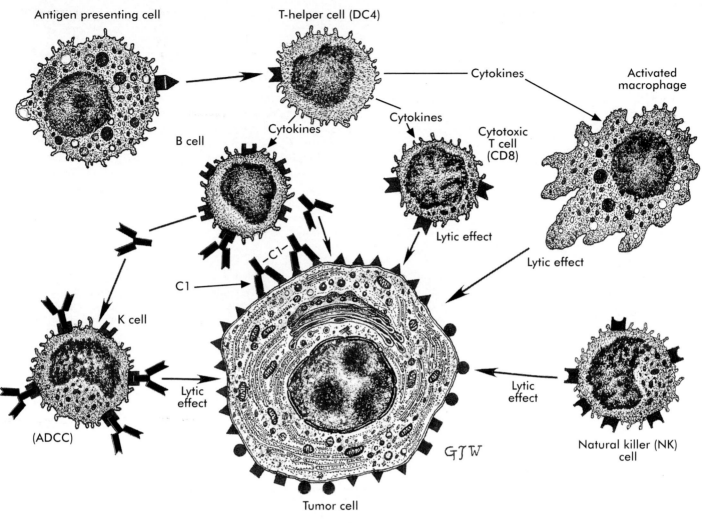

Antigen presenting cell

T-helper cell (DC4)

Cytokines

Activated macrophage

Cytokines

Cytokines

B cell

Cytotoxic T cell (CD8)

Lytic effect

Lytic effect

—C1—

C1

Lytic effect

K cell

Lytic effect

(ADCC)

Lytic effect

Tumor cell

Natural killer (NK) cell

ATTACK ON TUMOR CELL BY DIFFERENT RESPONSES OF IMMUNE SYSTEM

first indicators of the HIV epidemic in the United States. Previously KS appeared as skin lesions, mostly on the lower extremities, in older (>60 years of age) males of Mediterranean extraction and was characteristically indolent in clinical course. Among the HIV-infected population, however, KS appeared in younger men, involved virtually all organ systems, and behaved aggressively. Other forms of malignancies reportedly associated with HIV infection include lymphomas (especially non-Hodgkin's), anorectal malignancies, and female cervical disease.

Some viruses have been linked to increased risk of specific cancers. For example, certain subtypes of human papillomavirus (HPV) are implicated in the development of female cervical cancer and squamous cell anorectal cancers. In addition, the Epstein-Barr virus (EBV) is associated with Burkitt's lymphoma. Some clinicians believe, and evidence is accruing to support the theory, that Kaposi's sarcoma may be caused by an infectious agent.

HIV itself has not been implicated as the primary cause of malignant disease. Development of malignant diseases in persons with HIV infection may result from failure of the surveillance function of the immune system secondary to HIV infection. Epidemiologic data demonstrate significantly increased risk among HIV-infected persons for development of Kaposi's sarcoma and non-Hodgkin's lymphoma, and increased risk for anorectal and female cervical malignancies. See Table 10-1 for an overview of HIV-related malignancies.

Table 10-1 _____

OVERVIEW OF HIV-RELATED MALIGNANCIES

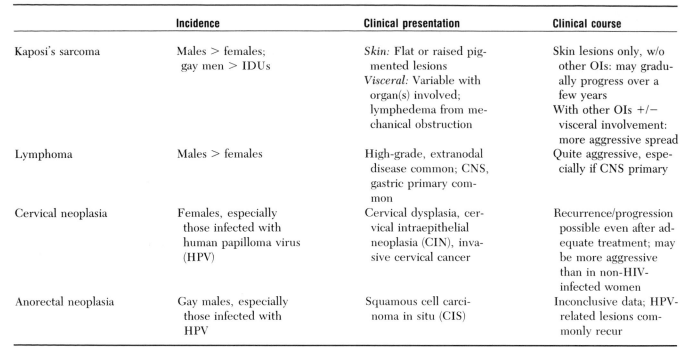

	Incidence	Clinical presentation	Clinical course
Kaposi's sarcoma	Males > females; gay men > IDUs	*Skin:* Flat or raised pigmented lesions *Visceral:* Variable with organ(s) involved; lymphedema from mechanical obstruction	Skin lesions only, w/o other OIs: may gradually progress over a few years With other OIs +/− visceral involvement: more aggressive spread
Lymphoma	Males > females	High-grade, extranodal disease common; CNS, gastric primary common	Quite aggressive, especially if CNS primary
Cervical neoplasia	Females, especially those infected with human papilloma virus (HPV)	Cervical dysplasia, cervical intraepithelial neoplasia (CIN), invasive cervical cancer	Recurrence/progression possible even after adequate treatment; may be more aggressive than in non-HIV-infected women
Anorectal neoplasia	Gay males, especially those infected with HPV	Squamous cell carcinoma in situ (CIS)	Inconclusive data; HPV-related lesions commonly recur

GENERAL PRINCIPLES OF CANCER TREATMENT

Treatment for HIV-related malignant disease may include surgery, radiation therapy, chemotherapy, and/or biotherapy. Unfortunately, HIV-related cancers tend to respond more poorly and/or more frequently recur after treatment than in those persons not infected with HIV. This does not mean that it is inappropriate to treat malignant disease in persons with HIV, but usual treatment approaches may need to be modified based on individual situations.

Surgery is used to remove bulky disease or relieve symptoms caused by space-occupying lesions. Surgical excision of early lesions can sometimes provide curative therapy, but in HIV-related cancers this is rare. The location, character, and extent of the cancer, the likelihood of recurrence, as well as the ability of the person to withstand the stress of surgery must also be considered when treating cancer in HIV-infected persons.

Radiation therapy can be administered through teletherapy, in which a beam of ionizing radiation is directed to a specific anatomic area of the body from an external source, or through brachytherapy, in which the source of radiation is implanted in the body. Like

surgery, radiation therapy is a localized treatment, producing benefit only in the area within the field exposed to the radiation. Exact calculations deliver the therapeutic dose at the tumor site, but normal tissue may receive some exposure as well, causing side effects. Different types of cells vary in their radiosensitivity. HIV-related cancers often recur following radiotherapy.

Chemotherapy can be administered as a systemic or, in some instances, a local treatment for cancer. Cytotoxic cancer chemotherapy agents have differing mechanisms of action and produce different side effect profiles. Most chemotherapy agents preferentially target cells that reproduce rapidly, such as malignant cells. Normal cells that also have a rapid rate of reproduction (e.g., hair follicles, oral or GI mucosa, bone marrow) may also be adversely affected by cytotoxic agents. Many cancer chemotherapy drugs are myelosuppressive (toxic to the bone marrow) and can cause neutropenia, which is of particular concern in patients whose immunity is already compromised by HIV infection.

Biotherapy involves administration of agents (biologic response modifiers, or BRMs) that occur naturally in the body or are reproduced, usually through recombinant technology, to manipulate the body's response to the presence of cancerous cells. BRMs can regulate or enhance the immune response or may attack cancerous cells directly. Biotherapy is the newest tool in the arsenal against cancer, and many of the substances used are considered experimental. Examples of biotherapeutic agents include interferon, interleukin, monoclonal antibodies, tumor necrosis factor, colony-stimulating factors, and tumor infiltrating lymphocytes.

The decision regarding which treatment approach(es) to use will be made based on the type and extent of cancer involved, the patient's overall status and ability to withstand side effects, and the likelihood of a significant therapeutic response.

Kaposi's Sarcoma

Kaposi's sarcoma (KS) is a soft tissue malignancy characterized by malignant growth cells of vascular or lymphatic endothelial origin. Prior to the HIV pandemic, KS was seen in fairly limited populations (Table 10-2). In the United States prior to the HIV pandemic, classic KS was seen in elderly males of Mediterranean extraction. The presentation of KS in this population involved purplish lesions on the lower extremities that responded readily to conventional treatment with radiation therapy. There is little morbidity with classic KS. In parts of central Africa, an aggressive form of KS (endemic KS) occurs in both children and adults, more often in males than in females. Various subtypes of KS occur, with nodular (most common in adults), exophytic, diffuse infiltrating, and lymphadenopathic (most common in children and young adults) types recognized.

Persons receiving immunosuppressive drugs following organ transplant face increased risk of developing KS, usually after 15 to 24 months of pharmacologic immunosuppression. Nodular KS is the most common presentation in this population; lesions may be seen in multiple organ systems. In many cases the KS symptoms regress spontaneously following withdrawal of immunosuppressive agents.

KS in HIV-infected persons (epidemic KS, or EKS) typically behaves much more aggressively than other forms and occurs mostly in men with HIV infection. While some cases of KS have been reported in HIV-infected women, this occurrence is rare. While skin lesions are the most commonly noted presentation, EKS presents and behaves quite aggressively, involving virtually all organ systems. Clinical presentation of EKS varies with the organ system involved (Table 10-3).

Definitive **diagnosis** of EKS is made by biopsy if obtaining a tissue sample is feasible. Histopathologic examination may reveal anaplastic, spindle-cell or, most commonly, mixed-cell forms. Once a tissue diagnosis has been established, clinicians may presumptively diagnose progressive disease. This is especially true in patients with known EKS who develop lesions in sensitive or inaccessible areas.

Prognosis for persons with HIV-related EKS relates to overall status. Persons with HIV diagnosed with KS alone survive longer than those diagnosed with other HIV-related illnesses. Median survival is less than 1

Table 10-2

COMPARISON OF HIV-RELATED AND OTHER FORMS OF KAPOSI'S SARCOMA

	Classic KS	Endemic (African) KS	Transplant-associated KS	Epidemic (HIV-related) KS
Age	40-70 yr	Children and adults	Variable	20-40 yr
Male/female ratio	10-15:1	2.5:1	2-3:1	Predominantly seen in males
Clinical course	Indolent	Variable	Relates to degree of immune suppression	Aggressive
Common sites	88% below knee	Variable	Variable	Virtually all organ systems

Table 10-3

CLINICAL PRESENTATION OF EPIDEMIC KAPOSI'S SARCOMA

Location of KS lesion	Common symptoms
Skin	Flat or raised lesions, pigmented purplish pink to red to brown; no blanching on pressure; nonpruritic, painless unless in sensitive area (e.g., sole of foot, between toes) or causing lymphedema; cosmetic disfigurement
GI tract	Malabsorption, diarrhea, obstipation, incontinence, painful elimination, early satiety
Lungs	Impaired gas exchange, hypoxemic fatigue, cacophonous breath sounds
Oral cavity	Lesions most common on palate, may also appear on gingiva or elsewhere in mouth or pharynx; may interfere with chewing, swallowing, or talking

Table 10-4

STAGING SYSTEM FOR KAPOSI'S SARCOMA

Stage I	Cutaneous, locally indolent
Stage II	Cutaneous, locally aggressive or without regional lymph nodes
Stage III	Generalized cutaneous and/or lymph node involvement
Stage IV	Visceral

Subtypes
  A. No systemic signs or symptoms
  B. Systemic signs: 10% weight loss or fever >100° F orally, unrelated to an identifiable source of infection lasting more than 2 weeks

From Krigel et al, 1983.

Table 10-5

STAGING CRITERIA FOR KAPOSI'S SARCOMA

	Good risk (0)	Poor risk (1)
Tumor (T)	Confined to skin and/or lymph nodes and/or minimal oral disease (nonnodular KS confined to the palate)	Tumor-associated edema, or ulceration Extensive oral KS Gastrointestinal KS KS in other nonnodal viscera
Immune system (I)	CD4+ cells >200/mm^3	CD4+ cells <200/mm^3
Systemic illness	No history of opportunistic infection or thrush No "B" symptoms (unexplained fever, night sweats, >10% involuntary weight loss, or diarrhea lasting >2 weeks); Karnofsky performance status >70	History of opportunistic infection and/or thrush B symptoms present Performance status <70 Other HIV-related illness (e.g., lymphoma, neurologic disease)

From Krown et al, 1989.

year for persons with prior or concurrent major opportunistic infections. See Tables 10-4 and 10-5 for two commonly used approaches to stage the disease by its extent and to predict a person's risk for disease progression.

Medical management of EKS does not remove the underlying problem of HIV infection. For EKS manifesting only as asymptomatic cutaneous lesions, treatment may be deferred until symptoms develop. Treatment for EKS is typically symptomatic or palliative and may include radiotherapy, systemic or intralesional chemotherapy, biotherapy, or limited surgery (local excision). Surgery may be used to remove symptomatic local lesions, such as those occurring on the gingiva. Radiotherapy may be used to reduce obstruction in the gastrointestinal tract, or for cosmesis when lesions appear on cosmetically sensitive areas. Duration of response is variable, and recurrence is common. Single-

agent (usually with vinca alkaloid agents) or combination systemic chemotherapy may be used for widespread disease or lesions inaccessible to other modalities. Vinca alkaloids, especially vinblastine, are used most often. Other agents commonly used include bleomycin, vincristine, methotrexate, doxorubicin, dacarbazine, and etoposide (VP-16). Response rates are higher in early disease. Biologic response modifiers may be used alone or in combination with other treatment. Interferon-alpha, with or without the antiretroviral zidovudine, has been approved for treatment of EKS. Recombinant colony-stimulating factors (CSFs) may be used to treat neutropenia secondary to cytotoxic chemotherapy. Because HIV is known to infect macrophages, and stimulation of macrophage production might increase HIV production, granulocyte CSF (G-CSF) is used more commonly than granulocyte-macrophage CSF (GM-CSF).

Lymphoma

Lymphoma is a neoplastic disease characterized by overproliferation of lymphoid cells. Hodgkin's disease (HD), a form of lymphoma characterized by the presence of large, multinucleated Reed-Sternberg cells, is thought to arise from cells of B lymphocyte, T lymphocyte, or macrophage cell lines. In persons with HIV disease, impaired T-cell–mediated immunoregulation, allowing polyclonal B-cell activity, might account for the high incidence of non-Hodgkin's lymphomas (NHD), usually B-cell types, though the incidence of HD may also be increasing among this population. Unusual primary sites (gastric, brain, and CNS) and extranodal involvement are common in this population.

Pathologic classification of lymphoma is made based upon the predominant cell type and degree of differentiation (Table 10-6). High-grade disease is common in persons with HIV infection and is associated with a poor prognosis. The Ann Arbor Staging System is frequently used (Table 10-7); persons with HIV-related lymphoma often present with advanced stage III or stage IV disease. So-called systemic "B symptoms" (fevers, chills, night sweats, diarrhea, unintentional weight loss) are poor indicators, but are even worse in persons with HIV infection because they may be due to opportunistic infections (e.g., mycobacterial infection) as well as symptoms of lymphoma.

Definitive diagnosis of lymphoma is made through

biopsy, although this may not always be feasible due to the location of the presenting lesion(s). This is particularly true in the case of brain lesions. Other conditions can cause space-occupying lesions in the brain, most notably toxoplasmosis, which has symptoms that may not be different from lymphomas. Radiologic evidence is not reliable in differentiating between cerebral toxoplasmosis and CNS lymphoma, though it does seem that multiple lesions are more characteristic of toxoplasmosis, while solitary or fewer lesions are associated with CNS lymphoma.

Medical management of HIV-related lymphoma provides multiple challenges. When a patient presents with a symptomatic space-occupying brain lesion and a positive toxo titer, many clinicians will begin presumptive therapy for toxoplasmosis (see Chapter 8). If no improvement is observed within 10 to 14 days, therapy (usually radiation therapy) is undertaken. In cases where tissue biopsy is feasible and lymphoma is diagnosed, treatment may consist of local radiation therapy for symptom control or systemic chemotherapy. Combination chemotherapy regimens are commonly used, but it is a challenge to manage the significant toxicities of such treatment regimens in the immunocompromised host. Primary CNS lymphoma is often resistant to intravenous chemotherapy, and intrathecal administration may be considered.

Table 10-6

CLASSIFICATION OF NON-HODGKIN'S LYMPHOMA (NHL)

Grade	Rappaport classification	Working formulation of NHL for clinical usage
Low	Diffuse lymphocytic, well differentiated	Small lymphocytic
	Nodular poorly differentiated lymphocytic	Follicular, predominantly small cleaved cell
	Nodular, mixed lymphocytic-histiocytic	Follicular, mixed small cleaved and large cell
Intermediate	Nodular histiocytic	Follicular, predominantly large cell
	Diffuse lymphocytic, poorly differentiated	Diffuse small cleaved cell
	Diffuse mixed lymphocytic-histiocytic	Diffuse, mixed small and large cell
	Diffuse histiocytic	Diffuse large cell
High	Diffuse histiocytic	Large cell immunoblastic
	Lymphoblastic convoluted/nonconvoluted	Lymphoblastic
	Undifferentiated, Burkitt's and non-Burkitt's	Small noncleaved cell

Table 10-7

ANN ARBOR STAGING SYSTEM FOR LYMPHOMAS

Involvement	Systemic symptoms	Stage
Single lymph node region	No	IA
	Yes	IB
Two or more lymph node regions on same side of diaphragm	No	IIA
	Yes	IIB
Lymph node regions on both sides of diaphragm	No	IIIA
	Yes	IIIB
Disseminated—extralymphatic disease with or without nodal involvement	No	IVA
	Yes	IVB

Gynecologic Malignancies

Immunocompromised women, despite the etiology of the compromise, are known to be at risk for lower genital tract neoplasia. As more women in the United States are identified as HIV infected and symptomatic, scientific understanding about these malignancies may increase. At present, invasive cervical cancer in the presence of HIV infection is included in the AIDS case definition. Cervical dysplasia and cervical intraepithelial neoplasia, precancerous conditions, are also more common in HIV-infected than in uninfected women.

Human papillomavirus (HPV) has been implicated as a potential oncogenic virus in cervical neoplasia, and herpes simplex virus (HSV) type 2 is also associated with this condition. Cervical neoplasia and HIV infection are associated with high-risk sexual behavior and genital HPV/HSV. Injection drug use is also associated with both HIV infection and high-risk sex. While the relationships among these various factors remain to be elaborated, clinical evidence suggests that HIV-infected women are more likely to exhibit cervical neoplasia, and cervical disease in this population tends to be more aggressive and refractory to treatment.

In some women cervical neoplasia may be the first indication of HIV infection. The degree of cervical neoplasia does not necessarily correlate with degree of immunosuppression or other opportunistic infection. High-grade presentation is common in HIV-infected women, as are multifocal lesions.

Diagnosis of cervical neoplasia can involve cytology (Pap smear), visualization on colposcopy, and biopsy.

Table 10-8

CLINICAL STAGING SYSTEM FOR CERVICAL CANCER (FIGO)

Stage	Description
0	Carcinoma in situ, intraepithelial carcinoma
I	Carcinoma confined to the cervix
IA	Preclinical carcinoma of cervix (diagnosed only by microscopy)
IA1	Minimal microscopically evident stromal invasion
IA2	Measurable microscopic lesion no more than 5 mm deep from epithelial base and no more than 7 mm wide
IB	Lesions greater than IA2, clinically seen or not
II	Involves vagina but not the lower third, or infiltration of the parametria but not out to the side wall
IIA	Involvement of vagina, no evidence of parametrial involvement
IIB	Infiltration of parametria but not out to side wall
III	Involves lower third of vagina or extension to pelvic side wall; all cases with hydronephrosis or nonfunctioning kidney unless known to be from other cause
IIIA	Involvement of lower third of vagina but not out to pelvic side wall
IIIB	Involvement of one or both parametria out to side wall or hydronephrosis or nonfunctioning kidney
IV	Extension beyond the true pelvis
IVA	Involvement of mucosa of bladder or rectum
IVB	Distant metastasis

The degree of dysplasia can range from carcinoma in situ or noninvasive disease (CIN) through advanced disease. Diagnosis of cancer is through biopsy. Evaluation of the extent of disease may entail cystoscopy, intravenous pyelography, sigmoidoscopy, proctoscopy, or barium enema examinations, as well as abdominopelvic imaging with ultrasound, CT, or MRI scans.

Medical management varies with stage of disease (Table 10-8). There is no consensus on optimal management of cervical disease in HIV-infected women. Preinvasive disease may be treated with local therapies such as excisional biopsy, cautery, cryotherapy, laser excision, or conization. Invasive disease may require more aggressive surgical intervention and radiation therapy using teletherapy and/or brachytherapy techniques. Recurrence is common in HIV-infected women, and regular follow-up is essential. Systemic chemotherapy may be indicated for recurrent or disseminated disease. As with other cancers in HIV-infected persons, administration of potentially myelosuppressive drugs must be undertaken with great care.

Anorectal Malignancies

The specific physiologic relationship between HIV infection and anorectal malignancies has not been demonstrated, but significant data suggest that anorectal dysplasia and malignancy may be related to infection with HPV and HIV-induced immunosuppression. Epidemiologic evidence suggests that homosexual men, especially those who practice receptive anal intercourse, are at increased risk for anorectal malignancies; this same behavior carries great risk for HIV infection as well. HPV, implicated as a possible oncogenic virus, is associated with development of anal condylomata (warts). In the presence of deficient surveillance of a person's immune status, oncogenic changes due to HPV—or other agents—could conceivably progress to clinical disease.

Abnormal anorectal cytology and anal intraepithelial neoplasia have been associated with advanced HIV-related immunosuppression. Identification and surveillance of persons at risk (through complete history taking and routine clinical evaluation) can identify disease earlier, when it is more easily treated.

1 ASSESS

ASSESSMENT	KS	LYMPHOMA	CERVICAL	ANORECTAL
History	Previous KS diagnosis	Weight loss, fevers, chills, night sweats, diarrhea, headache, seizure	Previous abnormal cervical cytology Age at first intercourse, number of lifetime sexual partners	Anal warts, prior HPV infection diagnosed, rectal STDs
Subjective symptoms	Dyspnea, change in bowel pattern, dysphagia, early satiety, nausea, vomiting, pain from lymphedema or mechanical irritation of lesions in sensitive areas	Fatigue, headache, personality changes, memory loss, difficulty concentrating, dysphagia	Usually none; dysuria in advanced disease	Painful defecation, rectal bleeding, bloody stool
Skin	Flat or raised lesions, pigmented pink to purple to brown anywhere on skin; edema—limbs, periorbital	Localized swelling, especially in lymph node regions	Vulvovaginal condyloma	Perianal warts, other growths
Oral cavity	Lesions on palate, gingiva, or mucosa	Swelling of gingiva, peritonsillar tissue	N/A	N/A
Abdomen	Distension, masses, hyperactive or hypoactive bowel sounds	Distension, masses, hyperactive or hypoactive bowel sounds	N/A	N/A
Respiratory	Dyspnea, cacophonous breath sounds	Dyspnea	N/A	N/A
Neurologic	N/A	Facial nerve or other weakness or paralysis; seizure	N/A	N/A

2 DIAGNOSE

NURSING DIAGNOSIS	SUPPORTIVE ASSESSMENT FINDINGS
Impaired skin integrity related to lymphedema, mechanical irritation of lesions, radiotherapy side effects	Swelling in areas where tumor growth impedes lymphatic drainage; taut, shiny skin, broken skin; broken skin in intertriginous areas, around belt line

NURSING DIAGNOSIS	SUPPORTIVE ASSESSMENT FINDINGS
Potential for social isolation and body image disturbance related to disfiguring lesions, lymphedema, weight loss	Verbalized feelings of distaste for appearance, neglect of appearance or failure to maintain personal grooming
Impaired mobility related to lymphedema, neurogenic weakness	Gait changes, ataxia, history or expressed fear of falling
Pain related to pressure from lesion, edema, mechanical irritation of lesions in sensitive areas, side effect of radiotherapy	Headache, guarding edematous limb, verbal complaints of pain, mucositis in radiated area
Altered thought process, potential for injury related to CNS lesions	Confusion, agitation, memory loss, inability to concentrate
Potential for infection related to myelosuppressive toxicity of treatment	Decreased WBC count

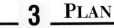 3 PLAN

Patient goals

1. Patient's skin will remain intact.
2. Patient will obtain relief from pain.

3. Patient will maintain/gain body weight.
4. Patient will maintain social contacts.
5. Patient will remain free of secondary infection.

4 IMPLEMENT

NURSING DIAGNOSIS	NURSING INTERVENTIONS	RATIONALE
Impaired skin integrity related to lymphedema, mechanical irritation of lesions, radiotherapy side effects	Assess areas of likely irritation—intertriginous, belt line, wherever clothes may rub. Elevate edematous limbs. Employ gentle skin care using water-based emollient lotion on radiated skin. Use alcohol-free products, soft toothbrush or swabs for mouth care.	To maintain integrity of skin.

→ › ›

NURSING DIAGNOSIS	NURSING INTERVENTIONS	RATIONALE
Potential for social isolation and body image disturbance related to disfiguring lesions, lymphedema, weight loss	Touch, make eye contact with patient. Teach or refer for teaching about ways to enhance appearance with use of concealing cosmetics, scarves to conceal edema or swollen lymph nodes, clothing styles appropriate to changing body mass. Acknowledge patient's efforts to enhance appearance.	To maintain optimal appearance, enhance self-image.
Impaired mobility related to lymphedema, neurogenic weakness	Elevate edematous limbs to promote drainage of lymphatic fluid. Avoid constrictive clothing (e.g., elastic), which can exacerbate edema. Provide mobility assist devices (cane, walker, wheelchair) as needed.	To maintain mobility, support independent functioning and safety.
Pain related to pressure from lesion, edema, mechanical irritation of lesions in sensitive areas, side effect of radiotherapy	Provide measures to decrease edema. Provide appropriate skin care to area in radiation field—use mild, nondeodorant soap, pat dry, and avoid brisk rubbing; avoid shaving area; no perfumes, water-based emollient lotions only; wear loose clothing of smooth, breathable material. Administer analgesic medications as required; assess effectiveness, obtain order for increased dose or change if relief is inadequate.	To reduce mechanical causes of pain, maintain patient comfort.
Altered thought process, potential for injury related to CNS lesions	Assess mental status, note changes. Observe for changes in neurologic function that affect gross or fine motor control, judgment, and ability to communicate. Provide environmental cues (calendar, clock, etc.) and frequent verbal orientation. If patient is confused, check frequently, consider arranging for companion care.	To avoid injury, maintain patient's orientation and sense of safety.
Potential for infection related to myelosuppressive toxicity of treatment	Monitor results of CBCs for neutropenia. Length of time to nadir (lowest point of WBC count) will vary with chemotherapeutic agent(s) used. Assess for other signs of infection—fever, increased respiratory rate, local inflammation, purulence—including IV sites. Teach patient appropriate neutropenic precautions.	To prevent infection or to identify and begin treatment of infection as early as possible.

NURSING DIAGNOSIS	NURSING INTERVENTIONS	RATIONALE
Inadequate nutritional intake related to mechanical obstruction of upper digestive tract, emetogenic toxicity of treatment, fatigue, inability to obtain or prepare food	Perform or refer for nutritional assessment. Assess for dysphagic symptoms, report/refer for treatment. Recommend appropriate nutritional supplements with instruction on how to obtain and use them. Refer for enrollment in nutrition program (e.g., home meal delivery) and/or homemaker assistance. Monitor for and treat nausea/vomiting. Instruct patient on techniques to reduce N/V or anorexia—lukewarm or cool rather than hot foods; small, frequent meals; avoid drinking large amounts of liquids at mealtime; keep handy ready-to-eat or easy to prepare foods.	To maintain adequate nutritional intake, body mass, and body stores of essential nutrients.

_ 5   EVALUATE

PATIENT OUTCOME	DATA INDICATING THAT OUTCOME IS REACHED
Patient's skin has remained intact.	Areas of lymphedema, KS lesions show no signs of broken or cracked skin.
Patient has obtained relief from pain.	Patient verbalizes relief from pain. Patient performs ADLs unimpaired by pain.
Patient has maintained/gained body weight.	Intake provides adequate nutrients, body weight is maintained or weight gained. Dysphagic symptoms are relieved or controlled.
Patient has maintained social contacts.	Patient engages in social activities as appropriate, utilizes available social services, has visitors, identifies persons who are available to provide assistance.
Patient has remained free of secondary infection.	Patient demonstrates no signs or symptoms of infection—acute fever, purulent drainage at IV site or elsewhere.

PATIENT TEACHING

1. Skin in area of radiation field should be treated delicately. Avoid use of harsh deodorant soaps, perfumes, and friction in the area. Cleanse gently with lukewarm water, mild soap; pat dry with soft cloth or let air dry. Apply only water-based lotions to the area. Protect the area from sun exposure. Wear loose, soft clothing over the area. If the oral cavity is being irradiated, avoid mouthwashes with alcohol. Plain water or saline, half-strength hydrogen peroxide, or commercially available alcohol-free products may be used. If the head is being irradiated, check with the radiation therapist about washing hair during treatment.

2. If nausea or vomiting occurs as a side effect of treatment, instruct patient on proper use of antiemetic medication. If unable to keep down oral antiemetic, consider using suppositories before going to parenteral route. Administer antiemetic 30 to 60 minutes before meals. Avoid greasy, spicy foods and foods with strong smells. Smaller, more frequent meals may be easier to handle than three large meals per day. See Patient Teaching Guide, page 256.

3. For flulike symptoms (fever, chills, malaise, myalgias, arthralgia), which may accompany treatment with interferon for KS, acetaminophen may be helpful, but do not self-medicate without reporting the occurrence of these symptoms. Aspirin should be avoided while receiving BRMs.

4. To increase nutritional intake, keep easy to prepare or ready-to-eat foods available. If the patient has been eating very little and commercial supplements are used, it may be necessary to start with a diluted form (add water), gradually decreasing the amount of water added to the formula as the patient tolerates.

5. If chronic pain is a problem, medications should be taken on a routine rather than "prn" schedule. Let the patient know that taking an analgesic before the pain worsens will likely provide better and longer lasting relief at a lower total dosage.

6. For all prescribed medications, provide verbal and legibly written instructions on the dose, schedule, and method of administration.

7. Commercially available makeup can be used to conceal KS lesions. If sensitivity reaction develops (itching, redness), other brands or hypoallergenic products may be tried.

8. If lymphedema develops, keep the limb elevated as much as possible to promote lymph drainage. Do not wear constrictive clothing (tightly buttoned, zipped, or elasticized) or jewelry on affected limbs.

9. Some chemotherapy agents are excreted in active forms in urine and feces. For patients receiving systemic chemotherapy, handle excrement (urine and feces) carefully (gloves, thorough handwashing, and rinsing of urinals and bedpans) for several days after administration of the drugs.

10. Vinca alkaloids can cause peripheral neuropathy. Report numbness or tingling sensations in extremities.

11. Fatigue can result from myelosuppression due to systemic chemotherapy or BRMs. Schedule frequent rest periods to conserve energy for ADL tasks and social activities.

12. New onset or increased level of fever and purulent drainage can indicate infection. Notify health care provider if these occur.

13. With CNS lymphoma, memory can become impaired. Keep written notes of appointments and medication schedules. Write down questions you want to ask at your next appointment as they occur to you. Keep a list of frequently used phone numbers near the phone, including health care providers and family/friends who provide assistance.

CHAPTER 11

Nursing Management

Nursing care of HIV-infected persons differs little from the care of persons with other acute and chronic health problems. Persons with HIV, for example, have the same nursing diagnoses as other patients and require the same nursing interventions. The major difference is that those with HIV infection may experience almost all of the diagnoses at some time during the course of the infection. There is also individual variation in the course of the infection. No two persons have the same constellation of problems at the same time. Nursing care must be flexible enough to respond to the specific needs of an individual patient and holistic enough to meet the complex needs of patients throughout the extended course of HIV infection.

_1 ASSESS

ASSESSMENT	OBSERVATIONS
History	HIV-positive test result or possible exposure to the virus; history of engaging in high-risk behaviors; diagnosis of STD, hepatitis B, persistent lymphadenopathy, or other infectious disease; reports use of multiple drugs, including prescribed, OTC, recreational, and unapproved drugs
General appearance	Cachectic, pale; slowed or impaired gait or movement
Subjective symptoms	Chronic fever, with or without chills; recurrent night sweats; malaise, weakness, severe fatigue; anorexia, weight loss; pain; difficulty sleeping
Psychosocial	Anxious appearance; history of recent loss of job and health insurance; alienation from significant others, changed living situation, and multiple life changes; expresses feelings of guilt, grief, powerlessness, or fear
Mental status	Behavior changes, expressions of anger or hopelessness; depressed affect, suicidal ideation, apathy, withdrawal, loss of interest in surroundings; reports selling or giving away possessions; disturbances in thought processes; impaired judgment; cognitive "slowing," memory loss, confusion; altered attention and concentration; impaired communication, aphasia, difficulty finding words; slurred speech; hallucinations, delusions
Head, ears, eyes, nose, and throat (HEENT)	Periorbital pain, photophobia, blurred or double vision, total loss of vision; diffuse hemorrhaging, exudates; headache; facial edema; tinnitus or hearing loss; white or red raised lesion(s) in oral cavity; ulcers on lips or in mouth, bleeding in mouth; dry mouth, voice changes; dysphagia; palpable lymph nodes; epistaxis
Neurologic	Altered pupillary reflexes, nystagmus; peripheral neuropathy; vertigo, imbalance, ataxia; neuromuscular incoordination; nuchal rigidity, severe headache; seizures, loss of consciousness; paraplegia, quadriplegia
Musculoskeletal	Muscle wasting; focal motor deficits; weakness and inability to perform ADLs
Cardiovascular	Tachycardia related to fever; hypotension related to dehydration; irregular heart rate, dizziness related to electrolyte imbalance; absent peripheral pulses and peripheral edema
Respiratory	Dyspnea, tachypnea, cyanosis; shortness of breath upon exertion; uses accessory muscles; positions self to facilitate respiration; productive or nonproductive cough; distant or decreased breath sounds upon auscultation
GI	Decreased food or fluid intake; reports oral pain (causing difficulty in eating); anorexia, nausea, vomiting, weight loss; diarrhea, incontinence; abdominal tenderness, cramping; hepatomegaly, splenomegaly, jaundice; bowel sounds (absent or hyperactive); anal lesions, rectal bleeding
Genitourinary	Lesions or exudate on genitalia; female reports pelvic pain; decreased urine output related to dehydration; incontinence
Integumentary	Reports dryness and pruritus, night sweats; rash or lesions anywhere on body; red-violet, raised lesions; petechiae; palpable lymph nodes; jaundice; poor skin turgor related to dehydration; skin warm and very moist to touch; markings from IV drug use

2   DIAGNOSE

Nursing diagnoses are organized as follows:

I. Diagnoses associated with systemic responses to HIV; these diagnoses are generally present throughout the course of HIV infection.

II. Diagnoses associated with psychosocial responses.

III. Diagnoses associated with specific body system responses (i.e., GI, respiratory, dermatologic, and central/peripheral nervous systems).

NURSING DIAGNOSIS	SUPPORTIVE ASSESSMENT FINDINGS
Systemic responses to HIV	
High risk for infection related to immunosuppression, effects of chemotherapy or radiation, frequent venipuncture, central lines, malnutrition, and high-risk life-style	History of high-risk life-style; laboratory findings of HIV infection and immunosuppression; reports recurrent fevers and night sweats, weight loss, fatigue; cachexia; pale skin color and poor skin turgor
High risk for transmitting infections related to HIV infection, life-style, and presence of nonopportunistic infections that can be transmitted	History of exposure to HIV; body secretions, excretions, or exudates contain viable pathogens; fever; lymphadenopathy; lesions; symptoms and/or diagnosis of pulmonary TB
Hyperthermia related to infections	Elevated temperature; hot, flushed skin; tachycardia, diaphoresis
High risk for poisoning related to toxic effects of drug therapy	Findings depend on drug; often mimic symptoms of CNS disease (i.e., confusion, disturbance in mood, sedation, loss of consciousness, dizziness, sensory disturbances); hypertension or hypotension, rashes, edema, hair loss, oral pain, nausea, vomiting, diarrhea
Activity intolerance related to weakness, CNS and neurologic involvement, altered O_2 exchange, malnutrition, fluid and electrolyte imbalance, fatigue	Reports fatigue, weakness, shortness of breath and tremors upon exertion; unable to perform ADLs; muscle atrophy; paralysis of limbs; exertional dyspnea and tachycardia; psychomotor incoordination
Chronic pain related to neurologic disease, pressure of KS lesions on nerves, lymphadenopathy, malignancies	Reports burning pain in extremities, severe headache or tenderness in areas of enlarged lymph nodes, diagnosis of malignancies, presence of lesions

→ ❯ ❯

NURSING DIAGNOSIS	SUPPORTIVE ASSESSMENT FINDINGS
Sleep pattern disturbance related to anxiety, night sweats, chills, and schedule of treatments	Reports inability to sleep, changing sleep patterns, and daytime fatigue
Self-care deficit in all ADLs related to deterioration of condition, opportunistic disease, exertional dyspnea, mental changes, neurologic impairment, depression, impoverishment	Reports being too tired to take care of self; stays in bed; decreases participation in self-care activities; appears to have neglected appearance
Impaired home maintenance management related to activity intolerance, inadequate finances, and lack of knowledge about sources of help	Reports living alone with limited or no help; limited finances; reports and demonstrates inability to care for self
Psychosocial responses	
Anxiety related to diagnosis, fear of treatment, hospitalization, pain, dying, death, and multiple losses associated with diagnosis of HIV	Expresses helplessness, anger, regretfulness, fear, denial, inability to sleep; demonstrates restlessness, agitation, pacing, poor eye contact, facial tension, increased perspiration, tachycardia, and tachypnea
Decisional conflict: treatment options related to lack of relevant information or previous experience and experimental nature of many HIV treatments	Expresses distress about making treatment choices; vacillates between alternatives; focuses on negative effects of alternatives; delays making decisions; "shops" for health care providers and treatments
Powerlessness related to poor prognosis of disease and perceived lack of control over disease outcome and health care decisions	Verbalizes having no control over life, future, or treatment; expresses anger, apathy, or passivity; increases dependence on others; demonstrates noncompliance with medical regimen; fails to keep scheduled appointments

NURSING DIAGNOSIS	SUPPORTIVE ASSESSMENT FINDINGS
Grieving and hopelessness related to multiple losses (health, attractiveness, job, insurance, family, friends, lovers) and lack of personal future	Has depressed affect, decreased communication; increases sleeping or staying in bed; sells or gives away all possessions; expresses anger, sorrow, suicidal ideation; demonstrates self-neglect
Social isolation related to others' fear of AIDS, family rejection, society's stigmatization, and patient's withdrawal from people and activities	Reports loss of job, living alone; withdrawn behavior; no visitors in the hospital; expresses loneliness
Ineffective family coping related to anxiety about loved one's condition, fear of infection or stigmatization, long-term dysfunctional relationships, and demands of providing care for the patient	Family/significant others demonstrate anxious or hostile behaviors; do not visit patient; patient expresses concern about how family/significant others are coping; patient expresses concern about being discharged from the hospital to be cared for by family/significant others

Central/peripheral nervous system

Altered thought processes related to CNS infection with HIV or other pathogens, malignancies, hypoxemia, drug reactions, depression	Reports forgetfulness, slowness in thinking and solving problems; demonstrates confusion, altered judgment, disorientation, personality change, memory loss, delusions and hallucinations; signs of meningitis; signs of self-neglect (e.g., failure to pay bills); laboratory or diagnostic findings of CNS infection or malignancy
High risk for injury related to CNS disease, mental status changes, generalized weakness, and neuromuscular impairment	Reports forgetfulness, unrealistic expectations of self, weakness, poor vision, altered feeling in extremities, falls; demonstrates impaired balance, gait, and muscle strength, signs of confusion; has seizures
Sensory-perceptual alterations (visual, auditory, and kinesthetic) related to CMV retinitis, otic infections, and HIV damage to CNS	Reports photophobia, loss of vision, impaired hearing; demonstrates ataxia, apraxia

→ › ›

NURSING DIAGNOSIS	SUPPORTIVE ASSESSMENT FINDINGS
Impaired verbal communication related to CNS disease	Demonstrates inability to recognize or understand written or spoken word; difficulty articulating words; unable to recall familiar words
Respiratory system	
Impaired gas exchange related to pulmonary infections or malignancies	Reports progressive shortness of breath, productive or nonproductive cough, fatigue, exertional dyspnea; demonstrates tachypnea, use of accessory muscles for respiration, distant or decreased breath sounds, circumoral cyanosis; laboratory and radiographic findings of respiratory disease
Gastrointestinal system	
Altered oral mucous membrane related to oral, pharyngeal, or esophageal infections or lesions; malnutrition	Reports soreness of mouth or throat, dysphagia, changes in taste; demonstrates inflammation, ulceration, or lesions of oral and pharyngeal mucosa; bleeding of gums or nose
Altered nutrition: less than body requirements related to decreased intake (associated with oral pain, dysphagia, anorexia, and nausea), increased metabolic needs (caused by infections), and decreased absorption of nutrients (caused by GI disease)	Reports inability to eat, decreased appetite, nausea, vomiting, diarrhea; weight loss of more than 20% of normal body weight, cachectic, pale; abdominal tenderness, abnormal bowel sounds, enlarged liver or spleen; laboratory findings indicate anemia, intestinal parasites, or malignancies
Diarrhea related to GI infection or malignancy, chemotherapy, radiation, or drug reactions	Up to 20 liquid stools a day; abdominal tenderness; hyperactive bowel sounds; incontinence of stool; laboratory and diagnostic findings indicate intestinal infections or malignancies
Fluid volume deficit related to nausea, vomiting, diarrhea, fever, and diaphoresis	Reports vomiting, diarrhea, decreased fluid intake, weight loss, dry mouth and skin, postural dizziness, profuse diaphoresis, poor skin turgor, hypotension, oliguria/anuria; laboratory findings of electrolyte and fluid imbalance
Dermatologic system	
Impaired skin integrity related to HIV, multiple skin infections, KS lesions, malnutrition, immobility, incontinence, and radiation therapy	Reports itching, burning; rash, lesions, or decubiti anywhere on the body; excoriated genital or perianal area; edema of extremities

NURSING DIAGNOSIS	SUPPORTIVE ASSESSMENT FINDINGS
Alteration in sexual patterns related to fear of transmission of HIV, presence of anal-genital lesions, alteration in self-concept, severed relationships, and activity intolerance	Reports changes in life-style and sexual activities, loss of significant persons in one's life; presence of anal-genital lesions

3

Patient goals

1. Patient will be free of opportunistic infections and their complications.
2. HIV infection will not be transmitted to patient contacts; health care workers will observe blood and body fluid precautions and other isolation procedures as indicated; patient will observe methods to prevent transmission of HIV or other pathogens.
3. Body temperature will be maintained within the normal range; comfort and safety will be maintained during fever.
4. Preventable drug reactions or allergic reactions will be avoided; patient will self-administer drugs as prescribed.
5. Patient will participate in energy-sparing activities as tolerated, and he or she will be free of dyspnea and tachycardia during activity.
6. Patient will obtain relief from pain.
7. Patient will obtain adequate rest and sleep.
8. Patient will have daily needs met by others during episodes of acute illness and will participate in self-care as tolerated.
9. Patient and significant others will be knowledgeable about community resources and services to facilitate home management.
10. Patient will verbalize anxiety and fears and will use individual strategies to cope with anxiety.
11. Patient will make and implement informed choices about treatment that are consistent with personal goals and values and presently approved therapies.
12. Patient will identify factors that he or she can control and will make informed decisions regarding personal, legal, and health care needs; patient will participate in decisions regarding treatment.
13. Patient will demonstrate beginning progression through the grieving process.
14. Patient will maintain significant relationships or will adapt to changes in relationships.
15. Family and significant others will strengthen and maintain mutual support system and adapt to changing demands on them.
16. Effects of altered thought process on patient's life will be minimized.
17. Patient will not experience accidental injury or falls.
18. Patient will not be confused or frightened by environmental stimuli; injury will not result from impaired vision, hearing, or kinesthetic activity.
19. Communication with patient will be maximized; patient will communicate needs by nonverbal methods if necessary.
20. Patient will demonstrate normal respiratory pattern, blood gas levels, and cellular oxygenation; patient will demonstrate ability to self-administer oxygen.
21. Damage to oral mucous membranes will be minimized; patient will experience maximum oral comfort.
22. Patient will have adequate calorie and protein intake to meet metabolic needs, and his or her weight will stabilize.
23. Patient will experience maximum comfort and control of diarrhea; complications of diarrhea will be minimized.
24. Fluid and electrolyte balance will be maintained.
25. Patient will be free of preventable and treatable skin lesions.
26. Patient or couple will be provided with support and counseling to enable resumption of safe sexual activity or alternative means of sexual satisfaction; patient will be treated for anal-genital lesions.

4 IMPLEMENT

NURSING DIAGNOSIS	NURSING INTERVENTIONS	RATIONALE
Systemic responses to HIV		
High risk for infection related to immunosuppression, effects of chemotherapy or radiation, frequent venipuncture, central lines, malnutrition, and high-risk life-style	Monitor and teach patient signs of new infection.	For early treatment.
	Use strict aseptic technique for any invasive procedure. Wash hands before giving care.	To avoid exposing patient to hospital-acquired pathogens.
	Instruct patient in methods to avoid exposure to environmental pathogens, particularly hand washing (see Patient Teaching). Give Patient Teaching Guides: "About Condoms," "The Female Condom," "Facts About HIV Infection and AIDS," "Food Safety," and, if indicated, "Care of the Hickman-Broviac Central Venous Catheter," "Care of the Implanted Port."	To prevent added infection burden.
	Obtain specimens for laboratory analysis as ordered.	To ensure accurate diagnosis and treatment.
	Administer antiinfectives as prescribed or teach self-medication. Give Patient Teaching Guides: "Use of Antiretroviral Drugs" and "Facts About Your Prescription."	To maintain therapeutic blood levels of drugs.
	Teach patient alterations in life-style (nutrition, rest, exercise, stress reduction, avoidance of recreational drugs, and excess alcohol use). Give Patient Teaching Guide: "When Your HIV Test Is Positive."	To promote optimum immune function.
High risk for transmitting infections related to HIV infection, life-style, and presence of nonopportunistic infections that can be transmitted	Instruct patient and significant others on methods of preventing transmission of HIV and other pathogens (see Patient Teaching). Give Patient Teaching Guides: "About Condoms," "The Female Condom," "Facts About HIV Infection and AIDS," "Facts About Sexually Transmitted Diseases," and "Tuberculosis."	Patient wants and needs this information.
	Use blood and body fluid precautions when caring for patient. Use other barriers, such as masks, as necessary.	Although the risk of transmitting HIV to health care workers is very small, it is real. The risk for transmitting hepatitis B or TB is greater.
Hyperthemia related to infections	Assess for signs of infection.	Infection is the most common cause of fever.
	Monitor temperature q 2 h.	To detect change associated with complications and resolution of infection.

NURSING DIAGNOSIS	NURSING INTERVENTIONS	RATIONALE
	Monitor for signs of dehydration; also monitor fluid and electrolytes, intake and output. Administer IV or oral fluids; provide high-calorie diet; provide for bed rest.	Significant fluid loss accompanies each degree centigrade increase in temperature. Fluids, sodium, and potassium are lost through sweating. Metabolic rate increases 12% with each degree centigrade increase in body temperature.
	Administer antipyretic agents or teach patient to self-administer antipyretics.	Antipyretic agents act to lower the set point in the hypothalamus; they may increase the patient's comfort.
	Assess for environmental factors. Adjust environmental temperature for patient's comfort. Provide fan or air conditioning. Remove excess clothing and bedding. Provide for frequent changes of clothing and bedding for patient who perspires heavily.	Excessive environmental heat or humidity may contribute to retention of body heat during fever. Body heat is lost through convection and evaporation of sweat.
	Apply hypothermia blanket, tepid sponge baths, and ice packs in areas of high blood flow. Control cooling efforts to avoid inducing shivering.	To facilitate heat loss through convection and conduction. Tepid water evaporates, permitting cooling of blood near surface of skin. Shivering induces heat production through muscle activity.
	Monitor for neurologic complications (altered consciousness, irritability, seizure activity). Institute seizure precautions.	Encephalopathy may result from infection, fever, dehydration, electrolyte imbalance, or a combination of factors.
	Teach patient and caregiver to monitor and care for fever. Give Patient Teaching Guide: "Fever."	Fever is a common symptom that HIV-infected persons must manage.
High risk for poisoning related to toxic effects of drug therapy	Instruct patient and significant other on all prescribed medications: their dosage, route of administration, action, side effects, and untoward reactions, and under what conditions to discontinue the drug and call a physician. Have patient keep a list of medications and time of administration. Give Patient Teaching Guides: "Facts About Your Prescription," "Dealing with the Effects of Immune and Bone Marrow Suppression," and "Use of Antiretroviral Drugs."	Patients with HIV are frequently taking multiple drugs, with an increased risk of drug reactions; patients with memory loss have increased risk of medication errors.
	Teach maintenance of IV line for patient receiving IV therapy at home. Give Patient Teaching Guides: "Care of the Hickman-Broviac Central Venous Catheter" or "Care of the Implanted Port."	To prevent complications.

→ ⟩ ⟩

NURSING DIAGNOSIS	NURSING INTERVENTIONS	RATIONALE
Activity intolerance related to weakness, CNS and neurologic involvement, altered O₂ exchange, malnutrition, fluid and electrolyte imbalance, fatigue	Monitor physiologic response to activity.	Tolerance varies from day to day.
	Monitor and treat underlying cause (e.g., infection).	Many of the causes of activity intolerance are treatable.
	Structure the environment to conserve patient energy; instruct on measures to use at home to conserve energy and prevent injury (e.g., ambulation aids, grab bars).	To decrease energy demands.
	Provide care that patient cannot provide for self.	Debilitation sometimes interferes with patient's ability to perform ADLs.
	Structure the nursing care to provide for uninterrupted rest.	Extra rest is necessary because of increased metabolic demands.
	Assist patient to develop a manageable schedule that balances activity with adequate rest periods.	Patient's quality of life will be improved if patient can continue with some activity.
Chronic pain related to neurologic disease, pressure of KS lesions on nerves, lymphadenopathy, malignancies	Assess patient's pain. Encourage patient to describe pain and measures used to relieve it.	To establish baseline data; to plan interventions for pain relief that are individualized.
	Intervene to relieve cause of pain, if possible, or refer patient to physician or dentist for treatment of cause of pain.	Many of the causes of pain, such as opportunistic infections, are treatable.
	Implement palliative measures (e.g., relaxation, back rubs). Instruct patient in alternative therapies or refer patient for instruction (e.g., guided imagery, relaxation, affirmation). Provide distracting activities. Give Patient Teaching Guide: "Managing Pain Without Drugs."	Promotes relaxation and sense of control over pain.
	Administer analgesics as prescribed.	To provide relief from pain.
Sleep pattern disturbance related to anxiety, night sweats, chills, and schedule of treatments	Assess sleep patterns; assist patient in maintaining bedtime rituals.	To plan care based on individual needs.
	Maintain quiet, calm environment; schedule nursing care to avoid interrupting sleep.	To induce uninterrupted sleep.
	Administer sleeping or antianxiety medication as ordered.	To relieve symptoms that may interfere with falling asleep and to promote relaxation.
	Teach patient to avoid alcohol, caffeine, and other stimulants before bedtime.	Stimulants promote wakefulness; alcohol interferes with normal sleep stages.

NURSING DIAGNOSIS	NURSING INTERVENTIONS	RATIONALE
Self-care deficit in all ADLs related to deterioration of condition, opportunistic disease, exertional dyspnea, mental changes, neurologic impairment, depression, impoverishment.	Assess patient's need for help with ADLs. Provide help with the activities that patient cannot do for self.	Patient's needs change with changes in patient's condition.
	Refer patient to occupational therapy for assistive devices and home equipment. Help patient make adaptations in home to facilitate ADLs.	To make it possible for patient to perform his or her own ADLs; this increases self-respect.
	Teach significant other to provide ADLs for patient.	So that care can be maintained at home.
Impaired home maintenance management related to activity intolerance, inadequate finances, and lack of knowledge about sources of help	Assess availability of someone in the home to help patient with shopping, meal preparation, simple housekeeping, and transportation. Assess adequacy of income to support living.	Patient's condition hinders his or her ability to maintain home's comfort and safety.
	Refer patient/family/significant other to community resources for help (e.g., food stamps, food pantries, transportation for handicapped, housekeeping services). Assist patient to alter living arrangements, if necessary.	Services are organized in most communities to help persons with HIV, low income, or special needs. Changing or simplifying one's living arrangements may make it possible to maintain independence in the home.

Psychosocial responses

NURSING DIAGNOSIS	NURSING INTERVENTIONS	RATIONALE
Anxiety related to diagnosis; fear of treatment, hospitalization, pain, dying, and death; multiple losses associated with diagnosis of HIV	Assess patient's coping skill. Be alert to signs of ineffective coping.	The patient may be using defenses (e.g., denial).
	Provide accurate, consistent information about condition and treatment.	To minimize fear of unknown.
	Allow patient to verbalize fears and anger. Recognize that anger is not directed toward health care worker. Reassure patient that feelings are normal.	Anger is a natural reaction; expressing it helps to control it.
	Provide quiet, nonthreatening environment.	To minimize anxiety-producing stimuli.
	Encourage interaction with support system. Refer to support groups.	To decrease feelings of isolation.
	Refer patient to mental health care or counseling. Administer antianxiety drugs as prescribed.	To intervene if anxiety becomes dysfunctional.
Decisional conflict: treatment options related to lack of relevant information or previous experience and experimental nature of many HIV treatments	Teach patients about treatments, side effects, etc. Give Patient Teaching Guides: "Clinical Trials—What Are They?" and "Use of Antiretroviral Drugs." Refer to "hotlines" and sources for information (see inside back cover).	To help patient clarify options and make personal choices.

→ › ›

NURSING DIAGNOSIS	NURSING INTERVENTIONS	RATIONALE
Powerlessness related to poor prognosis of disease and perceived lack of control over disease outcome and health care decisions	Respect patient. Provide for patient control of activities pertaining to care. Encourage patient's independent activities to improve health status. Assist patient to identify his or her strengths in coping with the disease. Reinforce behavior that demonstrates patient is planning for the future and taking control of his or her present situation. Assist patient in obtaining help in making wills, designating a power of attorney, etc.	This enhances feelings of self-worth and power over life.
Grieving and hopelessness related to multiple losses (health, attractiveness, job, insurance, family, friends, lovers) and lack of personal future	Encourage verbalization of feelings.	This shows recognition of the importance of losses and facilitates the grief process.
	Identify patient's lifetime coping mechanisms and reinforce the healthy ones; refer for alcohol or drug counseling if necessary.	Major coping mechanisms for some have been alcohol or drugs.
	Guide patient to think positively about what he or she can do to make life situation better.	Positive thinking leads to increased energy; allows constructive handling of grief.
	Refer to support groups.	To help with grieving, which may last a long time.
Social isolation related to others' fear of AIDS, family rejection, society's stigmatization, and patient's withdrawal from people and activities	Identify the important relationships in patient's life. Involve these people in patient's care, if patient desires. Encourage visitors and phone calls.	Encouraging interaction in the health care environment may stimulate continued interaction at home.
	Talk with patient frequently. Avoid wearing mask when there is no risk for splashes. Touch the patient whenever possible.	Mask is usually not required and adds an unnecessary barrier in communication. HIV is not transmitted by casual touching.
	Instruct patient and significant other on transmission.	To provide assurance that HIV is not transmitted casually.
	Refer to support groups and community AIDS resources (see inside back cover).	To facilitate patient's contact with people.
Ineffective family coping related to anxiety about loved one's condition, fear of infection or stigmatization, long-term dysfunctional relationships, and demands of providing care for the patient	Establish rapport with family and significant other; assess their strengths in coping with patient's illness and with caring for patient.	To begin a relationship for working constructively with the family and significant others.
	Allow them to verbalize their feelings (anger, withdrawal, blame).	They may have no one else with whom they can freely talk.
	Refer to family support groups.	Families benefit from interacting with others in a similar situation.

NURSING DIAGNOSIS	NURSING INTERVENTIONS	RATIONALE
	Teach family about disease and transmission.	To relieve anxiety about transmission by casual contact.
	Instruct on home care of patient; refer for respite care or for any other help they may need.	To enable family to provide care without excess stress.
Central/peripheral nervous system		
Altered thought processes related to CNS infection with HIV or other pathogens, malignancies, hypoxemia, drug reactions, depression	Assess mental and neurologic processes.	To establish baseline data.
	Monitor for infections, electrolyte imbalance, drug interactions, depression, hypoxemia; administer therapy as prescribed.	These conditions are treatable.
	Structure the environment and maintain comfortable and familiar stimuli.	To minimize disorienting stimuli.
	Encourage patient to have familiar objects nearby. Encourage presence of familiar people. Reorient patient to new occurrences in the environment. Provide clues for orientation (clocks, calendars).	Tangible reminders aid memory and orientation.
	Encourage patient to handle tasks in incremental steps; speak slowly and give simple, short instructions.	Requires less use of memory.
	Help patient obtain a power of attorney.	To handle legal and financial matters.
	Provide memory aids that help patient remember to take medication.	To avoid self-medication errors.
High risk for injury related to CNS disease, mental status changes, generalized weakness, and neuromuscular impairment	Structure environment for patient safety (e.g., provide safety bars and adequate lighting and eliminate clutter); instruct patient and significant other on home safety. Give caregiver Patient Teaching Guide: "Safety Tips for Caregivers of Persons with Confusion or Impaired Judgment." Counsel patient about driving a car; refer for alternative transportation. Supervise disoriented patient. Initiate seizure precautions for seizing patient. Supervise while patient smokes. Keep patient's belongings within reach. Encourage patient to ask for help when getting out of bed or ambulating.	To prevent accidents and injury.
	Refer for physical therapy evaluation.	Physical therapist will consult with patient about environmental aids and prosthetics to aid in mobility.

NURSING DIAGNOSIS	NURSING INTERVENTIONS	RATIONALE
Sensory-perceptual alterations (visual, auditory, and kines- thetic) related to CMV retinitis, otic infections, and HIV damage to CNS	Assess amount of sensory impairment.	To establish baseline data for care.
	Teach patient to report immediately any changes in vision to health care provider.	For early diagnosis and treatment of CMV retinitis.
	Orient patient to the environment; encour- age significant others to stay with patient.	To decrease fear and anxiety.
	Speak to and touch patient often.	To provide sensory stimulation.
Impaired verbal communication re- lated to CNS disease	Assess patient's verbal ability.	To establish baseline data for care.
	Provide alternative methods of communi- cating (e.g., picture boards).	To provide a means for patient to commu- nicate needs.
Respiratory system		
Impaired gas ex- change related to pulmonary infections or malignancies	Monitor breathing patterns and breath sounds.	To detect respiratory complications.
	Position patient to facilitate breathing and coughing; teach use of incentive spirom- eter; teach relaxation techniques and breathing through pursed lips.	To improve lung expansion.
	Provide chest physiotherapy; suction if nec- essary.	To aid in removal of secretions.
	Administer humidified O_2.	To reduce risk of hypoxemia.
	Provide preprocedural care and teaching for patient undergoing bronchoscopy.	To reduce anxiety.
	Teach patient about risk for TB (see dis- cussion of TB in Chapter 9). Give Patient Teaching Guide: "Tuberculosis."	For early diagnosis and treatment and to prevent opportunities for transmitting TB.
Gastrointestinal system		
Altered oral mucous membrane related to oral, pharyngeal, or esophageal infec- tion or lesions; mal- nutrition	Monitor status of oral cavity, throat, and lips.	To identify treatable conditions.
	Refer to dentist.	For care of periodontitis.
	Teach or provide oral hygiene (use of soft toothbrush, nonabrasive toothpaste, non- alcohol-based mouthwash). Encourage frequent rinsing of mouth with saline, hy- drogen peroxide, or Peridex solution; ap- ply lip balm.	Prevents trauma to mucosa, controls or- ganism growth and invasion, and pro- motes comfort.
	Administer antiinfectives as prescribed.	To control opportunistic infections in mouth.
	Counsel patient to avoid spicy and salty foods and foods of extreme temperature.	To prevent irritation.

NURSING DIAGNOSIS	NURSING INTERVENTIONS	RATIONALE
	Encourage oral fluid intake of at least 2500 ml.	To maintain hydration of mucous membranes.
Altered nutrition: less than body requirements related to decreased intake (associated with oral pain, dysphagia, anorexia, and nausea), increased metabolic needs (caused by infections), and decreased absorption of nutrients (caused by GI disease)	Monitor patient's chewing and swallowing.	Decreased intake is often related to oral and throat pain.
	Monitor weight and intake and output.	To establish baseline data.
	Assess availability of food in home and of someone to prepare food. Arrange for assistance, if needed.	Loss of job and income may be a problem. Patient may not have enough energy to shop for and prepare meals.
	Eliminate noxious stimuli, such as odors or unpleasant sights, from the environment.	They stimulate the gag reflex.
	Administer antiemetic as prescribed.	To reduce vomiting.
	Plan diet with patient and significant others.	To ensure that foods are offered that patient likes.
	See Patient Teaching for nutrition suggestions. Consult with a dietician. Give Patient Teaching Guides: "Food Safety" and "Dealing with Loss of Appetite, Nausea and Vomiting."	For additional suggestions tailored to patient's needs.
	Administer nasogastric tube feeding, TPN, or dietary supplements, as indicated.	For patient who cannot tolerate swallowing or cannot ingest enough calories or nutrients in food.
Diarrhea related to GI infection or malignancy, chemotherapy, radiation, or drug reactions	Assess consistency and frequency of stools and presence of blood.	To establish baseline data.
	Auscultate bowel sounds.	Hypermotility is common with diarrhea.
	Assess and refer for treatment for cause of diarrhea.	Most causes of diarrhea (e.g., drug reactions, infections) are treatable.
	Administer antimotility agents and psyllium (Metamucil) as prescribed.	Slows intestinal motility; psyllium acts to absorb fluid and form a more solid mass.
	Assess perianal area for excoriation; provide cleansing after every stool; apply A & D ointment, Vaseline, or zinc oxide.	To minimize burning of skin and decrease discomfort; heavy ointments act as barrier to keep moisture off skin.
Fluid volume deficit related to nausea, vomiting, diarrhea, fever, and diaphoresis	Monitor for signs of dehydration (e.g., poor skin turgor, postural hypotension, tachycardia, oliguria).	Fluid volume depletion is a common complication and can be corrected.
	Monitor intake and output and weight.	To establish baseline data and to detect rapid changes.
	Encourage intake of oral fluids.	To compensate for increased output.
	Administer IV and electrolytes as prescribed.	For patient who cannot tolerate oral fluids.

➜ ❯ ❯

NURSING DIAGNOSIS	NURSING INTERVENTIONS	RATIONALE
Dermatologic system		
Impaired skin integrity related to HIV, multiple skin infections, KS lesions, malnutrition, immobility, incontinence, and radiation therapy	Monitor status of skin and lesions daily.	To establish baseline data.
	Help patient keep skin clean and dry; apply moisturizing lotions; care for perianal area as described under diarrhea.	To prevent breakdown or cracking of skin.
	Change bed linen when soiled; reposition patient frequently; make use of air, water, or foam mattresses, sheep skin pads, and elbow and heel protectors.	To lessen pressure and shearing forces on skin to prevent pressure sores.
	Cover open areas with sterile dry or hydrocolloidal dressing.	To prevent entry of bacteria.
	Implement care of pressure sores as indicated.	To prevent further damage; it may be impossible to heal them.
	Elevate edematous extremities; elevate head of bed if face is edematous.	To help drain areas blocked by KS lesions.
Alteration in sexual patterns related to fear of transmission of HIV; presence of anal-genital lesions; presence of anal-genital lesions; alteration in self-concept; severed relationships; activity intolerance	Assess patient's and partner's concerns about sexual activity; provide complete information on transmission of HIV and on safe, safer, and unsafe sexual practices (see Patient Teaching). Give Patient Teaching Guides: "About Condoms," "The Female Condom," and "Facts About Sexually Transmitted Diseases."	To decrease the risk of further transmission of HIV and to reduce chance of acquiring other STDs, which would further weaken the immune system.
	Provide information on support groups or counselors.	To obtain long-term help with adjustment to effects of HIV on sexuality.
	Offer support to patient's partner.	Partner is likely to be confused and devastated by patient's diagnosis.

For additional nursing management of patients with HIV-related malignancies, refer to Chapter 10.

__ 5   EVALUATE

PATIENT OUTCOME	DATA INDICATING THAT OUTCOME IS REACHED
Patient is free of opportunistic infections and their complications.	There are no new signs of infection; laboratory findings indicate absence of opportunistic infection; temperature, pulse, and respirations are normal; lesions or exudates are absent.

PATIENT OUTCOME	DATA INDICATING THAT OUTCOME IS REACHED
HIV infection is not transmitted; health care workers observe blood and body fluid precautions and other isolation procedures as indicated; patient observes methods to prevent transmission of HIV or other pathogens.	Patient contacts and health care workers are not exposed to HIV—they do not test positive; health care workers are not infected with other pathogens, such as *M. tuberculosis*.
Body temperature is maintained within normal range; comfort and safety are maintained during fever.	Temperature is within normal limits; patient has no chills, flushing, or diaphoresis; clothing and bedding are dry; patient is free of headache and malaise.
Preventable drug reactions or allergic reactions are avoided; patient self-administers drugs as prescribed.	Patient completes full course of prescribed medications; if untoward reactions occur, patient discontinues medication and calls physician; patient informs health care provider of all drugs he or she is taking.
Patient participates in energy-sparing activities and is free of dyspnea and tachycardia during activity.	Environment is modified to accommodate patient's modified activity level; patient uses energy-saving methods and rests between activities.
Patient obtains relief from pain.	Patient rests, sleeps, and performs ADLs without apparent pain.
Patient obtains adequate rest and sleep.	Patient describes sleeping 7 to 9 hours a day and has energy upon waking.
Patient has daily needs met by others and participates in self-care as tolerated.	Patient participates in ADLs with assistance and with help of devices, or patient is fed, bathed, clothed, and toileted by a caregiver.

PATIENT OUTCOME	DATA INDICATING THAT OUTCOME IS REACHED
Patient and significant others are knowledgeable about community resources and services to facilitate home management.	Patient and significant other describe services that are available to provide help and how to arrange for help in the home; patient completes plans for adequate living situation.
Patient verbalizes anxieties and fears, and uses individual strategies to cope with anxiety.	Patient demonstrates decreased anxiety about hospitalization or treatment; he or she verbalizes understanding of condition and treatment and demonstrates methods to manage anxiety in productive ways.
Patient makes and implements informed choices about treatment options that are consistent with personal goals and values and presently approved therapies.	Treatment plan is in place and is appropriate to patient's needs and values; patient participates in developing and following the plan and informs health care provider of deviations from the plan.
Patient identifies factors he or she can control and makes informed decisions regarding personal, legal, and health care needs.	Patient participates actively in decisions about care and asks questions about treatment; patient verbalizes steps he or she will take to maintain present level of health and improve the quality of daily life; patient has considered and made decisions with regard to wills, living wills, and power of attorney.
Patient demonstrates beginning progression through the grieving process.	Patient expresses grief and describes the meaning of his or her losses; patient participates in planning for the future.
Patient maintains significant relationships or adapts to changes in relationships.	Patient has visitors, can identify people with whom he or she is close, and has names of people to call if help is needed.
Family and significant others strengthen and maintain mutual support system and adapt to changing demands on them.	Patient and family interact in constructive ways; family is supportive without denying patient power over decision making; family has information for obtaining help with home care of patient if needed.

PATIENT OUTCOME	DATA INDICATING THAT OUTCOME IS REACHED
Effects of altered thought processes on patient's life are minimized.	Patient is able to participate in ADLs without evidence of frustration; he or she has arranged for help with personal and legal affairs.
Patient does not experience accidental injury or falls.	Patient is adequately supervised and does not fall or sustain injury; he or she uses assistive devices safely; home environment is free of obstructions that could cause an injury; impaired person does not drive an automobile.
Patient is not confused or frightened by environmental stimuli; injury does not occur.	Patient is oriented to the environment, does not express fear of stimuli, and does not experience an injury.
Communication with patient is maximized.	Patient rests comfortably with needs met; he or she communicates in nonverbal manner without excess frustration.
Patient demonstrates normal respiratory pattern, blood gas levels, and cellular oxygenation; patient demonstrates ability to self-administer O_2.	Patient is free of dyspnea, cough, and cyanosis; bronchovesicular sounds are heard throughout the lungs; CO_2, Po_2, and Pco_2 levels are normal; patient engages in activity without shortness of breath.
Damage to oral mucous membranes is minimized, and patient experiences maximum oral comfort.	Mucous membranes are moist, with natural color and without bleeding or lesions; mouth is clean and free of food debris and exudates; lesions, if present, are being treated.
Patient has adequate calorie and protein intake to meet metabolic needs; weight has stabilized.	Nausea and vomiting are controlled; patient eats frequent meals of high-protein and high-calorie content; serum albumin and protein are within normal limits; weight is approaching pre-illness level.
Patient experiences maximum comfort and control of diarrhea; complications are minimized.	Abdomen is soft and nontender; stools are soft and normal colored and occur at pre-illness frequency; patient has relief from cramping; perianal area is free of tenderness.
Fluid and electrolyte balance is maintained.	Fluid intake equals output; skin turgor is normal; mucous membranes are moist; urine specific gravity is normal; serum sodium and albumin levels are normal.
Patient is free of preventable and treatable skin lesions.	Patient is free of decubiti and other skin breakdown or infection associated with patient's debilitated condition.

→ ⟩ ⟩

PATIENT OUTCOME	DATA INDICATING THAT OUTCOME IS REACHED
Patient or couple has been provided with support and counseling to enable resumption of safe sexual activity or alternative means of sexual satisfaction; patient is treated for anal-genital lesions.	Patient or couple describe methods for safe sexual expression and verbalize intent to use counseling resources as needed; patient is free of treatable anal-genital lesions.

PATIENT TEACHING

HIV testing

Persons who should be voluntarily tested: Anyone being treated for STDs or IV drug abuse, male and female prostitutes, women whose sexual partners are bisexual or have injected drugs, anyone who received a blood transfusion in the United States between 1978 and 1985, and anyone who considers himself or herself at risk.

Additional persons may be tested: Persons planning marriage or a long-term sexual relationship, those in correctional institutions, persons undergoing medical evaluation and treatment for infectious disease, and persons admitted to hospitals.

Pretest counseling

1. Discuss reasons the patient wants the test.
2. Inform the patient that if positive results are obtained with repeated ELISA tests, they will be confirmed with a second test (Western blot).
3. Assess the impact that the test results will have on the patient's life-style, risk behaviors, and psychologic state.
4. Determine whether the patient has a support system that will be available after the test results are obtained.
5. Discuss how the patient plans to handle the waiting time until the test results are available.
6. Instruct the patient to return for the test results; they should not be given over the phone.
7. Inform the patient of the laws in his or her state for reporting positive test results.
8. Give the Patient Teaching Guide, "HIV Testing."

Posttest counseling—negative result

Counsel the patient on behaviors to prevent transmission, even if the test results are negative:

1. Risk can be prevented by:
   Avoiding injecting drugs
   Avoiding vaginal, anal, or oral intercourse and any exchange of body secretions
2. Risk can be lessened, but not prevented totally, by:
   Maintaining a mutually monogamous sexual relationship
   Using latex condoms with 5% nonoxynol-9 from start to finish with each sexual encounter
   Avoiding passing or receiving body fluids (semen, vaginal secretions, blood) during sex
   Not sharing needles for drug use
3. Provide information on alcohol and drug treatment programs

Posttest counseling—positive result

A positive test result does not indicate AIDS but does indicate a 30% to 50% chance of developing AIDS within 7 years after infection. However, if the time of infection is unknown, the patient should be prepared to experience symptoms at any time.

1. Inform the patient that the virus can be transmitted at all phases after infection. Repeat the instructions for reducing the risk of transmission that were provided during pretesting. In addition, caution the patient to avoid sharing personal items that may be contaminated with blood, such as razors or toothbrushes, and to avoid donating blood, tissue, or sperm.
2. Encourage the patient to inform sexual and needle-sharing partners.
3. Counsel women to avoid pregnancy and breast-feeding if they wish to prevent the chance of transmission to offspring.
4. Provide the patient with information on additional counseling and community support services.
5. Counsel the patient to inform his or her physician and dentist of HIV status when seeking care.
6. The person with a positive test result is likely to hear nothing after being given the results of the test.

Schedule a repeat visit as soon as possible for follow-up counseling on maintaining the immune system and improving general health status.

7. Provide information on alcohol and drug treatment programs.

8. Give the Patient Teaching Guide, "When Your HIV Test Is Positive."

Follow-up counseling

1. Instruct the patient on the signs and symptoms of HIV-related illnesses.

2. Encourage the patient to keep a diary of illnesses, treatments, and medications used.

3. Counsel the patient to obtain regular medical care and early treatment of all HIV-related illnesses.

4. Remind the patient to update his or her immunization status.

5. Review basic principles for maintaining health status, such as diet, exercise, rest, avoidance of drugs and alcohol, cessation of smoking, and stress reduction.

6. Instruct the patient on methods to prevent exposure to pathogens:
   - Safe and "safer" sexual practices
   - Avoidance of needle sharing
   - Avoidance of contact with people with infections
   - Avoidance of food-borne infections through proper cooking and handling of food, particularly poultry and shellfish

7. Reteach the patient the proper use of a condom. Give the Patient Teaching Guides, "About Condoms" or "The Female Condom."

8. Respond to questions the patient may have about medical treatment to boost the immune system. Give the Patient Teaching Guide, "Use of Antiretroviral Drugs."

9. Instruct the patient on a balanced program of rest and activity.

10. Teach the importance of good oral hygiene—brushing and flossing after every meal and use of Peridex mouth rinse.

11. Instruct the patient on hygiene and skin care: Use mild soaps; rinse well; avoid powders or alcohol-based products that dry the skin; use lotions liberally; avoid scented products that may induce nausea.

12. Instruct the patient that nutrition is important. The patient should avoid fad diets that are nutritionally limited (e.g., the antiyeast diet and the macrobiotic diet) and avoid megadosing with vitamins, herbs, or other unproven products.

13. Depending on the patient's need for information, give Patient Teaching Guides, "Facts About HIV Infection and AIDS," "When Your HIV Test Is Positive," "Clinical Trials—What Are They?" "Facts About Sexually Transmitted Diseases," and "Food Safety."

Other teaching—depending on symptoms

1. Instruct the patient on prescribed medications, expected effects, dosages, route of administration, side effects, and untoward reactions.

2. Teach the patient these methods to minimize the effects of nausea: Clean the mouth before eating; avoid tepid foods; eat salty foods, which are sometimes less nauseating; avoid odors of food preparation area; eat small meals; eat dry foods in the morning; and avoid drinking liquids with meals. Sucking on hard candy or mints between meals may help prevent nausea.

3. Teach the patient these methods to manage a sore throat and mouth: Use a straw; begin a meal with cold fluids or juices; avoid highly seasoned or acid foods; and rinse the mouth frequently with water during meals.

4. Teach the patient these methods to improve the nutritional value of meals: Fortify meals with high-protein skim milk powder; add milk instead of water in recipes; fortify vegetable and pasta dishes with cheese or ground meat; eat puddings and custards for desert; eat foods with a high potassium content (e.g., bananas).

5. Teach the patient to eat when well-rested to ensure completing the meal.

6. Instruct the patient to prevent cramping by avoiding foods that cause gas, by eating small amounts of food often, and by chewing with the mouth closed to limit swallowing of air.

7. Teach the patient to prevent heartburn by not lying down after eating or by elevating the head of the bed.

8. Teach pursed-lip and diaphragmatic breathing to decrease respiratory effort; teach the patient how to use an incentive spirometer.

9. Depending on the patient's need for information, give Patient Teaching Guides: "Managing Pain Without Drugs," "Fever," "Dealing With Loss of Appetite, Nausea and Vomiting," "Dealing With the Effects of Immune and Bone Marrow Suppression," "Facts About Your Prescription," and "Tuberculosis."

CHAPTER 12

Issues Affecting Women and Injection Drug Users

Deborah L. Brimlow

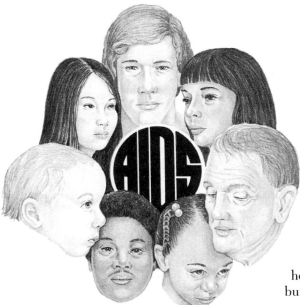

According to the Centers for Disease Control and Prevention (CDC), 58% of adults and adolescents with AIDS in the United States were infected through male-to-male sexual contact. The AIDS epidemic first emerged in the homosexual community, but it is now exploding in other groups; however, homosexual and bisexual men still bear the greatest burden of HIV infection.

In the United States most published research and clinical findings on HIV disease are based on cohorts of homosexual men. It has only been during the past few years that injection drug users (IDUs) and women have been enrolled in clinical trials. Medical management with educated, articulate, affluent, compliant gay men has served as the model for the past 10 years of the epidemic. This has led to difficulties in providing care to other HIV-infected groups, such as injection drug users and women, because they differ radically from gay men. This chapter will focus on HIV infection in women and injection drug users.

WOMEN

EPIDEMIOLOGY

In the United States, women have become the population with the fastest growing rate of HIV infection. As of December 1992, women accounted for 29,477 cases of AIDS reported to the CDC.[27] Women now make up 12% of all AIDS cases. AIDS is the fifth leading cause of death in women ages 25 to 44, and it is the leading cause of death for women in New York and New Jersey. Most women with AIDS are of childbearing age.

Since the beginning of the AIDS epidemic, almost 50% of women with AIDS acquired the infection through their own injection drug use; 35% were infected through heterosexual contact; and 21% acquired the virus through sex with an injection drug user (see the box below). In contrast, only 3% of men were infected heterosexually. Of the women who were reported as having AIDS in 1992, more were infected through heterosexual contact than through IDU for the first time.[27]

Women of color are disproportionately represented in reported AIDS cases, as shown in the box on this page. African-American women make up 53% of AIDS cases, and Hispanic women account for 21%. Injection drug use and heterosexual contact are the major risk behaviors for women of color.

Most women with AIDS live in large metropolitan areas, especially cities along the East Coast. However, the proportion of women with AIDS in rural areas increased from 22% to 28% in 1990.

Underreporting of AIDS cases remains problematic, and for women it is especially troublesome. Until the 1993 revisions, the CDC's AIDS case definition was not specific to women, and underreporting was estimated at 12% to 20%. The 1993 revisions include cervical cancer as an AIDS-defining condition (see inside front cover).

Almost no data are available on lesbian transmission, or female-to-female sexual transmission, of HIV. Lesbians account for less than 1% of AIDS cases in women reported to the CDC. Of these cases 95% occurred among IDUs, and the remainder are attributed to receipt of contaminated blood or blood products. The CDC's definition for a case of female-to-female transmission is particularly exacting. A lesbian must have had no sexual contact with a male since 1978. If she has had such contact, she is classified as bisexual. In attempting to rule out confounding factors, the CDC has created a standard that is almost impossible to meet.

Recent surveys by the CDC and state and local health departments suggest that female-to-female sexual transmission of HIV is probably rare, but that bisexual women run a higher risk of HIV infection.[127] Some case histories in the literature suggest that transmission between women can occur in connection with traumatic sex.

See Table 12-1 for information on factors associated with heterosexual transmission of HIV.

DISEASE MANIFESTATIONS AND PROGRESSION

Most of the current knowledge about the natural history of HIV disease is based on studies of large cohorts of gay men. Data on the natural history of HIV disease in women are urgently needed.

A number of reports suggest that particular AIDS-defining diseases are more common in women than in men. Case reports have identified wasting syndrome, esophageal candidiasis, *Mycobacterium avium* complex (MAC) infections, and herpes simplex virus infection as more common in women.[69,154] Kaposi's sarcoma (KS), an AIDS-defining illness, is rare in women. The few studies done on Kaposi's sarcoma in women with AIDS show that only an estimated 1% to 3% of HIV-positive women have developed KS in the United States or Europe.[99,105] In women Kaposi's sarcoma is diffuse and progressive and may be associated with severe immunodepression. Women with Kaposi's sarcoma more often report sexual contact with a bisexual man than do women with other AIDS-defining conditions.[12] See Table 12-2 for the top 10 presenting conditions for women with AIDS in the United States in 1992.

GYNECOLOGIC CONDITIONS

Across all stages of HIV infection, women commonly have non-AIDS-defining gynecologic conditions. One of the initial presenting symptoms for many HIV-infected

---

EPIDEMIOLOGY OF HIV IN WOMEN

- Number of women infected*:
  140,000 HIV infected
  29,477 with AIDS
- Race:
  75% women of color
  25% white
- Mode of transmission:
  50% injection of illicit drugs
  4% blood transfusions
  35% heterosexual contact†

Data from the Centers for Disease Control.[27]
*As of December, 1992.
†The fastest growing mode of HIV transmission.

Table 12-1

HETEROSEXUAL TRANSMISSION OF HIV: ASSOCIATED FACTORS

Factor	Male-to-female	Female-to-male
Lack of condom use	Yes	Yes
Anal intercourse	Yes	No
Sex during menses	No	Yes
Number of sexual contacts	Yes	Yes
Advanced disease state (as measured by CD4+ count, p24 antigen test, or AIDS diagnosis)	Yes	Yes
AZT*	Possibly	Unknown
Genital sores, infections, or inflammations	Yes	Yes
Oral contraceptives†	Yes	Unknown
IUD use	Possibly	Unknown
Cervical ectopy	Yes	Unknown

Adapted from Wofsy et al.[171]

*Possibly protective, because AZT decreases the viral load.

†Whether oral contraceptives are protective or increase the likelihood of transmission is controversial.

Table 12-2

WOMEN WITH AIDS: TEN MOST FREQUENTLY REPORTED AIDS-INDICATOR DISEASES*

Rank	Diagnosis	Percent of patients†
1	*Pneumocystis carinii* pneumonia	43
2	HIV wasting syndrome	21
3	Esophageal candidiasis	21
4	HIV encephalopathy	6
5	Herpes simplex infection	6
6	Toxoplasmosis of the brain	6
7	*Mycobacterium avium* complex (MAC)	6
8	Extrapulmonary cryptococcosis	4
9	Cytomegalovirus disease	3
10	Cytomegalovirus retinitis	3

From the Centers for Disease Control.[27]

*Reported in the United States in 1992.

†Some women had multiple diagnoses.

women is vaginal candidiasis. Chronic vaginal candidal infections have been reported among HIV-infected women with CD4+ counts over 500/mm³.[95] Viral infections, such as those caused by the herpes simplex virus (HSV) and the human papillomavirus (HPV), are commonly observed, as are pathologic conditions of the cervix. Other early signs of HIV in women may include any of the following: recurrent or severe pelvic inflammatory disease (PID), extensive genital warts, or an abnormal Pap smear.[91,110,127,139] The box on the next page presents potential indicators of HIV infection in women.

HIV-related immunosuppression has been associated with the human papillomavirus (HPV), resulting in increased clinical severity, disease recurrence, lack of disease regression, and shortened survival. It has also been associated with neoplasia of the lower genital tract (cervical, vulvar, and perianal cancer), as discussed in Chapters 6 and 10.

Menstruation

Data on the menstrual experience of HIV-infected women are scarce. Unpublished data from a pilot study

```
┌─────────────────────────────────────┐
│  POTENTIAL  INDICATORS  OF          │
│  HIV  INFECTION  IN  WOMEN          │
└─────────────────────────────────────┘
```

- Gynecologic infections*:
  Candidiasis
  Pelvic inflammatory disease (PID)
- Human papillomavirus (HPV) infection
- Genital ulcers
- Cervical dysplasias and genital warts (HPV)
- Opportunistic infections (OIs):
  Pneumocystis carinii pneumonia (PCP)
  Herpes simplex virus (HSV) infection
  Cytomegalovirus (CMV) infection
- Pneumonias
- Sepsis

*Includes changes in severity, frequency, and resistance to therapy.

of women attending a clinic in Brooklyn show that most of the women reported a variety of menstrual disorders, ranging from irregular, excessive, or painful bleeding to scanty or infrequent bleeding. In HIV-positive women, menstrual irregularities are caused by a variety of factors, which could include pregnancy and menopause, HIV itself, antiretroviral drugs such as zidovudine/AZT and ddI, drugs for opportunistic infections (OIs), cancer therapies, street drugs such as heroin and crack cocaine, methadone treatment, and chronic disease.

Heavy menstrual bleeding can increase the irregularities in blood that occur in HIV disease or as a side effect of zidovudine/AZT. As with HIV-negative women, it is important to conduct a thorough assessment that includes a menstrual history, complete blood count, and nutritional history.

If a woman with abnormal bleeding is over 35 years of age, a sample of cells from the lining of the uterus (the endometrium) should be taken in order to rule out the presence of abnormal cells that may cause cancer.[99]

Pregnancy

Perinatal transmission of HIV, also referred to as vertical transmission, is the transmission of HIV from mother to infant. There are three major routes of vertical transmission: (1) in utero, (2) perinatally during delivery, and (3) postnatally through breast-feeding. The estimates of the rate of vertical transmission in the United States and Western Europe range from 13% to 55%.[6,63] The rate is most commonly reported as 30%, which is the figure used in counseling HIV-infected women of childbearing age. Initially, all babies born to infected women test positive due to the presence of

maternal antibodies. True HIV infection of the infant is confirmed at approximately 15 months of age.

The risk factors for perinatal transmission are not well understood. Current research suggests that the rate of transmission may be related to the mother's stage of disease, with transmission more likely in the later stages. According to the clinical markers that are significant for HIV-infected pregnant women, low CD4+ counts and positive results on p24 antigen tests are associated with higher rates of perinatal transmission.[118]

Pregnancy has not been found to have an effect on the clinical progression of HIV disease when compared to the expected effect of time. The effect of repeated pregnancies on disease progression has yet to be determined.[6,63]

There is no evidence that a cesarean section delivery is safer than a vaginal delivery. Data from the 1992 European Collaborative Study suggest that a cesarean section may have a protective effect against vertical transmission.[63]

Several cases of HIV infection occurring through breast-feeding have been reported, and breast-feeding is contraindicated in HIV-infected women who have access to infant formula.[3,39]

Menopause

Premature menopause appears to be more common in immunosuppressed women. Hormone replacement may be necessary for severe symptoms of menopause such as hot flashes, vaginitis, urethritis, vaginal dryness, itch, and discomfort during urination. In HIV-infected women, symptoms such as hot flashes may be worse at night. Health care providers may mistake these for night sweats caused by tuberculosis or *Mycobacterium avium* complex (MAC). Vaginitis and urethritis may be wrongly diagnosed as thrush/candidiasis.[55]

Hormone Therapy in Transsexuals

Hormone therapy in preoperative and postoperative transsexuals is an issue that clinicians must consider. Transsexuals are frequently at risk of HIV infection if not already infected. Individuals may have had surgical castration with vaginal reconstruction and/or breast implants. Hormones are necessary to maintain the desired secondary sexual characteristics such as enlarged breasts, lack of facial hair, and change in voice quality. The prescribed estrogen doses are far greater than the estrogen doses found in oral contraceptives and estrogen replacement drugs. Denenberg suggests that the clinician supply hormone replacement and work to reach the minimal dosage needed to achieve desired effects.[55]

MANAGEMENT OF HIV INFECTION IN WOMEN
Diagnostic Considerations

It is extremely important to screen and treat HIV-infected women for sexually transmitted infections and other gynecologic infections, particularly vaginal candidiasis. Screening for cervical dysplasia and malignancy is also very important. Studies suggest that the prevalence of cervical dysplasia increases dramatically, especially in women with CD4+ counts below 200/mm^3. Regular pelvic examinations with Pap smears are indicated. Pap smears at 6-month intervals are suggested by some experts for women with low CD4+ counts.[117] In HIV-infected women the Pap test by itself may not reliably detect lower genital tract abnormalities such as neoplasia. Colposcopy with biopsy every 6 months is recommended by some clinicians experienced in treating HIV.

In women whose serostatus is unknown, referral for HIV counseling and testing is appropriate when any of the following conditions is present: persistent, recurrent, or unusually severe vaginal candidiasis; recurrent or unusually severe genital herpes simplex infection; genital ulcer disease (e.g., syphilis, chancroid); recalcitrant or multisite condyloma acuminatum; evidence on a Pap smear of moderate to severe cervical dysplasia, carcinoma in situ, or squamous cell carcinoma; persistent or recurrent PID; and pregnancy—regardless of the health care provider's or woman's perception of risk.[1] See the box below for suggestions on the management of HIV infection in women. Because half the cases of AIDS in women have occurred through injection drug use, a thorough history of drug use should be obtained on every woman diagnosed as HIV infected. Conversely, women reporting injection drug use should be counseled to receive HIV testing.

Treatment Considerations

Both therapy with zidovudine/AZT and prophylaxis against *Pneumocystis carinii* pneumonia (PCP) are recommended for pregnant, HIV-infected women whose CD4+ counts are below 200/mm^3.[117,149] Sperling and colleagues reported that zidovudine was well tolerated in a study of 43 pregnant women, and no adverse effects were observed in the infants.[150] Other antiretroviral drugs such as zalcitabine (ddC) and didanosine (ddI) have not been studied in pregnant women. See Table 12-3 for information on the use of therapeutic drugs during pregnancy.

Reducing the Risk of HIV Transmission

Current literature suggests that the fertility rates of HIV-infected women do not differ significantly from demographically similar uninfected women.[147] Barrier protection methods are promoted in most discussions of

---

MANAGEMENT OF HIV INFECTION IN WOMEN

- Assess the risk of HIV infection:
  Consider every woman a candidate
  Obtain sexual and gynecologic history
  Screen for high-risk behaviors
- Offer testing:
  Women with high-risk behaviors
  Women with potential indicators
- Provide pretest counseling:
  Confirm the presence of risk behaviors
  Confirm the presence of potential indicators
  Evaluate the availability of support systems (e.g., financial, emotional, medical) should the patient test positive
  Discuss confidentiality issues
  Set a time for the patient to return for test results
- Provide posttest counseling:
  Explain ways to avoid further HIV transmission
  Teach safer sex guidelines
  Provide guidance on whom to inform about the patient's condition
  Explain the nature and current management of HIV infection
  Explain how to maintain or obtain health insurance
- Offer early treatment with zidovudine to HIV-infected patients, whether symptomatic or asymptomatic, who have a CD4+ count of 500 cells/mm^3 or lower.

---

safer sex. However, for women who want protection from pregnancy, these barrier methods have a user failure rate that is markedly higher than that of several nonbarrier methods. HIV-infected women may request oral contraceptives in order to have more control in preventing pregnancy. However, use of the pill does not offer protection from HIV transmission; safer sex and the use of latex barrier protection (condoms and dental dams) are still necessary. Health care providers have been concerned about the effect of the method of contraception on the natural history of HIV disease. There are reports from outside the United States that prostitutes who use oral contraceptives are more likely to acquire HIV.[129] These data do not generalize to the population of HIV-infected women in the United States. No data are available on possible adverse interactions of the pill and antiretroviral drugs such as zidovudine/AZT.[117] However, the pill has been shown to interact with other drugs, such as antibiotics, barbiturates, anticonvulsants, Valium, oral antidiabetics, prednisone, antihypertensives, and acetaminophen.

Table 12-3 _____

MANAGEMENT OF HIV DISEASE IN PREGNANT WOMEN

Drug	FDA pregnancy category	Use in serious disease*
Acyclovir	C†	Yes
Amikacin	D	Traditionally avoided in early pregnancy
Amphotericin B	B	Yes
Ciprofloxacin	C	Avoid
Clindamycin	N/A	Yes
Clofazimine	C	No experience
Clotrimazole oral troche	C	Yes
Clotrimazole vaginal suppository cream	B	Yes
Dapsone	C	Yes
ddC (zalcitabine)*	C	No experience
Didanosine (ddI)*	B	No experience
Ethambutol	N/A	Yes
Fluconazole	C	No experience
Ganciclovir	C	No experience
Isoniazid	N/A	Yes
Ketoconazole	C	No experience
Pentamidine IV	N/A	Avoid in preference to alternatives
Pentamidine inhaled	C	Little systemic absorption; no experience
Primaquine	N/A	Avoid
Pyrazinamide (PZA)	N/A	Avoid
Pyrimethamine	C	Possibly
Rifampin	C	Yes
Sulfadiazine	N/A	Yes
Trimethoprim	C	Seldom indicated alone
Trimethoprim/sulfamethoxazole	C	Yes
Zidovudine (AZT)	C	Yes

Adapted from Wofsy.[171]
Updated 3/19/93 by Community Provider AIDS Training Program HIV Consultation Line (800) 933-3413.
*For life-threatening condition or serious indication.
†*N/A*, Classification not available. *A*, Controlled studies in women demonstrate no fetal risk. *B*, Animal studies demonstrate no fetal risk but there are no human trials, or animal studies demonstrate a risk not corroborated by human trials. *C*, Animal studies demonstrate fetal risk but there are no human trials, or neither human nor animal studies are available. *D*, Evidence exists for fetal risk in human—benefit may outweigh the risk. *X*, Evidence exists for fetal risk in humans—benefit clearly outweighed by risk.

For women with HIV disease, the usual precautions about the pill apply. For example, the pill should not be prescribed to women with liver dysfunction, because hormones are metabolized in the liver.

In addition to contraception, HIV-infected women may benefit from oral contraceptives in other ways. The pill is associated with regular, reasonably short and light menstrual periods. HIV-infected women who are anemic may benefit from this effect.

Longer acting hormonal contraceptives such as levonorgestrel implants (Norplant) and injections of medroxyprogesterone acetate (Depo-Provera) have not been evaluated for safety and potential drug interactions. There is no literature to suggest increased risk from their use in HIV-infected women.[99]

SOCIAL ISSUES

Women with AIDS/HIV: Vector or Vessel?

In our society women tend to be a forgotten group in the AIDS epidemic. Women differ from the groups initially affected by HIV and AIDS not only by gender, but also by race or ethnicity, socioeconomic status, and risk behaviors. Many people still think of AIDS as a disease that affects only two groups, men who have sex with men and injection drug users, but current AIDS statistics contradict that bias. From the beginning of the epidemic, women have been treated as vectors of disease who can transmit the virus to men and children, and as vessels who carry HIV-infected babies. The media often refer to HIV-infected children as innocent victims. This results in blaming the mother for the birth of an infected baby because of perinatal transmission.

Because HIV-infected women differ so much from other groups affected by HIV disease, they face an array of barriers to receiving care that are just now being recognized and addressed. For example, when women are infected by HIV, it is likely that the entire family is infected. Women are usually the caregivers in their families, often caring for their husbands and children while putting their own health care needs aside. They also face discrimination on the basis of gender and reproductive potential when they try to enroll in substance abuse treatment, HIV drug treatments, and clinical trials.

Until recently, women with HIV disease were studied only because of their potential to spread the virus to others. There were no natural history studies of HIV in women until 1992, when the CDC initiated a pilot study. The National Institutes of Health (NIH) funded natural history studies of HIV in women in 1993. Women were not enrolled in HIV-related clinical trials until Protocol 076 from the NIH was launched. This study looked at pregnant women and the use of zidovudine in attempts to avoid perinatal transmission. Until this study, women, particularly pregnant women, had been excluded from clinical trials because of their childbearing potential. The first study to exclusively involve women was one that viewed women as vessels. The focus of the research was the "innocent victim," the child.

Survival Rates in Women Versus Men

Higher mortality and lower survival rates have been reported for women with AIDS compared to men.[7,138] This may be partially explained by the higher proportion of IDUs among women, as discussed earlier in this chapter. In addition, women may be diagnosed later in the course of the disease than men, because physicians and other health care providers often do not consider AIDS as a possible diagnosis. Some studies suggest that HIV disease progresses more rapidly in women than in men. However, an alternative explanation is that women's decreased access to care and delayed treatment may account for this shorter survival. When access to health care is equal, HIV disease seems to progress at the same rate in both sexes. Until the 1993 revisions, the CDC's AIDS definition did not include illnesses that affect women earlier in the course of HIV disease. As a result, women who were diagnosed with

AIDS before 1993 may have been at a later stage of clinical and immunologic deterioration. This may account for the seemingly shorter survival following an AIDS diagnosis.

Women with HIV and AIDS have most of the same manifestations as men, but they also have high rates of gynecologic disorders. These gynecologic conditions frequently are not recognized by clinicians as being HIV related, and this lack of recognition can delay diagnosis and treatment. Because health care providers tend to avoid recommending HIV testing to women and fail to diagnose HIV disease in women, infected women do not receive early intervention that could prevent or slow the progress of the infection. The above factors, along with the demographic characteristics of HIV-infected women (predominantly poor and from racial or ethnic minority groups), have resulted in a disenfranchised, medically disadvantaged population.

Reproductive Rights and Responsibilities of HIV-Infected Women

The policy issues involving HIV-infected women and their reproductive rights and responsibilities continue to be debated. Hutchinson and Kurth outlined the following unspoken assumptions in current policy constructions regarding HIV and reproduction: (1) Women's reproductive decision making is understood well. (2) Reproductive decision making follows a cognitive model; thus, giving a woman the facts about HIV will lead to an "informed" decision. (3) Abortion is the "right" decision in the context of HIV. These researchers stress that clinicians may have strong beliefs about what an HIV-infected woman should do about a pregnancy, but clinicians should weigh the concept of pregnancy decision making as a woman's free choice against the alternatives of directive counseling, forced sterilization, or involuntary quarantine.[94]

INJECTION DRUG USERS

EPIDEMIOLOGY AND TRANSMISSION

Injection drug use accounts for almost one quarter of diagnosed AIDS cases in adults and adolescents in the United States and constitute the second largest transmission group. Heterosexual contact with an injection drug user can result in additional AIDS cases. Almost half of women with AIDS were infected with HIV through their own injection drug use, and more than 20% were infected through heterosexual contact with an injection drug user. Almost 60% of pediatric AIDS cases occur in children of injection drug users or their sexual partners. More than 80% of pediatric AIDS cases are children of color, either African-American or Hispanic.[27]

The term *injection drug use (IDU)* has replaced the term *intravenous drug use (IVDU)*, because researchers in the AIDS epidemic have discovered that drug users inject in a variety of ways—intravenously, intramuscularly, or subcutaneously. Needle drug use is not limited to illicit street drugs such as cocaine or heroin; steroids and amphetamines are also injected.

Transmission through injection drug use is related most often to intravenous injection of drugs. Cross-infection through needle sharing usually occurs as the result of a procedure called "booting," or "kicking." The drug user draws blood back into the barrel of the syringe and then injects. This procedure serves two functions. One, the drug user can determine if the needle is in the vein. Two, the blood drawn back into the syringe picks up whatever drug might remain in the syringe, and it is then injected. After this procedure is performed, both the needle and the syringe retain some of the user's blood, which will then be injected into the others who share the needle.

DISEASE MANIFESTATIONS AND PROGRESSION

Injection drug users, as well as other substance users, may have compromised immune systems. In people who already have compromised immune systems as a result of drug use, the introduction of HIV infection may accelerate the disease process. Immunosuppression in drug users may result from a number of variables. It may be due to the immunosuppressive properties of the drugs used, such as heroin, cocaine, or alcohol. Theoretically, ongoing antigenic stimulation and consequent immunosuppression may occur as a result of multiple infections associated with injection of nonsterile water, contaminated diluents, impure narcotics, and the use of needles contaminated with blood and dirt.[68] Also implicated are coinfections, such as viral hepatitis, and sexually transmitted diseases (STDs), such as gonorrhea, syphilis, chlamydia, and trichomoniasis. Substance users have higher rates of both sexually transmitted diseases and infections associated with injection drug use, such as endocarditis, tuberculosis, and hepatitis.[89]

Chemical immunosuppression may be due to physician-prescribed or self-medicating use of antibiotics for numerous infections. Additional factors that may compromise the immune system are sleep deprivation and chronic malnutrition. Drug use can suppress the appetite, and alcohol can impair absorption of food.[90]

It appears that the time from HIV infection to development of AIDS in IDUs is similar to that of other adult HIV-infected populations. Selwyn and colleagues reported that predictors of the progression to AIDS in IDUs included the presence of oral candidiasis or bacterial infections, declining CD4+ cell counts, and the absence of AZT therapy. In their study, beta$_2$-microglobulin was not an independent predictor of progression to AIDS, in contrast to findings in HIV-infected gay men. Flegg and coworkers have suggested that beta$_2$-microglobulin levels may be elevated in drug users, whether or not they are HIV infected, as a result of immune stimulation produced by the injection of foreign antigens and/or from increased infections. HIV-infected IDUs have a lower incidence of Kaposi's sarcoma, herpes simplex infection, and cytomegalovirus infection than do homosexual men.

Several studies have reported an association between continued intravenous drug use and an increased risk of disease progression for HIV-infected IDUs compared to IDUs who stopped using drugs.[162,163] However, Selwyn and colleagues found no consistent relation between continued use of injection drugs and the progression to disease.[146] Looking at other substance use, Brown and co-workers reported greater declines in CD4+ cells of cocaine users compared to nonusers.[23]

Survival following diagnosis of AIDS in IDUs is also similar to survival in other adult HIV-infected populations of the same gender and with the same AIDS-defining condition. Selwyn and colleagues identified bacterial infections as a significant cause of pre-AIDS morbidity and mortality among injection drug users.[146] Differences in availability and access to clinical care contribute to differences in survival rates.

WOMEN WHO ARE DRUG USERS

HIV-infected women who use drugs have many issues in common with other HIV-infected women, but they also have unique concerns. For example, female IDUs may have an infected needle-sharing sexual partner. They may also give birth to a baby who is either drug addicted or HIV infected, or both. These women tend to feel that mainstream society judges them harshly and treats them as throwaway people.

Contributing to this perception, some HIV-infected female IDUs support themselves, their habit, and their family by exchanging sex for either money or drugs. Traditionally this has been labeled prostitution; however, a better term might be survival sex. Because these women have no other marketable skills or means of support, they may continue to barter sex for money or drugs for as long as possible. Also, many people think only of women when they hear the term prostitution, but men and women, boys and girls trade their bodies for money or drugs. Treatment of the primary disease, drug addiction, and referral for social services may reduce the risk of transmission through prostitution.

For HIV-infected women who are drug users, reproductive and family planning issues are complicated.

When women are counseled that the odds of giving birth to an HIV-infected infant are about 30%, these odds may appear much better than what they experience in everyday life. The risk of having an HIV-infected baby may appear small when the desire to have a child is great. For women who already have children, some may have lost custody of them because of their drug use, abuse, or neglect. Child care and foster care may be unavailable or unaffordable for women who want to enter drug treatment programs or residential treatment facilities. Karan and Hoegerman provide an excellent discussion of the medical, psychologic, and social issues involved in understanding and working with the substance-using, HIV-infected woman.[98]

MANAGEMENT OF HIV-INFECTED IDUs

Health care providers are seeing increasing numbers of HIV-infected drug users in both inpatient and outpatient settings. The treatment and management of HIV-infected IDUs may be frustrating for health care providers for a number of reasons. Drug users tend to use services only when in crisis. Instead of seeking health care preventively or at the first sign of a problem, drug users may wait until the problem is overwhelming. Also, drug users are well known for being unreliable and noncompliant with appointments and treatment regimens. Finally, health care providers are concerned that taking care of drug users increases their own exposure to tuberculosis and HIV infection. They are especially concerned about noncompliance with tuberculosis treatment regimens (see Chapter 9) and with the increased risks involved in performing invasive procedures on intoxicated and/or combative patients.

IDUs are typically viewed by clinicians as manipulative, self-destructive, antisocial, violent, and drug seeking. As a result, drug users are frequently treated disrespectfully by health care providers. The emergence of HIV infection in IDUs has only worsened their treatment in many settings. It is this disrespectful treatment, even more than a lack of health insurance or funds, that makes the drug user reluctant to seek health care.

A number of excellent resources offer strategies for managing HIV-infected IDUs.[103,151,161] To work effectively with this group of patients, a nonjudgmental approach and good relationship skills are important. These skills include empathy, legitimation, respect, support, and partnership.[124]

Along with adopting a nonjudgmental or neutral stance, it is critical that the health care provider set limits. Patients in the clinical setting must be made aware that illicit drug use will not be tolerated. It is common for relatives or friends of the patient to bring drugs into the hospital setting. Additionally, violence,

threats of violence, and abusive or threatening language should not be tolerated. The patient should be informed that he or she will be discharged if this occurs. If the patient acts unacceptably, possible actions to implement include restricting the patient to the floor or room, limiting visitors, screening incoming packages, and performing urine toxicology screens.

The health care provider must try to avoid struggles over medications. The patient may request particular drugs in an attempt to continue his or her substance use. Wartenberg recommends that the health care provider order drugs that do not alter mood and are less addicting, such as nonsteroidal antiinflammatory drugs, and low-dose sedating antidepressants for sleep.[161] It is never a good idea to start a patient with a drug habit on methadone if he or she is not already enrolled in a methadone program. These approaches may have to be modified when dealing with a dying patient who needs pain control.

Dealing with the IDU's Self-Medication

Treatment of HIV-infected drug users is complicated by their tendencies to self-medicate. Problems occur when the nonprescribed drugs negatively interact with the prescribed drugs. These nonprescribed drugs can include antibiotics, benzodiazipines, methadone, cocaine, heroin, and others, which are bought on the street. Some drug users who cannot get into drug treatment programs may buy methadone on the street and attempt to treat themselves. Antibiotics are bought on the street in an attempt to treat abscesses or sexually transmitted diseases (STDs).

Excessive use or abuse of immunosuppressant drugs can affect the immune system. Many drugs are immunosuppressants, including alcohol, marijuana, tobacco, and steroids. In addition, drug users' lives are often chaotic and marked by poor nutrition, stress, lack of health care, and sleep deprivation.

Drugs That Interact with Methadone

Some medications prescribed for HIV-related diseases in drug users may interact with methadone treatment. Rifampin for tuberculosis and phenytoin for epilepsy are two examples of drug interactions that require methadone dosage adjustments. Zidovudine does not appear to interact with methadone.[44,145] Patients may confuse some zidovudine-associated side effects with similar symptoms of opiate withdrawal (e.g., insomnia, nausea). This may affect compliance with the treatment regimen.

Treating the IDU with Multiple Illnesses

In addition to HIV infection, drug users may have multiple illnesses. It is important for health care providers to recognize that the primary disease is drug addiction/

dependency. Drug users should be referred for specialized treatment and relapse prevention. Unless the underlying problem is addressed, all other treatment attempts will fail. IDUs and other drug users should be screened for STDs, hepatitis B, and tuberculosis. Dual diagnosis is frequently seen in drug users. Preexisting personality and affective disorders may be present. Cognitive deficits from years of drug use may be a problem as well.

Pain Management

Adequate pain management is essential for drug users, especially if they are HIV infected. Drug users are at higher risk of suicide if they have poorly controlled pain. The problems of unrelieved pain coupled with the punitive actions of health care providers can provoke suicide attempts and completions. Frequently, health care providers withhold pain medications from drug users because they are perceived to be manipulative around drugs, particularly narcotics. The health care provider may be attempting to set limits or is angrily asserting control over the drug-using patient. However, dosages of pain medications that may be adequate for other patients will not be enough for drug users with a current addiction. HIV disease can result in a painful death, which is made more agonizing by the lack of attention to pain control.

Risk Reduction

Drug use often results in disinhibition and impaired judgment. This can increase HIV-related risk behaviors such as unsafe sexual activity, needle sharing, and use of contaminated drug paraphernalia, including needles, syringes, rinse water, cottons, or cookers (spoons or bottle caps used to prepare or cook drugs). Engaging in risky behavior can lead to HIV exposure, infection, or reinfection.

Sometimes it is difficult to reach drug users with HIV information and education. One innovative and effective strategy has been to train indigenous outreach workers to provide information to drug users in their environment. Indigenous workers are often members of the same community who are of similar race or ethnic background; some are recovering drug users or addicts. For drug users who are in treatment, their best sources of information may be located in drug or alcohol treatment programs. HIV prevention and risk-reduction services such as risk assessment, counseling, and on-site HIV testing may be offered. Program staff can refer drug users for off-site HIV testing if necessary. Treatment program staff members are usually aware of clients who are HIV infected. They can help counsel and monitor clients who are struggling with drug dependency and HIV infection.

Counseling to prevent transmission of HIV through injection drug use

Although the easiest path to counseling injection drug users may appear to be advising them to quit or to seek substance abuse treatment, this is almost certain to fail. Most of the time, an injection drug user has a long history of drug use, as well as a physiologic and/or psychologic addiction. In addition, in many places substance abuse treatment is unavailable or unaffordable. Waiting lists, scarce resources, and indigence all act as barriers to drug treatment.

One clear message to give IDUs is that, if needle drugs are going to be used, the safest choice is to always use new sterile needles, syringes, and other injection equipment (cookers, cotton, etc.). Another safe choice is to never share equipment. To reduce HIV transmission among people who share injection drugs, instructions should be given about cleaning needles, syringes, and paraphernalia. Bleach disinfection is a method of reducing the risk of HIV infection from reusing or sharing needles and syringes. Recommendations on how bleach disinfection should be done were issued jointly by the CDC, the Center for Substance Abuse Treatment (CSAT), and the National Institute on Drug Abuse (NIDA).[53,116] These recommendations resulted from research that showed that a 10% dilution of household bleach (0.5% sodium hypochlorite) was not effective in removing blood from syringes using a 6-second rinse with bleach, followed by two 6-second rinses with water. Clotted blood was harder to clean from syringes than fresh blood.[48] The authors warn that cleaning needles and syringes with disinfectants, such as bleach, does not guarantee that HIV is inactivated. Disinfectants do not sterilize needles and syringes, but consistent and thorough cleaning of injection equipment with disinfectants such as bleach should reduce HIV transmission if equipment is shared.

Curran and colleagues offer the following provisional recommendations on the best procedures for bleach disinfection:

1. Clean needles and syringes twice—once immediately after use and again just before reuse.
2. Before using bleach, wash out the needle and syringe by filling them several times with clean water. (This will reduce the amount of blood and other debris in the syringe. Blood reduces the effectiveness of bleach.)
3. Use full-strength liquid household bleach (not diluted bleach).
4. Completely fill the needle and syringe with bleach several times (some suggest filling the syringe at least three times).
5. Allow the bleach to remain in the syringe for a time. The longer the syringe is completely full of

bleach, the more likely it is that HIV will be inactivated. (Some suggest the syringe should be full of bleach for at least 30 seconds.)

6. After using bleach, rinse the syringe and needle by filling them several times with clean water. Do not reuse the water used for the initial prebleach washing; it may be contaminated.

7. For every filling of the needle and syringe with prebleach water, bleach, and rinse water, fill the syringe completely (to the top).

8. Shake and tap the syringe while it is filled with prebleach wash water, bleach, and rinse water. Shaking the syringe should improve the effectiveness of all steps.

9. Take the syringe apart (remove the plunger); this may improve the cleaning and disinfection of parts (e.g., behind the plunger) that might not be reached by solutions in the syringe.

Health care providers can address a number of concerns for injection drug users. For example, carrying a bleach bottle does not constitute drug paraphernalia. However, IDUs should not be advised to carry clean needles at all times; this could result in arrests for possession of drug paraphernalia. IDUs can put together their own disinfection kits using small shampoo sample bottles, but they should make sure that the cap has a foil insert to prevent the bleach from weakening the cap.

It may be helpful to review local laws and regulations that affect needle and syringe availability and possession.[25] Access may be limited by federal and state laws, which include (1) prescription laws that require a physician's prescription as a condition for pharmacy sale of needles and syringes (in 11 states and the District of Columbia) and (2) drug paraphernalia laws that attach criminal penalties to the possession and distribution of needles and syringes (in about 44 states and the District of Columbia).

Referral for drug treatment

The most accessible resources for drug users may be 12-step programs such as Alcoholics Anonymous, Narcotics Anonymous, and Cocaine Anonymous. These programs are abstinence based and may prohibit methadone clients from attending.

Many urban areas have drug treatment programs or community-based organizations that work with drug users. HIV and AIDS services can frequently be found through these groups, which also may offer educational materials or programs. Health care providers can refer patients and clients to these programs or can request in-service programs from them. They may provide strategies for managing drug users.

Some cities, such as Seattle, have needle exchange programs that are run by Street Outreach Services. Injection drug users can exchange used needles for clean ones. New York City has experimented on a small scale with needle exchange programs. Currently, certain federal statutes prohibit using funds received from some federal programs to distribute needles or syringes for illegal drug use (e.g., Substance Abuse Prevention and Treatment Block Grant, 42 U.S.C. 300 × 31 and the Ryan White Comprehensive AIDS Resources Emergency Act, 42 U.S.C. 300 ff).

Drug users are often viewed as manipulative, self-destructive, violent, antisocial people. They are frequently blamed for their addiction and viewed as "guilty" victims of HIV and AIDS. Clinicians have to set aside these attitudes in order to successfully treat IDUs. Direct, nonjudgmental, nonmoralistic behaviors are most effective when working with drug users.

CHAPTER 13

Law, AIDS, and Nurses

Carl Hacker
Julie Watson

This chapter will examine the rights provided and duties imposed by the law for a nurse practicing where there are individuals infected with HIV. To identify these rights or duties in a particular circumstance, we look to two sources of law. One source, common law, is made by judges, who rely upon precedent, or past, cases to decide the outcome of the case before them. Common law can be used to anticipate the outcome of future lawsuits or court actions.

The second source of law, statutory law, is created by state or federal legislatures. These elected bodies derive their power from a constitution, which also places limits on the power of the legislature to direct individual actions. Because the U.S. Constitution prohibits the enacting of laws that make past actions unlawful, statutory law applies to the future. The activity proscribed by a statute and the range of penalties are known in advance.

This review begins with the questions that arise when the nurse is confronted with a patient infected with HIV. We then discuss the rights and duties that a nurse infected with HIV has relative to the uninfected patient and the nurse's employers. One must recognize that there are several kinds of nurses, several kinds of employers, and several kinds of patients, all of whom are subject to different state laws. Therefore, a short review cannot delve into all possible contingencies. This chapter is intended to familiarize the reader with the kinds of questions a nurse should ask in this area. It cannot, however, provide specific answers to all questions or be a comprehensive review of the law affecting nurses and the HIV infected.

THE NURSE AND THE HIV-INFECTED PATIENT

PROVIDING CARE TO HIV-POSITIVE PATIENTS

Many HIV-infected individuals have experienced discrimination by health care providers because of their infection. These individuals state that it is frequently difficult to obtain health care even when cost is not a factor. Some health care professionals are unwilling to expose themselves to the risks encountered from treating AIDS patients. This raises the question of whether a nurse must provide care to anyone seeking health care, or whether the nurse may be selective in deciding to whom he or she may provide care.

Under common law a nurse has no duty to render nursing care until there is a relationship to provide such care established between that patient and the nurse. This means, for example, that a nurse on encountering an accident is under no duty to stop and render aid to any of the victims, even if the nurse is specifically qualified in emergency treatment. Statutory law, however, may take precedence over common law.

There are both federal and state statutes guaranteeing civil rights to individuals that make it unlikely a health care worker will be completely free to exclude patients solely because they are HIV positive. For example, in *Minnesota v. Clausen*, a court of appeals in Minnesota ruled that a dentist was guilty of discrimination when he refused to provide a routine examination and teeth cleaning to a patient who was HIV positive. The patient was awarded $10,000 in damages and the dentist was assessed a $5,000 civil penalty, because the dentist violated the state's discrimination law.

The patient had been treated by the dentist from 1986 to 1990. When a new medical history given in 1989 disclosed the patient was HIV positive, the dentist referred the patient to the dental clinic at the university. The dentist argued that he transferred the patient to protect his employees' health and because of his lack of knowledge about the disease. Witnesses for the state testified that where a dentist used universal precautions, the evidence showed that risk was minimal. The court found that the dentist's reasons for transferring the patient to the university had little or no medical basis and were merely a pretext for discrimination.

The Minnesota statute that prohibits a dentist (and by extension other health care workers and health care institutions) from excluding patients who are HIV positive applies only to health care workers who practice in Minnesota. However, many other states have similar statutes. In addition, the Americans with Disabilities Act (the ADA), a federal statute, applies to virtually all health care workers no matter in what state they practice. This federal statute is intended to eliminate dis-

crimination against an individual because of his or her disability. HIV disease is explicitly named as a disability in the regulations promulgated under this statute. This statute is recent in its enactment and is intended and expected to have a major effect on employers. The ADA and its predecessor, the Rehabilitation Act of 1973, greatly limit the freedom of health care professionals to decide whom they will treat. These statutes will be discussed at greater length below when we look at the relationship between an HIV-positive nurse and the nurse's employer.

Where a nurse is working as an employee of a physician or health care institution, the employment contract will lay out the conditions of employment for the nurse. It is unlikely that a nurse would be able to negotiate a contract that excluded providing care to an HIV-infected patient. If the nurse's employer accepts patients who are HIV positive, then the nurse employee is required to provide care. The state and federal statutes discussed above require the likely employers of nurses to care for HIV-infected individuals. Therefore, because it will be very difficult to find a health care employer whose patients are all free of HIV, nurses probably will be unable to refuse to care for HIV patients.

GAINING A PATIENT'S INFORMED CONSENT FOR HIV TESTING

Most persons seeking health care recognize and expect that they will be asked to undergo one or more tests for diagnostic and treatment purposes. Nonetheless, all competent persons have a right to privacy, bodily integrity, and individual autonomy. These rights place a burden on health care providers to obtain an informed consent prior to carrying out any medical procedure. To provide an informed consent, a patient must have reasonably complete information about the proposed medical treatment. This means the patient must be warned of the risks associated with the treatment, the alternate methods of treatment, and the benefits of the treatment proposed. With respect to HIV testing, informed consent is particularly important. A person could have various reasons for refusing HIV testing. These reasons range from simply not wanting to know one's HIV status to fear of discrimination. Whatever the reason, gaining informed consent is an important concept.

Consent to a procedure need not be written and may even be implied, but a signed form seems to be a common practice in health care institutions today. These forms vary from giving general consent when a patient is admitted to a hospital to consenting to undergo a very specific surgery. A signed form stating that the patient consents to treatment might not always persuade a jury that the patient was giving an informed consent, so care must be taken in preparing these forms. This is especially true when testing the HIV status of a person.

For example, a person consenting to have blood drawn is usually not told that concentrations of several chemicals, as well as the activity of selected enzymes, will be measured, and that these may uncover a condition that is not apparent from the general symptoms the patient has reported. Whether the diagnosis comes back as diabetes or hemochromatosis, the patient, who is likely to be distressed by either one of these conditions, still is not likely to complain about not giving an informed consent. This may not be the case for a person who discovers, unexpectedly, that he or she is HIV infected. This is due to the consequences of infection being so devastating. Therefore, the prudent health care worker should get a written consent on a detailed form specifically requesting consent for HIV testing. This consent might have to be kept in a file that is separate from the general medical record so as to protect the patient's privacy. (See Chapter 2 for a more complete discussion of HIV testing.)

MANDATORY TESTING OF PATIENTS

Early during the AIDS epidemic, there was a call for mandatory testing of certain subgroups of the population. Such testing raises complex ethical and legal issues that continue to be debated by policymakers. Several states have enacted statutes that temper the common law of informed consent as it applies to HIV testing. These statutes affect what testing can be done and what must be done with the results of a test. Therefore, the health care worker must look to the law of the state where she or he is practicing when deciding whether and how to test a patient. Unfortunately, these statutes are not always a part of a comprehensive legislative scheme to deal with the AIDS epidemic, so they must be interpreted thoughtfully. In addition, the Centers for Disease Control has published guidelines and policies for testing that are regularly revised. These may be at variance with a state's statutes.

What if a health care provider refuses to provide medical care unless the patient undergoes HIV testing? Here again the health care worker should look to state law to determine if a statute or court decision provides an answer. For example, in New York, the state's Division of Human Rights ordered a dentist to pay $25,000 in damages to a patient for refusing to continue her treatment unless she had an HIV test. The patient had scheduled appointments for a root canal, but when the patient told the dentist's receptionist that her sister had died of AIDS, the dentist cancelled her appointment and refused to further treat her unless she had an HIV test. The Division of Human Rights held that suggesting an HIV test, with no legitimate medical reason for doing so, was discriminatory.

COUNSELING THE PATIENT

The relationship between health care worker and patient generally encompasses the ethical duty to provide counseling. Several states have imposed by statute an affirmative duty to counsel a patient when ordering an HIV test that goes beyond this general duty. For example, Texas law requires an immediate opportunity for individual, face-to-face counseling before a positive result can be released to a person. This counseling must include the meaning of the test result, the possible need for additional testing, measures to prevent the transmission of AIDS, the availability of appropriate health care services and social and support services in the geographic area of the person's residence, the benefits of partner notification, and the availability of partner notification.

PROTECTING THE CONFIDENTIALITY OF A PATIENT'S HIV STATUS

As a general rule, a patient's medical record is confidential. Only persons involved in the medical care of the patient should have access to the record. Anyone who allows an unauthorized disclosure of information from a patient's record may be liable to the patient under various causes of actions, the most likely being an invasion of privacy.

There are strong public policy concerns that support the protection of confidentiality rights of an HIV-positive individual. Assurance of confidentiality will encourage voluntary testing, so that individuals can learn of their status, make proper decisions regarding treatment, and adjust behavior that may place others at risk. Protecting confidentiality will also improve the professional relationship between the health care worker and the patient by encouraging open communication.

The consequences of disclosing a person's HIV status can cause prejudice and discrimination. The unauthorized disclosure could injure a person in major ways such as loss of employment, cancellation of insurance, eviction from a residence, and possible abandonment by family and friends. A health care worker has not only the usual moral, ethical, and legal duty not to disclose general medical information, but is also under a special obligation to protect confidentiality concerning the HIV status of a patient. This is not only because of the policy reasons mentioned above, but also because of the severe discriminatory consequences that may cause harm to the patient. Some states have statutes that provide further sources of protection against unauthorized disclosure of information about a patient's HIV status that go beyond a general right to privacy guaranteed by the U.S. Constitution and many state constitutions. Some of these statutes allow criminal damages to be assessed against the wrongdoer.

The New York case of *Doe v. Roe* illustrates how a

state statute protects the confidentiality of medical records. In *Doe*, the plaintiff, a flight attendant who was employed by a commercial airline, sought medical treatment for ear and sinus problems. In the course of the medical consultation, the plaintiff informed the physician that he was HIV positive. The plaintiff specifically asked the physician to protect the confidentiality of this fact, because he was concerned that its release would jeopardize his employment.

Several months later the plaintiff filed a claim for workmen's compensation, claiming that the problem for which he had sought treatment was work related. The physician submitted the plaintiff's medical records to the workmen's compensation board, and in the course of the investigation, information about the plaintiff's HIV status was disclosed. The plaintiff subsequently sued the physician for breach of confidentiality.

The New York court determined that the physician's disclosure of the plaintiff's HIV status violated the confidentiality provisions of New York public health laws. The court discussed at length the importance of confidentiality with regard to HIV and AIDS. It stated that the maximum confidentiality protection for information related to HIV infection and AIDS is an essential public measure.

Where the confidential relationship between a health care provider and patient has been breached, a court may sometimes allow an award of punitive damages. For example, in *Doe*, the court awarded punitive damages to the plaintiff even though the particular statute involved did not expressly authorize such damages. The court stated that the award of punitive damages advances the New York legislature's strong public policy of protecting the confidentiality of a patient's HIV status. Nonetheless, the court clarified this proposition by stating that punitive damages should be imposed only when it can be shown that a defendant's conduct is so reckless or grossly negligent that it amounts to a conscious disregard of another's rights.

Maintaining confidentiality is sometimes difficult. Staff workers are often curious and may gossip as they carry out their duties. Whereas a patient's diabetic condition does not raise much interest and may not have much potential for going beyond the staff, the HIV status of a patient raises many concerns, and knowledge of a patient's condition can quickly spread within an institution, even to the clerical staff, who have no direct contact with the patient.

The chances of breaching the confidentiality of a patient's condition can be greatly reduced by proper office and institutional policies regarding HIV testing. Developing such policies is not alone sufficient—they must be enforced. Failure to do so subjects individuals and institutions to liability. Health care workers must be informed of the civil and criminal liabilities that can follow the breaching of a confidential relationship.

DISCLOSING THE RESULTS OF AN HIV TEST

Although confidential, the results of an HIV test may, under appropriate circumstances, be disclosed to parties other than the patient. Generally, the staff of the health care institution who are involved in the care of the patient must know the patient's HIV status if that knowledge is necessary to the proper management of the patient's care. Care must be taken to make certain that this information is restricted to those who have a need to know. Gossip and idle conversation about HIV status do not benefit either the patient or the staff and open individuals and institutions to the very real possibility of being liable for damages.

Many states have reporting requirements imposed on those who order tests for HIV status. Twenty-five states now require the reporting, by name, of HIV-positive test results to public health authorities. The requirement of reporting by name allows health authorities to eliminate duplicate case reports. Other states require the number of positive tests, but not the names, to be reported. These results may be used for contact tracing, statistical reporting, and epidemiologic studies.

What might seem to be a simple reporting requirement by a state agency to aid in its tracking and study of the AIDS epidemic can give rise to complex legal issues and undesirable social outcomes. For example, the Pennsylvania Department of Health is currently asking medical laboratories to report names of patients who have blood cell counts low enough to signal a possible AIDS infection. This is an attempt by the state to keep track of the spread of the disease according to the revised 1993 CDC definition of AIDS. Critics of the state action have argued that reporting such cases by name will violate individual privacy rights and may have the effect of discouraging people from having testing done.

WARNING THIRD PARTIES

When a health care worker knows the patient is HIV positive, but the patient does not yet have the symptoms of the disease, the health care worker faces a difficult decision. If the health care worker reveals the patient's condition to others, the confidentiality of the health care worker/patient relationship is destroyed. It is foreseeable that the patient could possibly infect a third person, such as a spouse or sexual partner or other hospital workers who are in contact with the patient. What then is the duty of a health care worker to warn third parties about the HIV status of a patient?

Some state courts have found an exception to the general duty imposed on a health care worker to hold information about a patient in confidence. This exception typically arises when a therapist is treating a dangerous patient who might harm himself or a third party. The first case in this line is *Tarasoff v. Regents of the University of California*, where the California Supreme Court found that a psychiatrist treating a mentally ill patient has a duty to take reasonable care to warn third parties who might be threatened by foreseeable danger arising from his patient's condition.

Under what circumstances courts will find that being HIV positive forms a foreseeable danger to a threatened third party must await the development of case law. Some state legislatures have already addressed this issue. For example, in Texas, state law allows a health care worker to release the result of a positive test to the spouse of an HIV-positive person, but does not impose a duty to do so.

FOLLOWING THE PATIENT'S WISHES: LIVING WILLS AND DURABLE POWERS OF ATTORNEY

Living wills and durable powers of attorney are common examples of advance directives that individuals can use to make decisions pertaining to health care matters. They are legal instruments that allow individuals to express decisions regarding medical treatment should they become physically or mentally incapacitated. The majority of states recognize various forms of advance directives. In general, they are looked upon favorably by the law because they provide mechanisms to avoid conservatorship proceedings and give increased control over the decision-making process to the patient.

Living wills are legal instruments that allow a competent adult to designate the specific treatment he or she would wish to receive in the event of terminal illness or incompetence. A majority of the states have enacted statutes that recognize living wills. These laws are based on constitutional rights to privacy and individual autonomy. They are generally known as "right to die" laws.

Despite the benefits of living wills, they do have several disadvantages. The greatest drawback is that they can be inflexible and, in some circumstances, inadequate. The living will is unlikely to account for all the circumstances that may arise. If the living will does not provide for a specific situation that has in fact occurred, then the wishes expressed in the document may not be followed. It is very difficult, if not sometimes impossible, to foresee the specific situations that may arise as well as the specific treatment one would choose to have or forgo if terminally ill.

Another disadvantage of living wills is that they ordinarily will not become effective until the patient becomes terminally ill. This should be an important concern to an HIV-infected person, considering the many opportunistic infections the person could possibly encounter that may or may not result in incompetence or a terminal condition.

Yet another drawback to living wills is that a person's physician may be unwilling to carry out the intentions expressed. A living will has the effect of absolving a physician of criminal or civil liability for the act of withdrawing or withholding life-sustaining treatments, but it does not compel a health care worker to act. Some physicians, nonetheless, may be reluctant to comply with the patient's request because of personal ethical or moral beliefs.

Because of the disadvantages listed above, it is highly advisable to prepare a power of attorney for health care decisions along with the living will. Typically a power of attorney is a way of dealing with such matters as transactions for accounts at financial institutions, preparing and filing tax returns, buying and selling property, and general business transactions. Historically, a person was not able to delegate authority to others for decisions that were more personal in nature, such as medical decisions. Many states have bypassed this problem by creating laws that specifically authorize durable powers of attorney for health care decisions.

A durable power of attorney for health care decisions is an authorization for a person to act on behalf of another person. This power of attorney is termed "durable" because it remains valid despite the patient's incompetence. This legal document allows the patient to designate a person who can act as his or her agent for the patient's health care decisions. The agent steps into the shoes of the patient to make decisions on his or her behalf according to either the known desires or the best interests of the patient. The powers granted may be narrowly defined to cover specific treatments or may be very broad in nature. For example, the agent might be empowered to make decisions regarding life-sustaining treatment, invasive procedures, or access to medical records.

In states that do not have statutes recognizing a power of attorney for health care decisions, the power of attorney might still be used. Most health care providers will accept the proxy decision maker who has been designated by the incapacitated person. The patient's wishes, nonetheless, do need to be expressed clearly and unambiguously.

When preparing either a living will or durable power of attorney, one must be aware of the requirements of the state statute in one's particular state because these laws will vary. The execution of these documents requires certain formalities. For example, many state laws require the documents to be in writing and witnessed by disinterested persons. Some states require the use of a particular form. If the living will or durable power of attorney does not meet the particular requirements expressed by the state statute, it may be ineffective.

THE HIV-POSITIVE NURSE

In the first part of this chapter, we discussed several questions that arise when a health care worker cares for an HIV-infected patient. We now move to the perspective of the nurse as the person who is HIV positive and look at how this infection affects the nurse's rights and duties. We begin with the concerns of a patient being cared for by an HIV-positive nurse. We finish by considering the concerns that the nurse or the institution employing an HIV-positive nurse might have about rights and liabilities.

THE PATIENT AND THE HIV-POSITIVE NURSE

A nurse may have a common law duty to disclose his or her HIV status as well as a duty to be tested to determine this status. This duty could potentially be found in a lawsuit between an HIV-positive nurse and a patient where the nurse provided care without disclosing his or her HIV status. This area of the law is just beginning to emerge and bears close scrutiny.

In recent years members of both the American Medical Association and the CDC have deliberated the ethical and professional standards that would apply to infected health care workers. The CDC recommended in 1991 that health care workers who are infected with HIV should not perform exposure-prone procedures unless they have notified prospective patients of their seropositivity. From these deliberations a court could easily find that public policy imposes a duty upon health care workers both to know their HIV status and to obtain an informed consent before treating patients.

The law of informed consent requires a health care provider to tell the patient of any risks that may be material to the patient. A risk is material when a reasonable person would attach significance to the risk in deciding whether to forgo the proposed treatment. If the health care worker does not inform the patient of the risk of HIV transmission, a court might find that the health care worker acted negligently and, therefore, award damages to the patient for actual injuries.

A health care worker who does in fact know that he or she is HIV positive and who intentionally fails to inform the patient may be liable to the patient for battery and may be required to pay punitive damages. For example, in *Kerins v. Hartley*, a patient sued her surgeon after she discovered that the surgeon had performed her surgery while infected with HIV. The patient had specifically discussed with the surgeon her fear of con-

tracting AIDS from a blood transfusion and even stored some of her own blood in case it was needed. She additionally questioned the doctor about his health, at which time he failed to inform her of his HIV status. The court held that the surgeon's performance of an invasive surgical procedure, at a time when he knew he was HIV infected, constituted a technical battery, because there was an intentional deviation from the consent given.

In many states, courts will allow recovery for emotional distress arising from the fear of future disease. These courts focus their attention on the probability of developing a disease and the length of time involved before contracting the disease. To have a cause of action against a health care worker for emotional distress for the fear of contracting AIDS, a patient must prove (1) actual exposure to the AIDS virus, (2) actual physical injury, and (3) some form of physical manifestation of emotional distress. The majority of jurisdictions do not allow damages for this cause of action unless the plaintiff can further show it is more probable than not that one would actually develop the disease. Generally, in emotional distress lawsuits, the "physical manifestation" requirement has been used by the courts to thwart fraudulent claims. Courts deciding AIDS phobia–type cases have been more liberal in requiring a physical manifestation of disease.

To prevail on an emotional distress claim, the patient must present medical evidence or expert testimony establishing that the fear caused is reasonable. In determining the reasonableness of fear, courts do not require proof that the AIDS virus has been actually transmitted. Instead, the court will focus on the time period involved in which a patient could develop AIDS after exposure. If the patient subsequently tests negative, the court will look at the time period for a "reasonable window of anxiety." Specifically, this would be the time period from when the patient learns of the care provider's HIV-positive status to the time the patient receives his or her HIV-negative test results. For example, in the *Kerins* case the court pointed out that the fear of developing AIDS becomes unreasonable after the plaintiff has had sufficient opportunity to find, with reasonable medical certainty, that he or she has not been exposed to and/or infected with HIV.

In *Faya v. Almaraz*, two patients sued their HIV-positive surgeon, contending he breached a duty either to warn them of his infectious condition or to refrain from operating on them. The court held that they were entitled to seek damages for their fear of acquiring AIDS and did not have to prove actual transmission of the disease. The patients learned of the surgeon's HIV status approximately 1 year after the performed surgeries. At that time they were tested, and the results were negative. Because the court found the possibility of contracting AIDS beyond a year following exposure to be extremely unlikely, it held that the patients would be able to recover damages for their fear and its physical manifestations only for the period extending from when they learned of the surgeon's illness until they received their negative results.

To date these kinds of claims have involved health care providers who were performing exposure-prone invasive procedures. It is unresolved in the law whether a nurse performing noninvasive procedures would be required to inform a patient of his or her HIV status. Typically, to succeed on a claim for lack of informed consent or emotional distress, the patient would have to prove actual exposure to the AIDS virus. If a nurse is following universal precautions, such proof of actual exposure would be extremely difficult. Additionally, it has been shown that the risk of transmission of the AIDS virus during a patient's treatment is very low. Thus, courts should find that the fear of infection is speculative and unreasonable for noninvasive procedures.

THE EMPLOYER AND THE HIV-POSITIVE NURSE

Besides the issue of the nurse's liability for infecting patients, there is the issue of the liability of the nurse's employer following a nurse-to-patient transmission. The employer's liability for such an occurrence can be costly, so it would seem that employers who provide health care would want to reduce their risk by excluding HIV-positive persons from their staff. To do this, though, the employer must overcome several legal obstacles, the most significant of which are the Rehabilitation Act of 1973 and the Americans with Disabilities Act of 1990 (ADA). These statutes, which are intended to integrate those with handicaps and disabilities into the American work force and other institutions, have a major effect on many functions carried out by federal agencies and those receiving federal funds, and by employers generally. HIV infection is considered to be a condition that is covered by both of these statutes.

The Rehabilitation Act of 1973

The Rehabilitation Act of 1973 prohibits discrimination based upon a handicap or perceived handicap in a federally funded program or activity. To establish that an employer has violated the act, the nurse must claim (1) to be a handicapped individual under the statute, (2) to be otherwise qualified for participation in the program or activity, (3) to have been excluded from the program or activity solely by reason of a handicap, and (4) that the program or activity received federal financial assistance. As with most statutes, more than a simple reading of the act is necessary to apply the law, so we will examine now how several of these terms are defined and used.

Who must abide by the Rehabilitation Act?

The act applies to federal agencies, federal contractors, and programs that receive federal financial assistance of any kind. These programs include hospitals receiving Medicare funds, and independent contractors who provide services to, and have a close financial nexus with, a federally funded employer. Some private employers may also be covered by another section of the act that requires nondiscrimination and affirmative action by federal contractors and subcontractors to employ and advance individuals with disabilities. Given the present and projected federal involvement in health care financing, the act would seem to cover almost all employers of nurses.

Who is a handicapped person?

A handicapped person under this statute is any person who (1) has a physical or mental impairment that substantially limits one or more of the person's major life activities, (2) has a record of such impairment, or (3) is regarded as having such impairment. The Rehabilitation Act does not explicitly label HIV infection as a protected handicap, and before 1988 the courts were divided about whether HIV infection was considered to be a handicap under the Rehabilitation Act. In *School Board of Nassau County v. Arline*, a schoolteacher had been discharged from her job because she had tuberculosis. The U.S. Supreme Court held that the Rehabilitation Act prohibited discrimination based on the contagious effects of a disease. While the court did not consider whether a person with AIDS or HIV infection could be handicapped under the act solely based on contagiousness, cases from lower courts after *Arline* have held that these persons are handicapped under the act. In addition, a 1988 Department of Justice opinion stated that AIDS is a handicap, and an asymptomatic HIV carrier is protected under the Rehabilitation Act so long as the person is otherwise qualified.

What is meant by "otherwise qualified"?

To be considered "otherwise qualified" under the act, a person must be physically and mentally able to perform the essential functions of the activity with reasonable accommodation and must not create a health or safety risk to others that cannot be eliminated through reasonable accommodation. Reasonable accommodation can include physical adaptation of a facility to make it accessible to handicapped workers, job restructuring, reduced or modified work schedules, and equipment for handicapped workers. The nature and cost of these accommodations are also considered when deciding what is reasonable.

To determine whether the risk of contagion is significant enough to render a person not "otherwise qualified," the U.S. Supreme Court in *Arline* listed four factors that need to be considered: (1) the nature of the risk (how the disease is transmitted), (2) the duration of the risk (how long the carrier is infectious), (3) the severity of the risk (what is the potential harm to third parties), and (4) the probability that the disease will be transmitted and will cause varying degrees of harm. The court also stated that a person who poses a significant risk of communicating the disease to others is not "otherwise qualified" if the risk cannot be eliminated through reasonable accommodation.

The Rehabilitation Act would seem to prohibit most discrimination against an asymptomatic HIV carrier by an employer. An asymptomatic person would still be able to perform the essential functions of the position. Also, there is no significant risk of transmission in most employment circumstances. The same HIV-infected person would not be "otherwise qualified" as the disease progresses and there are frequent absences or significant diminution of physical or mental abilities.

A 1988 Department of Justice memorandum states that when there is a greater possibility that HIV infection could be transmitted, treating some HIV-infected employees differently may be justified. Where a legitimate concern for the health and safety of others exists, an HIV-infected person cannot be protected from discrimination based upon the handicap. The difficulty occurs in deciding what is legitimate.

When would discrimination occur "solely by reason of the handicap"?

To be covered by the Rehabilitation Act, the discrimination must occur "solely by reason of the handicap." Illustrative of this point is the Fifth Circuit case of *Leckelt v. Board of Commissioners of Hospital District No. 1.* Leckelt, a nurse, refused to submit his individual HIV test results to the hospital where he was employed. After being discharged Leckelt sued the hospital under the Rehabilitation Act. The court held that a plaintiff must show that the handicap was the *sole reason* for the termination decision. The hospital had a legitimate interest in maintaining infection control policies, and the plaintiff failed to comply with these policies. Therefore, Leckelt was not terminated *solely* because he was perceived to be infected with HIV.

How is the statute applied?

How this act is applied is illustrated by the case called *In the Matter of Westchester County Medical Center.* In this case a licensed pharmacist ("Doe") applied for and accepted a job with Westchester County Medical Center. As part of a preemployment examination, the examining physician discovered that Doe's medical records showed he was HIV positive. The doctor diagnosed Doe as suffering from AIDS-related complex and would not permit him to work for the hospital.

Doe filed a complaint with the New York Division of Human Rights, charging employment discrimination, and after an investigation, the division held that the hospital was discriminating against Doe. The hospital subsequently offered to hire Doe with restrictions, but Doe, unsatisfied with the restrictions placed upon the employment terms, filed a complaint with the U.S. Health and Human Services' Office of Civil Rights (HHS), claiming discrimination based on handicap, in violation of the Rehabilitation Act. The HHS asked Westchester to hire Doe back with no restrictions on his duties and with compensation for lost wages. The hospital refused, and HHS filed an administrative complaint against Westchester.

The judge found (1) that Westchester received federal financial assistance within the meaning of the Rehabilitation Act (in fact, 40% of Westchester's budget came from federal funding), (2) that Doe's HIV-positive status qualified him as an individual with a handicap within the criterion set by the statute, and (3) that he did not constitute a direct threat to the health and safety of others, nor would he be performing invasive procedures on patients (in fact, he would have no direct contact with patients at all). The judge then ruled that the hospital was required to treat Doe as it would treat any professional pharmacist on the staff. To ensure that this happened, the judge terminated all federal financial assistance to the hospital until Westchester satisfied HHS that it was in compliance with the Rehabilitation Act. The loss to the hospital was estimated to be about 40% of its annual budget. The hospital subsequently agreed to hire Doe without restriction. Under the agreement Doe was awarded damages for back pay, legal fees, and emotional distress.

The Americans with Disabilities Act

The Rehabilitation Act of 1973 left many disabled individuals unprotected from discrimination, because it applied only to federal agencies, those contracting with the federal government, and those receiving federal funds. Discrimination in most of the private sector was restricted only by state laws, and few states had antidiscrimination statutes when the Rehabilitation Act was passed. Some states soon enacted laws prohibiting discrimination based on handicap that covered both public and private sectors, but protection against discrimination was still limited and uneven. This led to support for comprehensive federal legislation in this area.

The Americans with Disabilities Act (ADA) was passed on July 12 and 13, 1990, and was signed into law by President George Bush on July 26, 1990. The ADA is a comprehensive antidiscrimination statute that combines the principles of nondiscrimination developed under the Rehabilitation Act with the remedies available under Title VII of the Civil Rights Act of 1964, which are intended to help induce compliance with the act. It is applicable to employment, public accommodations, transportation, and telecommunications.

The ADA is designed to remove barriers that prevent qualified individuals with disabilities from enjoying the same employment opportunities that are available to persons without disabilities. The act defines a qualified individual with a disability to be:

an individual with a disability who meets the skill, experience, education, and other job-related requirements of a position held or desired, and who, with or without reasonable accommodation, can perform the essential functions of a job.

The act ensures access to equal employment opportunities based on merit. It does not guarantee equal results, establish quotas, or require preferences favoring individuals with disabilities over those without disabilities. If a person has a disability and that disability creates a barrier to employment, the employer must consider whether reasonable accommodation could remove the barrier. The employer has to assess the disabled person's ability to perform the essential functions of the job, and the disabled person must be able to perform those essential functions.

The ADA enables disabled persons to compete based on the same performance standards and requirements that employers expect of nondisabled persons. If the person's disability impedes job performance, the employer must reasonably accommodate the person to overcome the impediment unless to do so would pose undue hardship on the employer. The accommodation should be tailored individually to the needs of the disabled person in order to accomplish the job's essential functions.

The U.S. Equal Employment Opportunity Commission (EEOC) is responsible for enforcement of the employment provisions of the ADA. The EEOC issues interpretive guidance materials to ensure that qualified individuals with disabilities understand their rights and also to encourage and facilitate compliance. An individual with a disability who feels he or she has experienced employment discrimination can file a claim with the EEOC. Remedies may include compensatory and punitive damages, back pay, front pay, restored benefits, attorney's fees, reasonable accommodation, reinstatement, and job offers.

Private employers, state and local governments, employment agencies, labor unions, and joint labor-management committees must comply with the employment provisions of the ADA. The definition of "employer" incorporates persons who are "agents" of the employer, such as managers, supervisors, foremen, or others who act for the employer. Thus, the employer is responsible for the actions of such persons who may violate the ADA.

What is a "disability" under the ADA?

Disability is defined as (1) a physical or mental impairment that substantially limits one or more of the major life activities of the individual, (2) a record of impairment, or (3) being regarded as having an impairment. Congress intended that the relevant case law developed under the Rehabilitation Act be generally followed under the ADA. As with the Rehabilitation Act, the terms in this definition require interpretation, which follows.

Physical or mental impairment. The phrase "physical or mental impairment" refers to any physiologic disorder or condition, cosmetic disfigurement, or anatomic loss affecting one or more of several body systems, or any mental or psychologic disorder. This includes a physiologic disorder or condition affecting hemic or lymphatic body systems. The legislative history of both the ADA and EEOC regulations explicitly identifies HIV infection and AIDS as disabling impairments.

An impairment that substantially limits one or more major life activities. An impairment is a disability if it substantially limits one or more of the individual's major life activities. Major life activities are those basic activities that the average person in the general population can perform with little or no difficulty. HIV limits an infected person's major life activities of procreation and intimate sexual relationships.

There is no laundry list of impairments under the ADA. An impairment may be disabling for one person but not for another. Multiple impairments that combine to substantially limit one or more of an individual's major life activities also constitute a disability. HIV infection is inherently substantially limiting. Temporary, nonchronic impairments of short duration are not disabilities.

To determine if an impairment is a disability, the following factors must be considered: (1) the nature and severity of the impairment, (2) the duration or expected duration of the impairment, and (3) the permanent or long-term impact of the impairment. These factors must be considered because, generally, it is not the name of an impairment or a condition that determines whether a person is protected by the ADA, but rather the effect of an impairment or condition on the life of a particular person. Some impairments, such as blindness, deafness, HIV infection, or AIDS, are by their nature substantially limiting. Many other impairments may be disabling for some individuals but not for others, depending on the impact on their activities.

The determination of an impairment is made individually without regard to mitigating measures such as medicines or prosthetic devices. The person does not have to be totally unable to work in order to be considered substantially limited in the major life activity.

Persons having a record of impairment. The ADA

covers persons who have recovered from an impairment or who have been misclassified as having an impairment. The intent of this provision is to ensure that people are not discriminated against because of a history of disability or because they have been misclassified as disabled. This category is not likely to apply to HIV-infected individuals, because testing for antibodies is relatively accurate. Conversely, an HIV test that falsely indicates HIV infection could cause an individual to be misclassified as disabled.

Persons being regarded as having an impairment. A person who is regarded by an employer as having an impairment that substantially limits a major life activity is a person with a disability. This applies even if the person does not have the impairment but is being stereotyped by the employer. If a person can show that an employer made an employment decision because of a perception of disability based on "myth, fear, or stereotype," the person will satisfy the "regarded as" part of the definition of disability. For example, if an employer discharged an employee based only upon a rumor that the individual was HIV positive, but the person did not have any impairment, then that person is being treated as though the person had a substantially limiting impairment.

Homosexuality and bisexuality are not considered impairments and so are not covered by the ADA. Nonetheless, if a gay person is regarded as being HIV-positive and is discriminated against on that basis, then the person is covered under the ADA.

There are three basic ways in which a person may satisfy the definition of "being regarded" as having a disability. First, the person may have an impairment that is not substantially limiting, but it is perceived by the employer as constituting a substantially limiting impairment. An example could be controlled high blood pressure. Second, the person might have an impairment that is only substantially limiting, but because of the attitudes of others toward the impairment, the person is regarded as having a substantially limiting impairment (for example, a facial scar, disfigurement, or involuntary jerk). Third, the person may have no impairment at all but is regarded by the employer as having a substantially limiting impairment. For example, a person is fired because of a rumor that the employee is HIV infected. This person would be considered an individual with a disability, because the employer perceived of this person to be disabled.

The disabled person must be a *qualified individual*

To be covered by the ADA, a person has to be qualified for the job. The ADA definition of qualified is "an individual with a disability who, with or without reasonable accommodation, can perform the essential functions of the employment position that such individual holds or desires." There is a two-step determination for deciding if an individual is qualified. First, it must be determined if the person has the prerequisites for the position. This encompasses a review of the person's educational background, employment experience, skills, and licenses. The person has to have the necessary educational background, employment experience, and skills to qualify for the job, regardless of the disability. Second, there must be a determination of whether the person can perform the essential functions of the position held or desired, with or without reasonable accommodation.

An employer cannot use employment standards or screening tests to screen out disabled individuals. The standards or tests have to be job related and consistent with normal business practices. Medical examinations or inquiries as to whether an applicant has a disability are not allowed by the ADA. The rationale of this restriction is to prevent inquiries unrelated to a legitimate business purpose. If an employer requires testing for AIDS, the employer would have to show that testing for HIV infection is job related and consistent with business necessity.

What are the "essential functions of the job"?

The person must be able to perform the essential functions of the position with or without reasonable accommodation. To determine which functions of the position are essential, the following factors should be considered: (1) whether the employer actually requires presently employed workers in the position to perform the functions, (2) whether others are available to perform that function, and (3) what degree of expertise or skill is required.

Evidence of an essential function can be established by the employer's own judgment. This could be a written job description prepared before seeking applicants for the job. The amount of time spent on the job performing the function, the consequences of not requiring the person to perform the function, the work experience of past employees in the job, and the current work experience of employees in similar jobs are all relevant in determining if the function is essential. Also, the terms of a collective bargaining agreement are important considerations.

What is a "direct threat to the health or safety of others"?

To be qualified under the ADA, the person must not pose a direct threat to the health or safety of other individuals in the work environment. The inquiry to be made is whether potential risks can be eliminated through reasonable accommodation. A "direct threat" refers to a "significant risk of substantial harm to the health or safety of the individual or others that cannot be eliminated or reduced by reasonable accommodation." The decision on whether a person poses a direct threat should be made individually. There should be an assessment based upon reasonable medical judgment that relies on the most current medical knowledge or on the best available objective evidence.

A health or safety risk can only be considered if it poses a significant risk of substantial harm. An employer cannot deny employment merely because of a slightly increased risk. Factors to consider should include the duration of the risk and the nature and severity of the potential harm. The likelihood that the potential harm will occur should also be taken into account. Additionally, the imminence of the potential harm should be considered. Consideration must rely on objective, factual evidence—not on subjective perceptions, irrational fears, patronizing attitudes, or stereotypes—about the nature or effect of a particular disability. For example, an employer may believe there is a risk in employing an individual with HIV disease as a teacher. Because there is little or no likelihood that employing this person as a teacher would pose a risk of transmitting this disease, an employer who uses this belief to decide not to hire this teacher would violate the act.

What is a "reasonable accommodation"?

The employer has to offer a "reasonable accommodation" to the disabled employee unless the employer can show the accommodation would impose an "undue hardship" on the operation of the business. An accommodation is any change in the work environment or in the way things are customarily done that enables a person with a disability to have equal employment opportunities. Reasonable accommodation includes making facilities accessible; restructuring jobs; reassigning disabled employees to vacant positions; modifying work schedules; acquiring or modifying equipment or devices; adjusting or modifying examinations, training materials, or policies; and providing qualified readers or interpreters.

Reasonable accommodation is unnecessary if it would pose an undue hardship for the employer. An undue hardship means, with respect to the accommodation, a significant difficulty or expense incurred by a covered entity. There is no bright-line test under the ADA as to what constitutes an undue hardship.

The accommodation will depend upon the person's physical condition and the nature of the employment position. Asymptomatic HIV-infected persons will be able to perform essential functions of most jobs, and an employer's claim of undue hardship is likely to fail. Yet, accommodating an individual with full-blown AIDS might cause undue hardship on an employer because of frequent absences or loss of mobility.

Reassignment to a vacant position is a potential form of "reasonable accommodation," but it is available only to current employees and not to applicants. An applicant for a position must be qualified for, and be able to perform the essential functions of, the position sought with or without reasonable accommodation. Reassignment should be considered only when accommodation within the person's current position would pose an undue hardship. An employer cannot reassign an individual to undesirable positions in an effort to circumvent the ADA. Only a reassignment to a comparable position is allowed. An employer does not have to promote an employee as an accommodation.

Association with a disabled person

The ADA protects against discrimination of a qualified person who associates with someone with a disability. It is unlawful for a covered entity to discriminate against a qualified person because of the known disability of a person with whom the qualified individual has a family, business, or social or other relationship. An example could be where a person who does volunteer work for AIDS victims is fired because the employer is afraid the employee may contract AIDS. Also, a person living with someone who has AIDS would be protected from discrimination by the ADA.

In summary, the ADA does not guarantee an HIV-infected nurse employment as a health care worker. It does prohibit an employer from dismissing or refusing to hire the HIV-positive nurse solely because of the infection. The nurse must be qualified for the job and be able to perform its essential functions, and the employer may need to make reasonable accommodation so that the nurse can carry out these functions. Fulfilling these requirements may be increasingly difficult as the course of infection progresses. For example, if the disease results in frequent tardiness or diminishment in mental capacity, the nurse will no longer be able to perform these functions nor will the employer be able to provide a reasonable accommodation.

The nurse's condition must not be a direct threat to the health and safety of others (i.e., it must not pose a significant risk or result in substantial harm). While there could be concern if a nurse is participating in an invasive procedure, other duties may not create an obstacle to continued employment. As the disease progresses and the HIV-infected nurse becomes symptomatic, the risk of error in performing medical procedures may be increased. An assessment of whether this increases the threat of substantial harm to others must be based on objective evidence. It must not be based on speculation or merely a slight increase in risk. Succinctly, under the ADA, deciding when an HIV-positive nurse may no longer be allowed to work as a health care worker must be done individually and with care.

Infection Control

Individuals who have HIV infection are highly likely to have infectious diseases, some of which could be transmitted to others, including health care workers. In addition, immunocompromised individuals can become seriously or even fatally ill from infectious agents that are benign, self-limiting, or easily treatable in the non-HIV-infected person. Preventing transmission of pathogens to patients is always desirable in the health care setting, but it is critical when caring for HIV-infected individuals.

The basic principles for controlling the spread of infectious diseases include (1) elimination of inanimate reservoirs of infection, (2) organizing barrier and environmental systems that prevent transmission of pathogens from infected to susceptible individuals, (3) strengthening the immune systems of individuals so that they are not susceptible to organisms, and (4) treating individuals so that they can be rendered free of infection before they transmit it to others. All of these approaches are used in the care of HIV-infected persons.

Careful cooking of food is an example of eliminating a reservoir. Implementing universal precautions is an example of organizing a barrier system to eliminate the transmission of organisms from patients to health care workers or from health care workers to patients. Encouraging good nutrition and immunizing a person, as recommended in Chapter 2, are examples of strengthening the immune system in order to prevent infectious diseases. Health care workers also must be current in their immunizations to avoid becoming ill and transmitting infection to patients, other staff, or families. Treating tuberculosis and sexually transmitted diseases is an example of controlling transmission by reducing the period of time during which a person is capable of transmitting a pathogen.

Individual chapters of this book discuss many of these approaches to preventing transmission of specific organisms. However, some universal approaches to prevention are reviewed here. These principles have been excerpted from infection control documents published by the Centers for Disease Control (see references 36, 37, 38, and 40 at the end of this book). They have been modified by the authors to meet the needs of this book.

GENERAL PRINCIPLES OF INFECTION CONTROL

NEEDLES AND SHARPS DISPOSAL

All health care workers must take precautions to prevent injuries caused by needles, scalpel blades, and other sharp instruments or devices during and following procedures. To prevent needle-stick injuries, needles should not be recapped, purposely bent or broken by hand, removed from disposable syringes, or otherwise manipulated by hand. Used disposable syringes and needles, scalpel blades, and other sharp items should be placed in puncture-resistant containers for disposal; the puncture-resistant containers should be located as close as practical to the work area.

HAND WASHING

Many hospital-acquired infections have been caused by failure of hospital staff to adequately wash their hands between patients. Immunocompromised patients are more susceptible to nosocomial infections and will be more difficult to treat if infected. Complete, thorough hand washing is essential when caring for HIV-infected individuals. This is true even if gloves are worn. Gloves sometimes leak, and hands can be contaminated when gloves are removed.

Health care workers also need to follow good hand-washing technique to protect themselves from organisms found in blood and other body fluids. Hands and other skin surfaces should be washed immediately and thoroughly if contaminated with blood, other body fluids to which universal precautions apply, or potentially contaminated articles. Hands should always be washed after gloves are removed, even if the gloves appear to be intact. Hands should be washed with soap and warm water using the appropriate facilities. When hand-washing facilities are not available, waterless antiseptic hand cleanser can be used, following the manufacturer's recommendations for use of the product.

HIV does not survive well outside the human body, and no environmentally caused case of transmission of HIV has been documented. Studies have shown that drying HIV causes a rapid reduction in viable virus, with 90% to 99% of the virus gone within several hours.

Studies have shown that HIV is inactivated rapidly after being exposed to commonly used chemical germicides at concentrations much lower than are used in practice. In addition to commercially available chemical germicides, a solution of sodium hypochlorite (household bleach) prepared daily is an inexpensive and effective germicide. Concentrations ranging from approximately 500 ppm sodium hypochlorite (1:100 dilution of household bleach) to 5,000 ppm (1:10 dilution of household bleach) are effective, depending on the amount of organic material (e.g., blood, mucus) present on the surface to be cleaned and disinfected. Commercially available chemical germicides may be more compatible with certain medical devices that might be corroded by repeated exposure to sodium hypochlorite, especially at the 1:10 dilution.

However, many of the pathogens that cause HIV-related opportunistic infections have much better survival characteristics in the environment. Therefore, instruments or devices that enter sterile tissue or the vascular system of any patient or through which blood flows should be sterilized before reuse. Devices or items that contact intact mucous membranes should be sterilized or receive high-level disinfection, a procedure that kills vegetative organisms and viruses but not necessarily large numbers of bacterial spores. Chemical germicides that are registered with the U.S. Environmental Protection Agency (EPA) as "sterilants" may be used either for sterilization or for high-level disinfection.

Standard sterilization and disinfection procedures for patient care equipment currently recommended for use in a variety of health care settings (including hospitals, clinics, hemodialysis centers, emergency care facilities, and long-term nursing care facilities) are adequate to sterilize or disinfect instruments, devices, or other items contaminated with blood or other body fluids from persons infected with blood-borne pathogens, including HIV.

Medical devices or instruments that require sterilization or disinfection should be thoroughly cleaned before being exposed to the germicide, and the manufacturer's instructions for use of the germicide should be followed. Furthermore, the manufacturer's specifications for compatibility of the medical device with chemical germicides should be followed closely. Information on specific label claims of commercial germicides can be obtained by writing to the Disinfectants Branch, Office of Pesticides, Environmental Protection Agency, 401 M Street, SW, Washington, D.C. 20460.

Environmental surfaces such as walls, floors, and other surfaces are not associated with transmission of infections to patients or health care workers. Therefore, extraordinary attempts to disinfect or sterilize these environmental surfaces are not necessary.

Cleaning schedules and methods vary according to the area of the hospital or institution, the type of surface to be cleaned, and the amount and type of soil present. Horizontal surfaces (e.g., bedside tables and hard-surfaced flooring) in patient care areas are usually cleaned on a regular basis, when soiling or spills occur, and when a patient is discharged. Cleaning of walls, blinds, and curtains is recommended only if they are visibly soiled. Disinfectant fogging is an unsatisfactory method of decontaminating air and surfaces and is not recommended.

Disinfectant-detergent formulations registered by the EPA can be used for cleaning environmental surfaces, but the actual physical removal of microorganisms by scrubbing is probably as important as any antimicrobial effect of the cleaning agent used. Therefore, cost, safety, and acceptability by housekeepers can be the main criteria for selecting any such registered agent. The manufacturers' instructions for appropriate use should be followed.

CLEANING AND DECONTAMINATING SPILLS OF BLOOD OR OTHER BODY FLUIDS

Chemical germicides that are approved for use as "hospital disinfectants" and that are tuberculocidal when used at recommended dilutions can be used to decontaminate spills of blood and other body fluids. Strategies for decontaminating spills of blood and other body fluids in a patient care setting are different than for spills of cultures or other materials in clinical, public health, or research laboratories. In patient care areas, visible material should first be removed, and then the area should be decontaminated. With large spills of cultured or concentrated infectious agents in the laboratory, the contaminated area should be flooded with a liquid germicide before cleaning, and then decontaminated with fresh germicidal chemical. In both settings, gloves should be worn during the cleaning and decontaminating procedures.

LAUNDRY

Although soiled linen has been identified as a source of large numbers of certain pathogenic microorganisms, the risk of actual disease transmission is negligible. Rather than rigid procedures and specification, hygienic and common-sense storage and processing of clean and soiled linen are recommended. Soiled linen should be handled as little as possible and with minimum agitation to prevent gross microbial contamination of the air and of persons handling the linen. All soiled linen should be bagged at the location where it was used; it should not be sorted or rinsed in patient care areas. Linen soiled with blood or body fluids should be placed and transported in bags that prevent leakage. If hot water is used, linen should be washed with detergent in water at least 71° C (160° F) for 25 minutes. If low-temperature (<70° C [158° F]) laundry cycles are used, chemicals suitable for low-temperature washing at proper concentration should be used.

INFECTIVE WASTE

There is no epidemiologic evidence to suggest that most hospital waste is any more infective than residential waste. Moreover, there is no epidemiologic evidence that hospital waste has caused disease in the community as a result of improper disposal. Therefore, identifying wastes for which special precautions are indicated is largely a matter of judgment about the relative risk of disease transmission. The most practical approach to the management of infective waste is to identify waste with the potential for causing infection during handling and disposal and for which some special precautions appear prudent. Hospital waste for which special precautions appear prudent include microbiology laboratory waste, pathology waste, and blood specimens or blood products. Although any item that has had contact with blood, exudates, or secretions may be potentially infective, it is not usually considered practical or necessary to treat all such items as infective. Infective waste, in general, either should be incinerated or should be autoclaved before disposal. Bulk blood, suctioned fluids, excretions, and secretions may be carefully poured down a drain connected to a sanitary sewer.

ISOLATION

There is no need to isolate a person simply because he or she has HIV infection. The virus is not spread in such ways that isolation procedures would prevent transmission. However, HIV patients may have other diseases that require isolation. The box beginning on the next page indicates the degree of isolation required for specific infectious diseases.

PRODUCT SELECTION

Whenever possible, equipment that minimizes the chances of health care workers coming into contact with body fluids should be available. Resuscitation devices with one-way valves are a good example of such equipment. When dealing with the potential for contamination with pathogens, single-use, disposable items are usually preferred. New products that minimize the risk of exposure to blood and body fluids are being tested and marketed. Examples include the self-covering hypodermic needle pictured in Figure 14-1, page 202.

UNIVERSAL PRECAUTIONS

The risk of HIV transmission from patients to health care workers is quite low. Hundreds of thousands of HIV-infected patients in the United States have undergone tens of millions of procedures performed by hundreds of thousands of health care workers. In spite of this widespread potential for transmission, less than a hundred documented cases of HIV transmission from patient to health care worker have been reported in the United States. Nonetheless, the consequences of HIV

CATEGORY-SPECIFIC ISOLATION SYSTEM

Strict isolation

Strict isolation is an isolation category designed to prevent transmission of highly contagious or virulent infections that may be spread by both air and contact.

Specifications for strict isolation

1. Private room is indicated; door should be kept closed. In general, patients infected with the same organism may share a room.
2. Masks are indicated for all persons entering the room.
3. Gowns are indicated for all persons entering the room.
4. Gloves are indicated for all persons entering the room.
5. Hands must be washed after touching the patient or potentially contaminated articles and before taking care of another patient.
6. Articles contaminated with infective material should be discarded or bagged and labeled before being sent for decontamination and reprocessing.

Diseases requiring strict isolation

Diphtheria, pharyngeal
Lassa fever and other viral hemorrhagic fevers, such as Marburg virus disease*
Plague, pneumonic
Smallpox*
Varicella (chickenpox)
Zoster, localized in immunocompromised patient or disseminated

Contact isolation

Contact isolation is designed to prevent transmission of highly transmissible or epidemiologically important infections (or colonization) that do not warrant Strict Isolation.

All diseases or conditions included in this category are spread primarily by close or direct contact. Thus masks, gowns, and gloves are recommended for anyone in close or direct contact with any patient who has an infection (or colonization) that is included in this category. For individual diseases or conditions, however, 1 or more of these 3 barriers may not be indicated. For example, masks and gowns are not generally indicated for care of infants and young children with acute viral respiratory infections; gowns are not generally indicated for gonococcal conjunctivitis in newborns; and masks are not generally indicated for patients infected with multiply-resistant microorganisms, except those with pneumonia. Therefore some degree of "over-isolation" may occur in this category.

Specifications for contact isolation

1. Private room is indicated. In general, patients infected with the same organism may share a room. During outbreaks, infants and young children with the same respiratory clinical syndrome may share a room.

2. Masks are indicated for those who come close to patient.
3. Gowns are indicated if soiling is likely.
4. Gloves are indicated for touching infective material.
5. Hands must be washed after touching the patient or potentially contaminated articles and before taking care of another patient.
6. Articles contaminated with infective material should be discarded or bagged and labeled before being sent for decontamination and reprocessing.

Diseases or conditions requiring contact isolation

Acute respiratory infections in infants and young children, including croup, colds, bronchitis, and bronchiolitis caused by respiratory syncytial virus, adenovirus, coronavirus, influenza viruses, parainfluenza viruses, and rhinovirus
Conjunctivitis, gonococcal in newborns
Diphtheria, cutaneous
Endometritis, group A *Streptococcus*
Furunculosis, staphylococcal in newborns
Herpes simplex, disseminated, severe primary or neonatal
Impetigo
Influenza, in infants and young children
Multiply-resistant bacteria, infection, or colonization (any site) with any of the following:
1. Gram-negative bacilli resistant to all aminoglycosides that are tested. (In general, such organisms should be resistant to gentamicin, tobramycin, and amikacin for these special precautions to be indicated.)
2. *Staphylococcus aureus* resistant to methicillin (or nafcillin or oxacillin if they are used instead of methicillin for testing).
3. *Pneumococcus* resistant to penicillin.
4. *Haemophilus influenzae* resistant to ampicillin (beta-lactamase positive) and chloramphenicol.
5. Other resistant bacteria may be included if they are judged by the infection control team to be of special clinical and epidemiologic significance.
Pediculosis
Pharyngitis, infectious, in infants and young children
Pneumonia, viral, in infants and young children
Pneumonia, *Staphylococcus aureus* or group A *Streptococcus*
Rabies
Rubella, congenital and other
Scabies
Scalded skin syndrome, staphylococcal (Ritter's disease)
Skin wound or burn infection, major (draining and not covered by dressing or dressing does not adequately contain the purulent material) including those infected with *Staphylococcus aureus* or group A *Streptococcus*
Vaccinia (generalized and progressive eczema vaccinatum)

*A private room with special ventilation is indicated.

Continued.

CATEGORY-SPECIFIC ISOLATION SYSTEM—cont'd

Respiratory isolation

Respiratory isolation is designed to prevent transmission of infectious diseases primarily over short distances through the air (droplet transmission). Direct and indirect contact transmission occurs with some infections in this isolation category but is infrequent.

Specifications for respiratory isolation

1. Private room is indicated. In general, patients infected with the same organism may share a room.
2. Masks are indicated for those who come close to the patient.
3. Gowns are not indicated.
4. Gloves are not indicated.
5. Hands must be washed after touching the patient or potentially contaminated articles and before taking care of another patient.
6. Articles contaminated with infective material should be discarded or bagged and labeled before being sent for decontamination and reprocessing.

Diseases requiring respiratory isolation

Epiglottitis, *Haemophilus influenzae*
Erythema infectiosum
Measles
Meningitis
   Haemophilus influenzae, known or suspected
   Meningococcal, known or suspected
Meningococcal pneumonia
Meningococcemia
Mumps
Pertussis (whooping cough)
Pneumonia, *Haemophilus influenzae*, in children (any age)

Tuberculosis isolation (AFB isolation)

Tuberculosis isolation (AFB isolation) is an isolation category for patients with pulmonary TB who have a positive sputum smear or a chest x-ray that strongly suggests current (active) TB. Laryngeal TB is also included in this isolation category. In general, infants and young children with pulmonary TB do not require isolation precautions because they rarely cough, and their bronchial secretions contain few AFB, compared with adults with pulmonary TB. On the instruction card, this category is called AFB (for acid-fast bacilli) isolation to protect the patient's privacy.

Specifications for tuberculosis isolation (AFB isolation)

1. Private room with special ventilation is indicated; door should be kept closed. In general, patients infected with the same organism may share a room.
2. Masks are indicated only if the patient is coughing and does not reliably cover mouth.
3. Gowns are indicated only if needed to prevent gross contamination of clothing.
4. Gloves are not indicated.
5. Hands must be washed after touching the patient or potentially contaminated articles and before taking care of another patient.
6. Articles are rarely involved in transmission of TB. However, articles should be thoroughly cleaned and disinfected or discarded.

Enteric precautions

Enteric precautions are designed to prevent infections that are transmitted by direct or indirect contact with feces. Hepatitis A is included in this category because it is spread through feces, although the disease is much less likely to be transmitted after the onset of jaundice. Most infections in this category primarily cause gastrointestinal symptoms, but some do not. For example, feces from patients infected with poliovirus and coxsackieviruses are infective, but those infections do not usually cause prominent gastrointestinal symptoms.

Specifications for enteric precautions

1. Private room is indicated if patient hygiene is poor. A patient with poor hygiene does not wash hands after touching infective material, contaminates the environment with infective material, or shares contaminated articles with other patients. In general, patients infected with the same organism may share a room.
2. Masks are not indicated.
3. Gowns are indicated if soiling is likely.
4. Gloves are indicated if touching infective material.
5. Hands must be washed after touching the patient or potentially contaminated articles and before taking care of another patient.
6. Articles contaminated with infective material should be discarded or bagged and labeled before being sent for decontamination or reprocessing.

CATEGORY-SPECIFIC ISOLATION SYSTEM—cont'd

Diseases requiring enteric precautions

Amebic dysentery

Cholera

Coxsackievirus disease

Diarrhea, acute illness with suspected infectious etiology

Echovirus disease

Encephalitis (unless known not to be caused by enteroviruses)

Enterocolitis caused by *Clostridium difficile* or *S. aureus*

Enteroviral infection

Gastroenteritis caused by

    Campylobacter species

    Cryptosporidium species

    Dientamoeba fragilis

    Escherichia coli (enterotoxic, enteropathogenic, or enteroinvasive)

    Giardia lamblia

    Salmonella species

    Shigella species

    Vibrio parahaemolyticus

    Viruses—including Norwalk agent and rotavirus

    Yersinia enterocolitica

    Unknown etiology but presumed to be an infectious agent

Hand, foot, and mouth disease

Hepatitis, viral, type A

Herpangina

Meningitis, viral (unless known not to be caused by enteroviruses)

Necrotizing enterocolitis

Pleurodynia

Poliomyelitis

Typhoid fever (*Salmonella typhi*)

Viral pericarditis, myocarditis, or meningitis (unless known not to be caused by enteroviruses)

Drainage/secretion precautions

Drainage/secretion precautions are designed to prevent infections that are transmitted by direct or indirect contact with purulent material or drainage from an infected body site. This newly created isolation category includes many infections formerly included in Wound and Skin Precautions, Discharge (lesion), and Secretion (oral) Precautions, which have been discontinued. Infectious diseases included in this category are those that result in the production of infective purulent material, drainage, or secretions, unless the disease is included in another isolation category that requires more rigorous precautions. For example, minor limited skin, wound, or burn infections are included in this category, but major skin, wound, or burn infections are included in Contact Isolation.

Specifications for drainage/secretion precautions

1. Private room is not indicated.
2. Masks are not indicated.
3. Gowns are indicated if soiling is likely.
4. Gloves are indicated for touching infective material.
5. Hands must be washed after touching the patient or potentially contaminated articles and before taking care of another patient.
6. Articles contaminated with infective material should be discarded or bagged and labeled before being sent for decontamination and reprocessing.

Diseases requiring drainage/secretion precautions

The following infections are examples of those included in this category provided they are not (a) caused by multiply-resistant microorganisms, (b) major draining (and not covered by a dressing or dressing does not adequately contain the drainage) skin, wound, or burn infections, including those caused by *S. aureus* or group A *Streptococcus*, or (c) gonococcal eye infections in newborns. See Contact Isolation if the infection is one of these three.

    Abscess, minor limited

    Burn infection, minor limited

    Conjunctivitis

    Decubitus ulcer, infected, minor or limited

    Skin infection, minor or limited

    Wound infection, minor or limited

From CDC.[40]

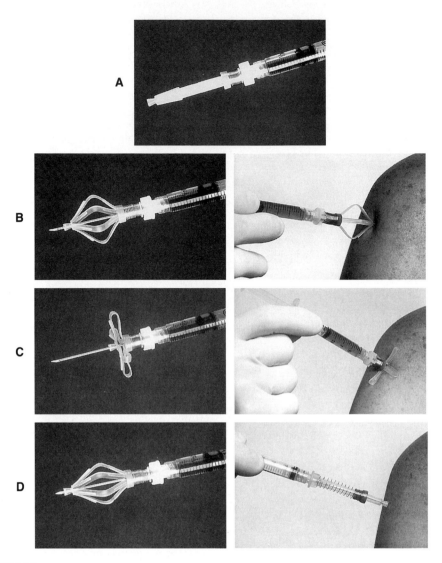

FIGURE 14-1
The Protector Self-Covering Hypodermic Needle by InjectiMed, Inc. **A,** Ready. Needle with protector covering ready for use. **B,** Plunge. Needle tip is exposed only when spring cover is compressed during use. **C,** Inject. **D,** Withdraw from injection site. Protector passively covers the needle.

are so severe that major efforts have been made to reduce the likelihood of such transmissions. These efforts have been termed "universal precautions" and are summarized in the box on the next page.

It is important to remember that these precautions are to be followed for all patients, not just for those known to be HIV positive. The epidemiology of HIV infection (see Chapter 2) clearly indicates that no population group is free of HIV infection. The disease is not the exclusive property of any population. Even knowing that someone has recently tested negative is not protective. Presently utilized laboratory screening tests identify the presence of HIV antibodies—not the virus. Antibodies may not be detectable for up to 6 months af-

ter infection. Unfortunately, that period between infection and the appearance of antibodies is characterized by high levels of viremia. Thus individuals who test negative but are in this early period of infection may be more infectious than those who test positive. Therefore, given that there is no effective way of determining who is infected and who is not, universal precautions apply for all patients.

The circumstances under which various levels of universal precautions should be used are described in Table 14-1, page 204. Although the table does not cover every circumstance and all body fluids, it gives good direction as to the situations in which the various forms of barrier protection should and should not be employed.

UNIVERSAL BLOOD AND BODY FLUID PRECAUTIONS

1. All health care workers should routinely use appropriate barrier precautions to prevent skin and mucous membrane exposure when contact with blood or other body fluids of any patient is anticipated. Gloves should be worn for touching blood and body fluids, mucous membranes, or nonintact skin of all patients, for handling items or surfaces soiled with blood or body fluids, and for performing venipuncture and other vascular access procedures. Gloves should be changed after contact with each patient. Masks and protective eyewear or face shields should be worn during procedures that are likely to generate droplets of blood or other body fluids to prevent exposure of mucous membranes of the mouth, nose, and eyes. Gowns or aprons should be worn during procedures that are likely to generate splashes of blood or other body fluids.

2. Hands and other skin surfaces should be washed immediately and thoroughly if contaminated with blood or other body fluids. Hands should be washed immediately after gloves are removed.

3. All health care workers should take precautions to prevent injuries caused by needles, scalpels, and other sharp instruments or devices during procedures; when cleaning used instruments; during disposal of used needles; and when handling sharp instruments after procedures. To prevent needlestick injuries, needles should not be recapped, purposely bent or broken by hand, removed from disposable syringes, or otherwise manipulated by hand. After they are used, disposable syringes and needles, scalpel blades, and other sharp items should be placed in puncture-resistant containers for disposal; the puncture-resistant containers should be located as close as practical to the use area. Large-bore reusable needles should be placed in a puncture-resistant container for transport to the reprocessing area.

4. Although saliva has not been implicated in HIV transmission, to minimize the need for emergency mouth-to-mouth resuscitation, mouthpieces, resuscitation bags, or other ventilation devices should be available for use in areas in which the need for resuscitation is predictable.

5. Health care workers who have exudative lesions or weeping dermatitis should refrain from all direct patient care and from handling patient-care equipment until the condition resolves.

6. Pregnant health care workers are not known to be at greater risk of contracting HIV infection than health care workers who are not pregnant; however, if a health care worker develops HIV infection during pregnancy, the infant is at risk of infection resulting from perinatal transmission. Because of this risk, pregnant health care workers should be especially familiar with and strictly adhere to precautions to minimize the risk of HIV transmission.

Implementation of universal blood and body fluid precautions for **all** patients eliminates the need for use of the isolation category of "Blood and Body Fluid Precautions" previously recommended by the CDC for patients known or suspected to be infected with blood-borne pathogens. Isolation precautions (e.g., enteric and "AFB") should be used as necessary if associated conditions, such as infectious diarrhea or tuberculosis, are diagnosed or suspected.

Precautions for invasive procedures

In this document, an invasive procedure is defined as surgical entry into tissues, cavities, or organs or repair of major traumatic injuries in (1) an operating or delivery room, emergency department, or outpatient setting, including both physicians' and dentists' offices; (2) cardiac catheterization and angiographic procedures; (3) a vaginal or cesarean delivery or other invasive obstetric procedure during which bleeding may occur; or (4) the manipulation, cutting, or removal of any oral or perioral tissues, including tooth structure, during which bleeding occurs or the potential for bleeding exists. The universal blood and body fluid precautions listed above, combined with the precautions listed below, should be the minimum precautions for **all** such invasive procedures.

1. All health care workers who participate in invasive procedures must routinely use appropriate barrier precautions to prevent skin and mucous membrane contact with blood and other body fluids of all patients. Gloves and surgical masks must be worn for all invasive procedures. Protective eyewear or face shields should be worn for procedures that commonly result in the generation of droplets, splashing of blood or other body fluids, or the generation of bone chips. Gowns or aprons made of materials that provide an effective barrier should be worn during invasive procedures that are likely to result in the splashing of blood or other body fluids. All health care workers who perform or assist in vaginal or cesarean deliveries should wear gloves and gowns when handling the placenta or the infant until blood and amniotic fluid have been removed from the infant's skin and should wear gloves during postdelivery care of the umbilical cord.

2. If a glove is torn or a needlestick or other injury occurs, the glove should be removed and a new glove used as promptly as patient safety permits; the needle or instrument involved in the incident should also be removed from the sterile field.

Table 14-1

EXAMPLES OF RECOMMENDED PERSONAL PROTECTIVE EQUIPMENT FOR WORKER PROTECTION AGAINST HIV AND HBV TRANSMISSION*

Task or activity	Disposable gloves	Gown	Mask†	Protective eyewear
Bleeding control with spurting blood	Yes	Yes	Yes	Yes
Bleeding control with minimal bleeding	Yes	No	No	No
Emergency childbirth	Yes	Yes	Yes, if splashing is likely	Yes, if splashing is likely
Blood drawing	Yes‡	No	No	No
Starting an intravenous (IV) line	Yes	No	No	No
Endotracheal intubation, esophageal obturator use	Yes	No	No, unless splashing is likely	No, unless splashing is likely
Oral/nasal suctioning, manually cleaning airway	Yes§	No	No, unless splashing is likely	No, unless splashing is likely
Handling and cleaning instruments with microbial contamination	Yes	No, unless soiling is likely	No	No
Measuring blood pressure	No	No	No	No
Measuring temperature	No	No	No	No
Giving an injection	No	No	No	No

*The examples provided in this table are based on application of universal precautions. Universal precautions are intended to supplement rather than replace recommendations for routine infection control, such as hand washing and using gloves to prevent gross microbial contamination of hands (e.g., contact with urine or feces).

†Refers to protective masks to prevent exposure of mucous membranes to blood or other potentially contaminated body fluids.

‡Although not strictly required, almost all institutions follow policy.

§Although not clearly necessary to prevent HIV or HBV transmission unless blood is present, gloves are recommended to prevent transmission of other agents (e.g., herpes simplex virus).

TUBERCULOSIS PRECAUTIONS

Individuals who are HIV infected are prone to development of active tuberculosis. This can be from new infection or from reactivation of old tuberculosis that may have been latent for many years (see Chapter 9). In either event, individuals with active tuberculosis pose a significant threat to health care workers and patients. The CDC recommends that five principles be followed for controlling TB in health care facilities.[36]

FIRST PRINCIPLE: PREVENT GENERATION OF INFECTIOUS DROPLET NUCLEI CONTAINING MYCOBACTERIA

In order to accomplish this, health care facilities must do the following:

Identify and Provide Early Preventive Therapy for Persons with Tuberculosis Infection

Persons at increased risk of tuberculosis (see the following box) or those for whom the consequences of tuberculosis may be especially severe should be screened for

---

INDIVIDUALS AT HIGH RISK FOR TUBERCULOSIS INFECTION

- HIV-infected individuals
- Close personal contacts of infectious tuberculosis cases
- Persons with medical conditions that increase the risk for tuberculosis
- Foreign-born persons from high-prevalence areas of the world (e.g., Asia, Africa, the Caribbean, and Latin America)
- Low-income populations, including high-risk minorities
- Alcoholics and injection drug users
- Residents of long-term care facilities (including prisons)
- Health care workers

tuberculous infection with a tuberculin skin test, utilizing the following methods: The Mantoux technique—intradermal injection of 0.1 ml of purified protein derivative (PPD) containing 5 tuberculin units (TU)—is used to detect tuberculous infection. Although tuberculin skin tests are less than 100% sensitive and specific for detection of infection with *Mycobacterium tuberculosis*, no better screening method has been devised. Tuberculin skin tests should be interpreted as significant when an individual who previously tested negative on the PPD test shows a positive result, according to the following guidelines:

>5 mm induration is positive for HIV-infected individuals or those who have recently been exposed to tuberculosis

>10 mm is positive for high-risk groups (see the box on p. 204) and health care workers who have been in clinical situations where exposure is possible

>15 mm is positive for all others

A negative skin test does not rule out tuberculosis disease or infection. Because of the possibility of a false-negative result, the tuberculin skin test should never be used to exclude the possibility of active tuberculosis among persons for whom the diagnosis is being considered, even if reactions to other skin-test antigens are positive. Persons with HIV infection are more likely to have false-negative skin tests than are persons without HIV infection. The likelihood of a false-negative skin test increases as the stage of HIV infection advances. For this reason, a history of a positive tuberculin reaction is meaningful, even if the current skin-test result is negative.

Identify and Treat Persons With Active Tuberculosis

This provides an effective means of preventing tuberculosis transmission by preventing the generation of infectious droplet nuclei. Tuberculosis may be more difficult to diagnose among persons with HIV infection because of atypical clinical or radiographic presentation and/or the simultaneous occurrence of other pulmonary infections (e.g., *Pneumocystis carinii* pneumonia [PCP]). The difficulty in making a diagnosis in HIV-infected persons may be further compounded by impaired responses to tuberculin skin tests, low sensitivity of sputum smears for detecting AFB (acid-fast bacilli), or overgrowth of cultures with *Mycobacterium avium* complex (MAC) among patients with both MAC and *M. tuberculosis* infections.

A diagnosis of tuberculosis should be considered for any patient with a persistent cough or other symptoms compatible with tuberculosis, such as weight loss, anorexia, or fevers. Diagnostic measures include history, physical examination, tuberculin skin test, chest radiograph, microscopic examination, and culture of sputum or other appropriate specimens. Other diagnostic methods, such as bronchoscopy or biopsy, may be indicated. The probability of tuberculosis is increased by a positive reaction to a tuberculin skin test or a history of a positive skin test, a history of previous tuberculosis, membership in a group at high risk for tuberculosis (see the box on p. 204), or a history of exposure to tuberculosis. Active tuberculosis is suspected if the diagnostic evaluation reveals AFB in sputum, a chest radiograph is suggestive of tuberculosis, or the person has symptoms associated with TB (e.g., productive cough, night sweats, anorexia, and weight loss).

The radiographic presentation of pulmonary tuberculosis among patients with HIV infection may be unusual. Typical apical cavitary disease is less common among persons with HIV infection. They may have infiltrates in any lung zone, often associated with mediastinal and/or hilar adenopathy, or they may have a normal chest radiograph.

Smear and culture examination of three to five sputum specimens collected on different days is the main diagnostic procedure for pulmonary tuberculosis. Sputum smears that fail to demonstrate AFB do not exclude the diagnosis of tuberculosis. Studies indicate that 50% to 80% of patients with pulmonary tuberculosis have positive sputum smears. Sputum smears from patients with HIV infection and pulmonary tuberculosis may be less likely to reveal AFB than those from immunocompetent patients, a finding believed to be consistent with the lower frequency of cavitary pulmonary disease observed among HIV-infected persons.

A positive sputum culture, with organisms identified as *M. tuberculosis*, provides a definitive diagnosis of tuberculosis. Conventional laboratory methods may require 4 to 8 weeks for species identification; however, the use of radiometric culture techniques and genetic probes facilitates more rapid detection and identification of mycobacteria. Mixed mycobacterial infection (either simultaneous or sequential) may occur and may obscure the recognition of *M. tuberculosis* clinically and in the laboratory. The use of genetic probes for both MAC and *M. tuberculosis* may be useful for identifying mixed mycobacterial infections in clinical specimens.

Determine Infectiousness of Tuberculosis Patients

The infectiousness of a person with tuberculosis correlates with the number of organisms that are expelled into the air, which, in turn, correlates with the following factors: (a) anatomic site of disease, (b) presence of coughed or other forceful expirational maneuvers, (c) presence of AFB in the sputum smear, (d) willingness or ability of the patient to cover his or her mouth when coughing, (e) presence of cavitation on chest radiograph, (f) length of time the patient has been on adequate chemotherapy, (g) duration of symptoms, and (h) administration of procedures that can enhance coughing (e.g., sputum induction).

The most infectious persons are those with pulmonary or laryngeal tuberculosis. Those with extrapulmonary tuberculosis are usually not infectious, with the following exceptions: (a) nonpulmonary disease located in the respiratory tract or oral cavity or (b) extrapulmonary disease that includes an open abscess or lesion in which the concentration of organisms is high, especially if drainage from the abscess or lesion is extensive. Although the data are limited, findings suggest that tuberculosis patients with AIDS, if smear positive, have infectiousness similar to that of tuberculosis patients without AIDS.

Infectiousness is greatest among patients who have a productive cough, pulmonary cavitation on chest radiograph, and AFB on sputum smear. Infection is more likely to result from exposure to a person who has unsuspected pulmonary tuberculosis and who is not receiving antituberculosis therapy, or from a person with diagnosed tuberculosis who is not receiving adequate therapy because of patient noncompliance or the presence of drug-resistant organisms. Administering effective antituberculosis medications has been shown to be strongly associated with a decrease in infectiousness among persons with tuberculosis. Effective chemotherapy reduces coughing, the amount of sputum, and the number of organisms in the sputum. However, the length of time a patient must be on effective medication before becoming noninfectious varies; some patients are never infectious, whereas those with unrecognized or inadequately treated drug-resistant disease may remain infectious for weeks or months. Thus, decisions about terminating isolation precautions should be made on a case-by-case basis.

In general, persons suspected of having active tuberculosis and those with confirmed tuberculosis should be considered infectious if cough is present, if cough-inducing procedures are performed, or if sputum smears are known to contain AFB; these patients should also be considered infectious if they are not undergoing chemotherapy, have just started chemotherapy, or have a poor clinical or bacteriologic response to chemotherapy. A person with tuberculosis who has been on adequate chemotherapy for at least 2 to 3 weeks and has had a definite clinical and bacteriologic response to therapy (reduction in cough, resolution of fever, and progressively decreasing quantity of bacilli on smear) is probably no longer infectious. Most tuberculosis experts agree that noninfectiousness in pulmonary tuberculosis can be established by finding sputum free of bacilli by smear examination on 3 consecutive days for a patient on effective chemotherapy. Even after isolation precautions have been discontinued, caution should be exercised when a patient with tuberculosis is placed in a room with another patient, especially if the other patient is immunocompromised.

SECOND PRINCIPLE: PREVENT SPREAD OF INFECTIOUS DROPLET NUCLEI THROUGH SOURCE CONTROL

Certain techniques can be applied in high-risk settings to prevent or reduce the spread of infectious droplet nuclei into the general air circulation. The application of these techniques, which are called source-control methods because they entrap infectious droplet nuclei as they are emitted by the patient, or "source," is especially important during performance of medical procedures likely to generate aerosols containing infectious particles.

Use Local Exhaust Ventilation

Local exhaust ventilation removes airborne contaminants at or near their sources. The use of booths for sputum induction or administration of aerosolized medications (e.g., aerosolized pentamidine) is an example of local exhaust ventilation for preventing the spread of infectious droplet nuclei generated by these procedures into the general air circulation. Booths used for source control should be equipped with exhaust fans that remove nearly 100% of airborne particles during the time interval between the departure of one patient and the arrival of the next.

The exhaust fan should maintain negative pressure in the booth with respect to adjacent areas, so that air flows into the booth. Maintaining negative pressure in the booth minimizes the possibility that infectious droplet nuclei in the booth will move into adjacent rooms or hallways. Ideally, the air from these booths should be exhausted directly to the outside of the building (away from air intake vents, people, and animals, in accordance with federal, state, and local regulations concerning environmental discharges). If direct exhaust to the outside is impossible, the air from the booth could be exhausted through a properly designed, installed, and maintained high-efficiency particulate air (HEPA) filter; however, the efficacy of this method has not been demonstrated in clinical settings.

Implement Other Source-Control Methods

A simple but important source-control technique is for infectious patients to cover all coughs and sneezes with a tissue, thus containing most liquid drops and droplets before evaporation can occur. A patient's use of a properly fitted surgical mask or a disposable, valveless particulate respirator also may reduce the spread of infectious particles. However, since the device would need to be worn constantly for the protection of others, it would be practical in only very limited circumstances (e.g., when a patient is being transported within a medical facility or between facilities).

THIRD PRINCIPLE: REDUCE THE MICROBIAL CONTAMINATION OF AIR

Once infectious droplet nuclei have been released into room air, they should be eliminated or reduced in number by ventilation, which may be supplemented by additional measures (e.g., trapping organisms by high-efficiency filtration or killing organisms with germicidal ultraviolet [UV] irradiation [100 to 290 nanometers]). Health care workers may also reduce the risk of inhaling contaminated air by using personal respirators.

Ventilation and, to a lesser extent, UV lamps and face masks have been used in health care settings for the past few decades to prevent tuberculosis transmission. Few published data, however, are available to evaluate their effectiveness or to draw conclusions about the role each method should play. None of the four methods (ventilation, UV irradiation, high-efficiency filtration, and face masks) used alone or in combination can completely eliminate the risk of tuberculosis transmission. However, when used with the other infection-control measures outlined in this chapter, they can substantially reduce the risk.

Each area to which an infectious tuberculosis patient might be admitted should be evaluated for its potential for the spread of tuberculosis bacilli. Modifications to the ventilation system, if needed, should be made by a qualified ventilation engineer. Individual evaluations should address factors such as the risk of tuberculosis in the patient population served, special procedures that may be performed, and ability to make the necessary changes.

Too much ventilation in an area can create problems. In addition to the incurring of additional expense for marginal benefits, occupants bothered by the drafts may elect to shut down the system entirely. Furthermore, if the concentration of infectious droplet nuclei in an area is high, the levels of ventilation that are practical to achieve may be inadequate to completely remove the contaminants.

FOURTH PRINCIPLE: DECONTAMINATE EQUIPMENT THAT MAY CONTAIN TB BACILLI

Procedures for sterilizing, disinfecting, and cleaning were discussed earlier in this chapter. For application of these methods in TB control, medical devices, equipment, and surgical materials can be divided into three categories: critical items, semicritical items, and noncritical items.

Critical items are instruments (e.g., needles, surgical instruments) that are introduced directly into the bloodstream or into other normally sterile areas of the body. These items should be sterile at the time of use.

Semicritical items (e.g., noninvasive flexible and rigid fiberoptic endoscopes or bronchoscopes) are items that may come in contact with mucous membranes but that do not ordinarily penetrate body surfaces. Although sterilization is preferred for these instruments, a high-level disinfection procedure that destroys vegetative microorganisms, most fungal spores, tubercle bacilli, and small, nonlipid viruses may be used. Meticulous physical cleaning before sterilization or high-level disinfection is essential.

Noncritical items are those either that do not ordinarily touch the patient or that touch intact skin (e.g., blood pressure cuffs). These items do not transmit tuberculous infection. Washing with a detergent is usually sufficient.

Decisions about decontamination processes should be based on the intended use of the item and not on the diagnosis of the patient for whom the item was used. The selection of chemical disinfectants depends on the intended use, the level of disinfection required, and the structure and material of the item to be disinfected.

Although microorganisms are normally found on walls, floors, and other surfaces, these environmental surfaces are rarely associated with transmission of infections to patient or health care workers. This is particularly true with organisms such as tubercle bacilli, which generally require inhalation by the host for infection to occur. Therefore, extraordinary attempts to disinfect or sterilize environmental surfaces are rarely indicated. Routine cleaning with a hospital-grade, EPA-approved germicide/disinfectant is recommended for all hospital rooms, including AFB isolation rooms.

FIFTH PRINCIPLE: MONITOR FOR TUBERCULOSIS TRANSMISSION TO HEALTH CARE PERSONNEL

A tuberculosis screening and prevention program should be established for protecting health care workers and patients. Personnel with tuberculous infection and without evidence of current (active) disease should be identified as soon as possible after infection, because preventive treatment with isoniazid may be indicated. Regular screening of health care workers also enables public health personnel and the health care facility to evaluate the effectiveness of current infection-control practices.

The basic elements of the screening program should include the following:

a. Surveillance and reporting

- Health care facilities providing care to patients at risk for tuberculosis should maintain active surveillance for tuberculosis among patients and health care facility personnel and for skin test conversions among health care facility personnel. When tuberculosis is suspected or diagnosed, public health authorities should be notified so that appropriate contact investigation can be performed. Data on the occurrence of tuberculosis and skin test conversions among patients and health care facility personnel should be collected and analyzed to estimate the risk of tuberculosis transmission in the facility and to evaluate the effectiveness of infection-control and screening practices.
- At the time of employment, all health care facility personnel, including those with a history of bacillus of Calmette and Guerin (BCG) vaccination, should receive a Mantoux tuberculin skin test unless a previously positive reaction can be documented or completion of adequate preventive therapy or adequate therapy for active disease can be documented.
- Initial and follow-up tuberculin skin tests should be administered and interpreted according to current guidelines.
- Health care facility personnel with a documented history of a positive tuberculin test or adequate treatment for disease or preventive therapy for infection should be exempt from further screening unless they develop symptoms suggestive of tuberculosis.
- Periodic retesting of PPD-negative health care workers should be conducted to identify persons whose skin tests convert to positive. In general, the frequency of repeat testing should be based on the risk of developing new infection. Health care facility workers who may be frequently exposed to patients with tuberculosis or who are involved with potentially high-risk procedures (e.g., bronchoscopy, sputum induction, or aerosol treatments given to patients who may have tuberculosis) should be retested at least every 6 months. Health care facility personnel in other areas should be retested annually. Data on skin test conversions should be periodically reviewed so that the risk of acquiring new infection may be estimated for each area of the facility. On the basis of this analysis, the frequency of retesting may be altered accordingly.

b. Evaluation of health care facility personnel after unprotected exposure to tuberculosis

- In addition to periodic screening, health care facility personnel and patients should be evaluated if they have been exposed to a potentially infectious tuberculosis patient for whom the infection-control procedures outlined in this document have not been taken. Unless a negative skin test has been documented within the preceding 3 months, each exposed health care facility worker (except those already known to be positive reactors) should receive a Mantoux tuberculin skin test as soon as possible after exposure and should be managed in the same way as other contacts. If the initial skin test is negative, the test should be repeated 12 weeks after the exposure ended. Exposed persons with skin test reactions ≥ 5 mm or with symptoms suggestive of tuberculosis should receive chest x-rays. Persons with previously known positive skin test reactions who have been exposed to an infectious patient do not require a repeat skin test or a chest x-ray unless they have symptoms suggestive of tuberculosis.

c. Evaluation and management of health care facility personnel with positive skin tests or symptoms that may be due to tuberculosis

- Health care facility personnel with positive tuberculin skin tests or with skin test conversions on repeat testing or after exposure should be clinically evaluated for active tuberculosis. Persons with symptoms suggestive of tuberculosis should be evaluated regardless of skin test results. If tuberculosis is diagnosed, appropriate therapy should be instituted according to published guidelines. Personnel diagnosed with active tuberculosis should be offered counseling and HIV antibody testing.
- Health care facility personnel who have positive tuberculin skin tests or skin test conversions but do not have clinical tuberculosis should be evaluated for preventive therapy according to published guidelines. Personnel with positive skin tests should be evaluated for risk of HIV infection. If HIV infection is considered a possibility, counseling and HIV antibody testing should be strongly encouraged.
- All persons with a history of tuberculosis or positive tuberculin tests are at risk for contracting tuberculosis in the future. These persons should be reminded periodically that they should promptly report any pulmonary symptoms. If symptoms of tuberculosis should de-

velop, the person should be evaluated immediately.

d. Routine and follow-up chest x-rays

- Routine chest films are not required for asymptomatic, tuberculin-negative health care facility personnel. After the initial chest x-ray is taken, personnel with positive skin test reactions do not need repeat chest x-rays unless symptoms develop that may be due to tuberculosis.

e. Work restrictions

- Health care facility personnel with current pulmonary or laryngeal tuberculosis pose a risk to patients and other personnel while they are infectious; therefore, stringent work restrictions for these persons are necessary. They should be excluded from work until adequate treatment is instituted, cough is resolved, and sputum is free of bacilli on three consecutive smears. Health care facility personnel with current tuberculosis at sites other than the lung or larynx usually do not need to be excluded from work if concurrent pulmonary tuberculosis has been ruled out. Personnel who discontinue treatment before the recommended course of therapy has been completed should not be allowed to work until treatment is resumed, an adequate response to therapy is documented, and they have negative sputum smears on 3 consecutive days.
- Health care facility personnel who are otherwise healthy and receiving preventive treatment for tuberculous infection should be allowed to continue usual work activities.

- Health care facility personnel who cannot take or do not accept or complete a full course of preventive therapy should have their work situations evaluated to determine whether reassignment is indicated. Work restrictions may not be necessary for otherwise healthy persons who do not accept or complete preventive therapy. These persons should be counseled about the risk of contracting disease and should be instructed to seek evaluation promptly if symptoms develop that may be due to tuberculosis, especially if they have contact with high-risk patients (i.e., patients at high risk for severe consequences if they become infected).

f. Consultation

- Consultation on tuberculosis surveillance and screening, as well as other methods to reduce tuberculosis transmission, should be available from state health department tuberculosis-control programs. Facilities are encouraged to use the services of health departments in planning and implementing their surveillance and screening programs.

Controlling transmission of tuberculosis in a health care facility is complex and requires adherence to the five principles described. Previous experience has demonstrated that failure to follow any of the five principles greatly increases the chances of a breakdown in the control system, resulting in preventable disease, suffering, and, occasionally, death. These preventable problems are not restricted to the health care environment, but can spread to health care workers' families and communities.

Therapeutic Procedures

Kristen K. Ownby

Aerosolized Pentamidine

Pneumocystis carinii pneumonia (PCP) remains one of the most common causes of morbidity and mortality in the patient with AIDS. Several drugs have been identified as agents that prevent the reactivation of the organism, thus preventing pneumonia. One such drug is pentamidine. Pentamidine is administered intravenously for the treatment of acute pneumonia and is administered through inhalation therapy for the prevention of PCP. The pentamidine is aerosolized through a nebulizer to produce particles small enough to reach the lung parenchyma. Aerosolized pentamidine (AP) is considered secondary prophylaxis, used when a patient is unable to tolerate the first-line therapy, trimethoprim-sulfamethoxazole.

INDICATIONS

PCP prophylaxis is recommended for patients meeting one of several criteria:

- CD4+ counts of less than 200 cells/mm^3 or below 20%
- An acute episode of *Pneumocystis carinii* pneumonia
- Having had another opportunistic infection

CONTRAINDICATIONS

Aerosolized pentamidine is generally well tolerated. The most common side effect from this therapy is bron-

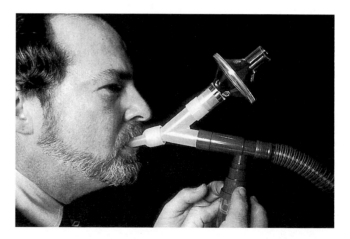

FIGURE 15-1
Respirgard II nebulizer for pentamidine inhalation therapy.

chospasms. In most cases this side effect is alleviated with the administration of bronchodilators, such as albuterol. However, in extreme cases the patient will not respond to bronchodilators, and another type of drug will have to be used as PCP prophylaxis. Aerosolized pentamidine offers no protection against extrapulmonary pneumocystis. If the patient develops an extrapulmonary site, a drug that acts systemically must be administered.

COMPLICATIONS

Bronchospasms are the most common complication seen with the administration of nebulized pentamidine. Most patients respond to bronchodilators administered prior to receiving the pentamidine treatment. If the patient continues to have bronchospasms despite the administration of a bronchodilator, a different drug may have to be considered for PCP prophylaxis.

SAFETY ISSUES FOR HEALTH CARE WORKERS

The safety of the health care worker and other patients needs to be considered with the administration of pentamidine. Droplets produced during the administration of pentamidine contain particles of the drug and possible infectious microorganisms, such as tuberculosis. These droplets create a health hazard to all persons in the treatment room. Health care workers should always wear particulate respirator masks and goggles during the administration of the drug. If possible, the treatment should be administered in individual rooms or booths to minimize exposure to other persons. The rooms should have negative pressure ventilation to adjacent areas with exhaust directly to the outside environment. This exhaust needs to be away from all the windows and air-intake ducts. Before starting the treatment for another patient, the nurse needs to allow adequate time for the room air exchange to occur and clear. (Also see Chapter 14.)

NURSING CARE

Pretreatment

- Before administering aerosolized pentamidine prophylaxis, conduct a thorough assessment of the patient's health status. Assess for any symptoms or illnesses that would contraindicate administering aerosolized pentamidine to the patient. This allows the nurse to individualize treatment for each patient.
- Assessment includes identifying any active pulmonary symptoms or illnesses, including tuberculosis, emphysema, bronchitis, and asthma. If the patient has a history of tuberculosis, assess that the patient has received adequate treatment. If the patient has obstructive airway disease, alter the treatment plan to include administration of a bronchodilator. If the patient has a past history of TB, a medical evaluation for active TB is appropriate. This includes chest radiograph and a PPD with an anergy panel. If the patient is suspected of having TB, also collect sputum for AFB.
- Assess for previous or current use of tobacco products, or for smoking crack or marijuana. The patient may not tolerate the administration of aerosolized pentamidine, and will need to be monitored closely for adverse reactions.
- Assess whether a woman of childbearing age is pregnant or breast-feeding, because aerosolized pentamidine may be contraindicated.
- Assess whether the patient has a past history of PCP. If the patient has received IV pentamidine in the past, evaluate how well the patient tolerated treatment, and determine whether the patient experienced hypoglycemia or hypotension.

Treatment

- Wash hands to maintain asepsis.
- Gather all equipment: 300-mg vial of pentamidine, one 10-cc vial of sterile water (preservative free), one 10-cc syringe with an 18-gauge needle, nebulizer (Respirgard II or Fisoneb), a bronchodilator, if prescribed by physician, and a gas source (compressed air or oxygen).
- Wear protective garb to protect from occupational exposure to aerosolized pentamidine or infectious microorganisms.
- Assess the patient's vital signs.
- Reconstitute the pentamidine by injecting 6 cc of sterile water into the vial. Shake the vial gently to dissolve all particles.
- Assemble nebulizer, following package instructions.
- Place reconstituted drug into the nebulizer reservoir. There are two types of nebulizers: the Respirgard II, which uses 300 mg pentamidine, and the Fisoneb, which uses 60 mg pentamidine.
- Attach the nebulizer to the chosen gas source. The flow rate of oxygen or compressed air should be 5 to 7 liters per minute.
- Position the patient in the supine position to promote even distribution of the drug through all the lung fields.
- Auscultate the lungs during administration of the drug to detect wheezing. If wheezing occurs, a bronchodilator can be administered.
- Continue administering the treatment until the reservoir of the nebulizer is empty (about 30 to 40 minutes for the Respirgard II and 20 minutes for the Fisoneb).

Posttreatment

- Reevaluate the patient's vital signs. Assess for hypotension, increased respiratory rate, and tachycardia.
- Discard equipment. The Respirgard II is disposed of. The Fisoneb is saved and reused.
- Document the procedure. Documentation includes: how well the patient tolerated the procedure, the type of nebulizer used, the drug used, the dose administered, the time and date the drug was administered, if a bronchodilator was administered, and if there were any side effects.

PATIENT TEACHING

- Instruct the patient on the proper breathing techniques to be done during the procedure. The patient breathes through the mouth only, so that any exhaled drug or microorganism will be trapped by the nebulizer's exhalation filter. Some patients have difficulty breathing through their mouths only. A nasal clip can be used to prevent nasal breathing.
- Instruct the patient to exhale all the air from the lungs every minute or so, then to inhale deeply. The patient then holds his or her breath for a few seconds before exhaling. This ensures better inhalation of the drug.
- If the patient needs to take a break from the aerosol therapy, the patient turns off the oxygen source before removing the mouthpiece, to prevent environmental contamination.
- If the patient experiences coughing, instruct to place a tissue over his or her mouth to prevent the transmission of microorganisms to other patients or health care workers. If coughing is a problem, instruct patient to sip liquids throughout the treatment.

- If the patient experiences shortness of breath, dizziness, or lightheadedness, frequent rest periods can be planned.
- A metallic taste is a side effect of the aerosolized pentamidine treatment. If this occurs, instruct the patient to suck on hard candies. Oral hygiene before and after each treatment also helps to reduce the metallic aftertaste. If appetite is disturbed by the treatment, encourage the use of nutritional supplements.
- For those patients who complain of fatigue after the pentamidine treatment, schedule their appointments in the evenings.
- If the patient has a history of hypoglycemia, ensure that the patient has eaten at least one meal prior to the treatment.
- Instruct the patient that aerosolized pentamidine treatments are scheduled every month. Missing an appointment could result in reactivation of the pneumonia.
- Instruct patient to notify nurse if the patient develops difficulty breathing. A bronchodilator may need to be administered.

Chemotherapy

Chemotherapeutic agents are drugs that are used to cure, control, and palliate different types of cancers. Although these drugs differ from one another in many ways, they all share two important features: the chemotherapeutic agents work by interrupting or altering DNA synthesis, and they are more effective in killing cells that are preparing to enter or are actively undergoing cellular replication. There are five main classifications of chemotherapeutic drugs and one miscellaneous group, as shown in the box on the next page. These drugs are classified based on whether they damage a cell during a specific phase of the cell cycle or during any phase of the cell cycle. The agents that can cause damage and death to cancer cells are known as cell cycle–nonspecific agents. The various drugs within a classification may have side effects that differ.

The first classification of antineoplastic agents is the *alkylating agents*. These drugs destroy cancer cells by producing breaks and cross-links in the strands of DNA. These agents are cell cycle nonspecific because

they cause damage to both dividing and nondividing cells. The *nitrosoureas* are a subcategory of the alkylating agents, because they have some additional properties. They not only produce breaks in the DNA strand, but also inhibit DNA repair. Another unique property of these drugs is that they are able to cross the blood-brain barrier. The *antitumor antobiotics* are another classification of antineoplastic agents that are cell cycle nonspecific. They act by binding directly with the DNA, causing changes to the DNA configuration, and preventing normal duplication of the DNA. The *antimetabolites* are antineoplastic agents that are chemically similar to the essential cellular component known as metabolites. These agents destroy tumor cells by fooling cells into believing that they are the normal metabolites of the body. Once they are incorporated into the cell, they interrupt the synthesis of DNA by blocking the production of the nitrogenous bases. These agents also interrupt enzymatic actions. The last of the five classifications of chemotherapeutic agents are the

---

CLASSIFICATION OF CHEMOTHERAPEUTIC AGENTS

Alkylating agents

Busulfan (Myleran)
Carboplatinum (Paraplatin)
Chlorambucil (Leukeran)
cis-diamminedichloroplatinum (cisplatin)
Cyclophosphamide (Cytoxan)
DTIC (dacarbazine)
Ifosfamide (Ifex)
Mechlorethamine (nitrogen mustard)
L-Phenylalanine (Alkeran, Melphalan)
Triethylenethiophosphoramide (Thiotepa)

Antitumor antibiotics

Actinomycin-D (Dactinomycin D)
Bleomycin (Blenoxane)
Daunorubicin (Daunomycin)
Doxorubicin (Adriamycin)
Mitomycin-C (mitomycin)
Mitoxantrone (Novantrone)
Plicamycin (mithramycin)

Antimetabolites

5-Azacytidine (Azacitidine)
Cytosine arabinoside (ARA-C, Cytosar)
5-Fluorouracil (5-FU, fluorouracil)
6-Mercaptopurine (6-MP)
Methotrexate (MTX, Mexate)
6-Thioguanine (6-TG, thioguanine)

Vinca alkaloids

Vincristine (Oncovin)
Vinblastine (Velban)
Vindesine (Eldisine)
VP-16 (Etoposide)

Miscellaneous

Procarbazine (Matulane)
Hydroxyurea (Hydrea)
L-Asparaginase (Elspar)

Hormones

Adrenocorticosteroids
    Dexamethasone (Decadron)
    Hydrocortisone sodium succinate
    (Solu-Cortef)
    Methylprednisolone sodium succinate
    (Solu-Medrol)
    Prednisone (Meticorten)
Androgens
Estrogens
Progestins

Nitrosoureas

BCNU (Carmustine)
CCNU (Lomustine)
Streptozocin (Zanosar)

---

plant alkaloids, which are extracted from the periwinkle plant. These agents are cell cycle specific and damage cells by binding with microtubular proteins that are essential for mitotic spindle formation during cell division. They disrupt cellular division during metaphase.

Steroidal hormones are beneficial in treating certain types of tumors, including many types of lymphomas. The mechanism of action varies for the different drugs used. Some hormones alter the permeability of the cell membrane, thus interfering with cell growth. Others are thought to bind with a receptor protein and then undergo transfer to DNA, where the transcription of RNA is altered.

INDICATIONS

Several cancers have been identified as occurring in fairly large numbers among patients with AIDS as compared to the general population. These include Kaposi's sarcoma, non-Hodgkin's lymphomas, primary CNS lymphomas, cervical cancer, and Hodgkin's lymphomas. Some of these tumors are sensitive to chemotherapy, with the individual usually responding well to this treatment modality.

CONTRAINDICATIONS

Particular lab values need to be monitored carefully in the patient receiving chemotherapy. If the patient becomes neutropenic or thrombocytopenic, those agents that are myelosuppressive need to be held until the blood counts recover. Many of the drugs that the patient with AIDS is prescribed are also myelosuppressive. Drugs such as zidovudine, ganciclovir, and trimethoprin-sulfamethoxazole may be changed to agents that do not have the same side effect as the chemotherapeutic agents. Renal and hepatic dysfunction can prevent the patient from receiving certain chemotherapeutic agents or cause the physician to modify the dose of the drug the patient will receive. Assessment for cardiac and pulmonary function is necessary before administering certain antineoplastic agents such as bleomycin or adriamycin. If the patient has compromised pulmonary or cardiac status, these agents may be dose reduced or not used in the treatment.

SAFETY ISSUES FOR HEALTH CARE WORKERS

Many of the chemotherapeutic agents are known mutagenic agents. Although the potential risks to health care workers when handling and administering chemotherapeutic agents are not known, it is important for the nurse to protect himself or herself from exposure to these agents. It has been suggested that health care workers may be exposed to antineoplastic agents through inhalation of particles or through absorption from skin exposure.

The drugs must be prepared under a vertical laminar airflow hood that vents exhausted air to the outdoors. The nurse preparing the drugs wears latex gloves and a closed-front gown with knit cuffs. Polyvinyl gloves do not provide adequate protection. After preparing the drugs and removing gloves, the nurse must wash his or her hands.

Before administering the drugs, the nurse needs to be aware of the institution's policy regarding the cleanup of spills. Small spills are those that are less than 5 ml or 5 g of a cytotoxic agent. The person cleaning up a spill wears a gown, double latex gloves, and eye protection. Absorbent gauze pads are used to wipe up liquid spills, and damp gauze pads are used for solid cleanup. For large spills the nurse wears the same protective gear. A respirator mask is added, since a large spill cleanup may generate airborne particles. Absorbent sheets or spill pads are used to clean up the spill.

All spill areas are cleaned three times with a detergent solution followed by water. The area of the spill is restricted until the spill is completely cleaned. The equipment used to clean up the spill is discarded into a cytotoxic drug waste container.

When administering the antineoplastic agents, the nurse wears latex gloves, a closed-front gown with knit cuffs, and goggles if splashing is possible. After administering the drugs, the nurse disposes of the syringes, IV bags, needles, and gloves in a leak- and puncture-proof container that can be incinerated, and washes his or her hands.

If the nurse comes into contact with a chemotherapeutic agent, the skin must be washed thoroughly with soap and water. If the exposure occurs in the eye, the eyelid is held open and flushed well for 15 minutes. Employee health services needs to be informed of all exposures.

Personnel caring for patients who have recently received chemotherapy need to know how to handle and dispose of body fluids to protect themselves and their patients from potential exposure. Latex gloves and disposable gowns are to be worn when handling the blood, vomitus, or body excreta of patients who have received cytotoxic drugs within the previous 48 hours. The linen of a patient who has received chemotherapy in the last 48 hours may be contaminated. Contaminated linen should be placed in designated laundry bags, which are placed in a second, leak-proof bag for separate washing. Contaminated wash is then added to the routine laundry for a second wash.

NURSING CARE

There are several steps that the nurse should follow when administering chemotherapy to ensure safety for the patient.

- Become familiar with the type of vascular access device the patient has and the procedures that are necessary to access and administer medications through the device. If the patient does not have a vascular access device, initiate a peripheral IV. The veins located in a joint, such as in the antecubital fossa, and veins on the dorsal surface of the hands are contraindicated for the administration of chemotherapy, especially vesicant agents.
- If the institution has a consent form for the administration of chemotherapy, verify that the patient has signed the form.
- Review the chemotherapy orders for the name of the drugs, dosage, route of administration, and date and time of drug administration. Be familiar with the mechanism of action of the drugs, as well as their potential acute and long-term side effects.
- Prior to the administration of the chemotherapeutic agents, review the most recent laboratory reports, including the complete blood count with a differential and platelet count, liver function tests, BUN, and creatinine. If any of these labs are abnormal, the drugs should not be administered until the physician is notified.
- Review the orders as to what companion drugs are to be administered with the chemotherapy. Many drugs, such as antiemetics, are administered to prevent some of the acute side effects associated with chemotherapy.
- Assess the patient for any physiologic or psychologic conditions that might contraindicate administration of chemotherapy.

- Weigh the patient at every visit and calculate a body surface area (BSA). The BSA is calculated with a special ruler, using the patient's weight and height to calculate the body surface area in square meters. With this information the accuracy of the dosage calculations can be checked with the physician.
- Verify the physician's orders and the dosage calculations with another nurse.
- Review the recommended procedure for administration of the drugs and the extravasation procedures used when administering a vesicant agent. Ensure that the appropriate drugs are available to treat a patient if an extravasation occurs. Review the policy regarding the treatment of anaphylaxis and have available the necessary medications.
- Teach the patient about the potential side effects and toxicities of the various chemotherapeutic agents before chemotherapy is administered. Also teach the patient the interventions he or she can do to prevent or minimize the side effects of chemotherapy. Provide the patient with written literature, made available through organizations such as the American Cancer Society.
- After accurately identifying the patient by looking at his or her arm band or asking the patient's name and confirming the information with the patient's name on the label on the chemotherapy, administer the drugs according to the written policies and procedures of the institution.
- Verify that the vascular access device or peripheral IV is patent by checking for a blood return. If

no blood return is obtained, withhold the treatment and notify the physician of the problem if the patient has a vascular access device. If the patient has a peripheral IV, restart the IV.
- Do not allow anyone to interrupt the process of preparing and administering the drugs.
- Dispose of the intravenous supplies according to the OSHA guidelines and the institution's policies and procedures.
- Document the drug administration in the patient's chart; include the name of the drugs, doses, route of administration, time and date the drugs were administered, how the patient tolerated the procedure, and patient teaching. Also document the type of vascular access device the patient had or if an IV was started and where it was placed.
- Observe the patient for any adverse reactions.

PATIENT TEACHING

Providing information to the patient receiving chemotherapy can help to alleviate the patient's fear of the unknown and allow the patient to take an active role in his or her care. Prior to the patient's receiving chemotherapy, instruct the patient about the type of drug, how it is administered, and the potential side effects and toxicities. During administration of the agents and afterward, reinforce the information provided to the patient. Many written materials are available at no charge to provide to patients receiving chemotherapy. After the patient receives treatment, provide written information concerning the names of the drugs and their doses, the names and phone numbers of the physician and other resource personnel, and the next appointment date and time for follow-up visits, including laboratory visits to monitor blood counts.

Total Parenteral Nutrition

Total parenteral nutrition (TPN) is a form of nutritional support administered through a central venous catheter. TPN, also known as hyperalimentation, is composed of intravenous fluids containing proteins such as amino acids, hypertonic glucose, and additives such as vitamins, minerals, electrolytes, and trace elements. TPN can provide the patient with calories, maintain positive nitrogen balance, and supply or replace

needed essential minerals, vitamins, and electrolytes. It preserves lean body mass. Fat emulsions or intralipids may also be included as a source of parenteral fats. Fats supply essential fatty acids that are used as energy.

INDICATIONS

Four general types of patients benefit from TPN support: (1) patients who are unable to eat for prolonged periods of time because of trauma or coma; (2) patients who are unable to absorb nutrients because of a primary gastrointestinal obstruction, fistula, or disease; (3) patients who are malnourished preoperatively or postoperatively because of problems such as malignancies; and (4) patients who require bowel rest because of diseases such as acute pancreatitis or inflammatory bowel disease. TPN is recommended for those patients who have compromised gut functioning and will require long-term supplemental or total nutritional support. Long-term support is defined as longer than 10 days. The patient with AIDS can develop opportunistic infections that alter the ability of the gastrointestinal tract to absorb nutrients and can lead to cachexia. Opportunistic infections such as cryptosporidiosis or microsporidiosis can render the gut dysfunctional for the duration of the patient's life.

CONTRAINDICATIONS

TPN is contraindicated in those patients who have normal gut function and are able to consume their daily calories, protein, and other nutrients either through oral or enteral feedings. Patients who have limited gut dysfunction and require short-term supplemental therapy are not candidates for TPN. Short-term therapy is less than 10 days. Whenever the patient is able to take in nutrients through the oral or enteral route, these routes should be utilized before using the parenteral route.

Intralipids are contraindicated in those patients who have a disturbance of normal fat metabolism, such as in acute pancreatitis or jaundice.

COMPLICATIONS

There are many complications from TPN, and patients must be monitored closely for these potential problems. First, the patient may experience problems related to the venous catheter. Air emboli and infection are two problems related to catheter complications. Air emboli can occur when IV tubing becomes disconnected or when a syringe, tubing, or injection cap is removed from the hub of the catheter without the clamp being closed on the catheter. Infection is a common catheter-associated complication. This can occur without TPN being infused into the catheter; however, TPN, due to its hypertonic glucose, is a culture medium for microorganism growth. Infection results from poor aseptic technique or contaminated tubing.

Complications related to TPN itself include hyperglycemia, hypoglycemia, hepatic dysfunction, hypertriglyceridemia, and protein-, fat-, and micronutrient-related complications. Hyperglycemia can occur when the amount of glucose infused exceeds that which the body can metabolize. When the TPN solution is infused

too rapidly, hyperglycemia can occur. Infection can also cause hyperglycemia. Hypoglycemia can result from TPN fluids stopped abruptly, too much insulin in the TPN solution, or decreased flow rate of the solution. Hepatic dysfunction occurs because of toxicity of components within the TPN. Essential fatty acid deficiency and excessive calorie intake can lead to hepatic dysfunction. Hypertriglyceridemia results from excessive delivery of intravenous fat emulsions. Cases of cholestasis during extended periods of TPN support have been reported. Protein-related complications of TPN therapy include azotemia. Azotemia results from increased urea production that sends an increased solute to the kidneys for excretion. TPN can cause osmotic diuresis and glycosuria. Acid-base imbalances can occur, especially in patients with renal or pulmonary dysfunction. Amino acid imbalance is a problem that needs to be monitored in the patient with hepatic dysfunction, since these patients may have decreased ability to metabolize the amino acids. Vitamin deficiencies can result in scurvy and rickets.

Complications from intralipids may result from the body not clearing the fat from the system. A lipoprotein lipase is responsible for clearance of fat from the circulation. If it is not activated, there can be an excess accumulation of fat. This is manifested by increased triglyceride levels, fever, chills, nausea and vomiting, headaches, backache, chest pain, and muscle aches. Other adverse reactions to the administration of intralipids include dyspnea, cyanosis, urticaria, and hypercoagulability. Long-term administration of intralipids can result in hepatomegaly, splenomegaly, thrombocytopenia, leukopenia, transient increases in liver function tests, and overload syndrome.

NURSING CARE

Prior to initiating TPN, perform a nutritional assessment to identify any patient whose nutritional status is or may be potentially compromised. *A nursing history examines the patient's nutritional status and practices and includes:*

- Admission weight and height
- Normal weight
- Recent weight loss
- Amount or frequency of oral intake
- Recent change in dietary intake or habits
- Food preferences, including personal, ethnic, and religious considerations

A physical assessment includes:

- Observation of condition of hair, nails, skin, mucous membranes, teeth, and mouth
- Body systems pertinent to nutritional assessment

- Laboratory tests: complete blood count with differential, serum albumin, transferrin, cholesterol, triglycerides, liver function tests, creatinine, BUN, and electrolytes, including calcium and magnesium

Practice the following recommendations when initiating TPN:

- Ensure that the solution is refrigerated at 4° C until used.
- Verify the solution label with the physician's order and check the expiration time and date.
- Inspect the solution to ensure clarity to prevent infusion of possible contaminates or precipitants.
- Begin with a slower infusion rate, and after determining that the patient tolerates the therapy, increase the infusion rate to 125 cc/hr.
- When attaching the IV tubing to the catheter, prevent the air from entering the central venous catheter by clamping the catheter. If no clamp is available, then the patient can lie flat in bed, performing a Valsalva maneuver.
- Secure the tubing junctions by taping them or with Luer-Lok connectors.
- Label the IV tubing with the time and date indicating when the administration set should be changed.
- Use a pump to control the rate of the infusion.
- TPN is to hang no longer than 24 hours and fat emulsions no longer than 12 hours. Discard solutions after the allotted time.
- The routine discontinuation of TPN involves a gradual and systematic decrease in the flow rate of the solution, to minimize the risk of rebound hypoglycemia.
- Change the dressing covering the central venous catheter every 3 days or more frequently if indicated.
- Do not use the lumen of the venous catheter designated for the infusion of TPN for any other functions such as blood sampling, blood infusions, or the administration of medications or IV fluids.

Monitor the patient closely because of the many complications associated with the administration of TPN.

- Monitor the patient's temperature and record it at least every 8 hours. A temperature of 38.0° C or greater may indicate an infection.
- Test urine for sugar and acetone every 6 hours.
- Patient weight, measured at the same time each day on the same scale, is obtained and recorded.
- Measure and record fluid intake and output every 8 hours.

- Monitor and record vital signs every 8 hours.
- Observe patient's skin turgor.
- Assess for generalized edema.
- Laboratory tests are drawn and sent daily and monitored for abnormalities.

Preparing for Home Care with TPN

For the patient who will receive TPN at home, the nursing staff at the hospital needs to initiate the teaching necessary to prepare the patient and caregivers to administer hyperalimentation. Instruction includes how to store TPN, how to access the bag of TPN with the IV tubing, how to operate the pump, the potential side effects of TPN therapy, and how to monitor for side effects.

A home health nursing agency needs to assess the patient's home for the suitability of the environment to provide TPN safely. In many situations a refrigerator is provided for the patient to store the TPN. The nurse will assess if the patient is able to maneuver from his or her bedroom to the bathroom without disconnecting the infusion. If this is not possible, then arrangements are made for the patient to have a urinal and bedside commode. The nurse representing the home health agency contacts the patient while still in the hospital. The nurse should arrange with the hospital staff to observe the patient and primary caregiver performing the necessary procedures to administer TPN before the patient is discharged home.

Once the patient is discharged home, a home health nurse will assist in the administration of TPN for several weeks, until the patient and primary caregiver are comfortable and proficient with the procedures. The nurse will need to review the other medications the patient is receiving and schedule these drugs so as to prevent incompatibilities. The home health nursing agency will have a nurse visit the patient periodically to evaluate the patient and to draw laboratory tests. Arrangements are made between the pharmacy at the home health agency and the patient to deliver TPN and intralipids to the home.

Once the patient is able to manage the TPN therapy and his or her lab values are normal, the nurse will decrease visits to the home to once a week, to evaluate the patient and draw laboratory tests. The laboratory tests that are monitored include glucose level, electrolytes, BUN, creatinine, albumin, total protein, calcium, magnesium, phosphorus, CBC, serum osmolarity, transferrin, and liver enzymes, including SGOT, SGPT, and bilirubin. Triglyceride levels are also obtained if the patient is receiving intralipids. These tests will be monitored throughout the duration of the TPN administration.

PATIENT TEACHING

- Provide the patient with information about the rationale behind the use of TPN.

- Prepare the patient for administration of TPN at home if indicated. This includes teaching the patient the information necessary to care for his or her catheter. Catheter care involves dressing changes to the exit site, flushing the catheter, and assessing the catheter exit site for redness, tenderness, swelling, and warmth.

- Instruct the patient to use a clamp to close the catheter system if there is breakage or damage to the catheter.

- Before beginning the process of preparing the IV pump for the TPN infusion, instruct the patient to check the label of the TPN bag to verify that the bag is for the patient and to verify the expiration date. Teach the patient not to use outdated solution and to notify the nurse or pharmacy.

- Instruct the patient on how to operate the IV infusion pump, including how to prime the tubing, load the reservoir and tubing into the pump, and set the rate of the infusion. Explain about pump alarms and how to identify and correct problems with the pump.

- Many patients receive what is known as cyclic TPN, which is a process where patients receive TPN for a 12-hour period instead of as a continuous 24-hour infusion. Teach these patients the purpose behind this method of infusion of the TPN and how to initiate and stop the infusion. Cyclic TPN infusion begins with a slower infusion rate for the first 2 hours of the infusion, and then the rate is increased to the prescribed rate. If the patient does not have a pump that readjusts the infusion rate automatically, instruct the patient on the procedure to change the rate of the infusion. This same process is done 2 hours prior to the completion of the infusion.

- Teach the patient to prepare the TPN. Instruct him or her to clear off a clean, dust-free surface and to prepare the TPN using aseptic technique. Preparation of the TPN includes adding any additives to the solution. Vitamins and insulin are added to the solution just prior to starting the infusion.

- Teach the patient that one potential risk associated with the administration of TPN is infection. TPN solution is not to hang for more than 24 hours. IV tubing is changed every 24 hours. Teach the patient the signs and symptoms of infection, including monitoring for fever by taking the temperature several times a day. Instruct the patient who has a temperature of 38.0° C (100.4° F) or more to notify the nurse.

- If the TPN is to be administered through a filter, teach the patient how to prime the filter and attach it to the IV tubing, the rationale behind the use of the filter, and to discard the filter after 24 hours.

- If the patient is to receive intralipids with the TPN therapy, instruct the patient to examine the bottle for opacity and consistency in color and texture. If the solution is discolored, the bottle should not be used. The bottle of intralipids should not be shaken excessively, since this can disrupt the physical stability of the fat globules.

- Intralipids are also a source for potential infection. Intralipids can hang for no more than 12 hours. If the intralipids are added to the TPN solution, then the fats are stable for up to 24 hours.

- If intralipids are piggybacked into the TPN intravenous tubing, instruct the patient on how to prime the tubing, wipe the injection port on the main IV tubing with alcohol pad, and attach the secondary IV into the port. Instruct the patient that 10% fat emulsions are infused over 4 hours, and 20% fat emulsions are infused over 6 hours.

- Provide the patient with phone numbers to reach a nurse or pharmacist when questions or a problem arises. This includes being able to reach someone at any time of the day or night. The patient should also have the phone number of the pump manufacturer so that pump malfunctions can be addressed.

- Instruct on potential complications associated with the infusion of TPN. These include signs and symptoms of fluid, electrolyte, and glucose imbalances.

- Instruct the patient to monitor urine for its glucose content. This includes how to collect urine and how to use the strips used to read the level of glucose in the urine. Glucose is monitored an hour after the start of the TPN infusion and a half hour after the infusion is completed. Instruct the patient to notify the nurse if the glucose level is over 0.5%. Signs and symptoms of hyperglycemia include weakness, increased thirst, nausea, excessive urination, and headache.

- Hypoglycemia is a potentially life-threatening complication of TPN therapy. Instruct the patient on the signs and symptoms of this problem, including sweating, pale skin, palpitations, nausea, headache, a shaky feeling, feeling of hunger, and blurred vision. Instruct the patient to keep orange juice, cake frosting in a tube, or hard candy available. If the patient develops one of these symptoms, he or she can ingest one of these foods and should immediately notify the nurse or physician.

- Instruct the patient to weigh himself or herself daily and notify the nurse if he or she gains more than ½ pound in a day.

Vascular Access Devices

IMPLANTED PORTS

Long-term intravenous therapy is delivered through one of three different types of vascular access devices: implanted ports, long-term central venous catheters, or external catheters. All three types of vascular access devices are used for the administration of intravenous fluids and medications, blood and blood products, hyperalimentation and intralipids, and chemotherapy. They are also used as an access for blood sampling.

The implanted port contains a self-sealing injection port housed in a plastic or metal case and is connected to a silicone venous catheter. The port is surgically placed in the anterior upper chest wall, where it rests in a subcutaneous pocket in the infraclavicular fossa. The catheter is placed in a large vein and threaded into the right atrium. The port can be easily palpated to determine its placement.

Another type of implanted port is the PAS port. It is a port that is implanted below the antecubital fossa. The catheter is placed in either the cephalic or basilic vein, and the catheter is threaded to the right atrium. Its care is similar to that of the implanted port located in the upper anterior chest wall, with the following exceptions: The port is accessed with a Huber needle, which is a ½-inch long, 20- or 22-gauge needle. The patient cannot have blood pressure monitored from that arm, nor can blood samples be drawn from that arm unless drawn from the port.

INDICATIONS

There are many factors to consider when selecting an implanted port for a patient. Ports are indicated for those patients who have poor or limited venous access sites. For patients who are concerned with cosmesis, the port provides an alternative to the central venous catheter, since the port is hidden underneath the skin. For patients who have a disability that impairs their ability to care for an indwelling catheter, the port offers an alternative, since care of the port is less involved than care of an external catheter or a central venous catheter. Ports are ideally used when the patient requires intermittent venous access for blood sampling, administration of blood or blood products, or short-term IV therapy.

CONTRAINDICATIONS

Use of the implanted port is contraindicated for patients who receive chemotherapeutic agents that are

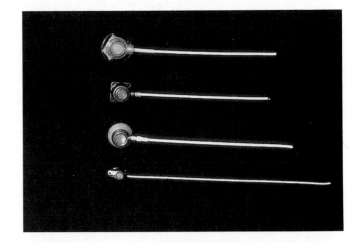

FIGURE 15-2
Implanted ports: Infus-a-Port, PortAcath, Hickman port, and PAS port.

known vesicants. There are many reports of catheters becoming dislodged from the port, with subsequent leakage of IV fluids into the body cavity. A vesicant agent that has leaked into subcutaneous tissue could cause severe tissue necrosis. The implanted port is also contraindicated in those patients who require access of the port for periods longer than a month. Patients receiving cyclic hyperalimentation should not have an implanted port as their vascular access device. Unless the needle is left in place, the patient receiving cyclic hyperalimentation will have to have the port accessed daily with a needle. This leads to irritation and breakdown of the skin over the port site.

COMPLICATIONS

There are several potential complications associated with implanted ports. A common complication is that of occlusion, where the patency of the catheter is lost. Many times, this is due to blood clot formation in the catheter. In some cases this is reversible with the use of urokinase, an agent that dissolves blood clots. Medication precipitants can also cause occlusion of the catheter. Some hospitals will use a weak hydrochloric acid solution to dissolve drug precipitants. Another potential complication of the implanted port is infection. Many patients who receive these ports are immunocompromised due to their disease or the side effects of their treatments. The port provides an access for microorganisms to enter the patient's body, causing an infection. Antibiotics are instituted when this occurs. If the port is identified as the source of the infection and antibiotics do not eradicate the infection, then the port is removed.

Other complications with implanted ports include erosion of the subcutaneous tissue over the port site, venous thrombosis, and dislodgement of the needle from the port. There are reports of the port separating from the catheter, rendering the system useless. The catheter can migrate from the right atrium into another vein. Another problem is the development of what is called portal sludge, where, after continuous use, blood and medication precipitants collect inside the port. After time, the port becomes nonfunctional.

NURSING CARE

Accessing the Implanted Port

- Wash hands to maintain asepsis.
- Gather all equipment: sterile gloves, povidone-iodine swabs, alcohol pads, a noncoring needle (Huber needle) attached to an extension tubing or a syringe.
- Palpate the site to identify the port and to become familiar with the position of the port underneath the skin.
- Don sterile gloves to maintain asepsis.
- Palpate the site to locate the implanted port again.
- Starting over the port, cleanse a 2-inch area with a povidone-iodine swab, moving outward in a spiral motion. Always move from an area of clean to dirty.
- Repeat the process two more times using a new povidone-iodine swab each time. Allow each application to dry 30 seconds before each step. Cleansing the skin with povidone-iodine eradicates microorganisms.
- Cleanse the port site with an alcohol swab, starting on top of the port and moving in a spiral outward motion, cleansing a 2-inch area. Alcohol removes the povidone-iodine and removes fats and oils from the skin.
- Access the port using the appropriate noncoring needle attached to a syringe or an extension tubing. Noncoring needles are used because they do not core out pieces of the portal septum when inserted and removed. Use a straight needle to access the port when drawing blood, giving an IV push medication, or flushing the port. If the port is being accessed for long-term use, access with a bent (90-degree) noncoring needle. Always access the port with a syringe or IV tubing attached to the needle to prevent an air embolus.
- Push the needle firmly through the skin and portal septum until the needle makes contact with the bottom of the portal chamber. Change the noncoring needle every 7 days.

Blood Sampling From the Implanted Port

- Wash hands to maintain asepsis.
- Gather all equipment: sterile gloves, povidone-iodine swabs, alcohol swab, noncoring needle attached to an extension tubing with a slide clamp, 10-cc syringe with normal saline, several syringes, Band-Aid, and a heparinized syringe.
- Attach the extension tubing to a noncoring needle. Attach a 10-cc syringe and prime the extension tubing with the normal saline. Clamp the extension tubing to prevent an air embolus.
- Follow the prior procedure to access the port.
- Flush the port with 5 cc of the normal saline to ensure patency and to clear heparin from the system.
- Withdraw 5 cc of blood/solution. The blood/solution initially withdrawn may alter laboratory results. If blood cultures are drawn, the first 5 cc is used.
- Clamp the extension tubing to prevent air emboli, and remove the syringe. Discard the syringe with blood in the appropriate waste receptacle.
- Attach a new syringe to the clamped extension tubing. Depending on the volume of blood needed for lab tests, several syringes may be needed. Always clamp the extension tubing when removing and attaching a syringe.
- Open the clamp and remove the desired amount of blood.
- Close the clamp and remove the syringe.
- Attach a 10-cc syringe that is filled with normal saline to the extension tubing. Open the clamp and flush the clamp with the saline. This clears the port and catheter of blood, thus preventing clotting and subsequent occlusion of the port.
- Close the clamp and remove the syringe.
- Attach a syringe filled with heparinized saline and open the clamp; then flush the port with heparin. (To avoid reflux of blood into the catheter, maintain positive injection pressure while closing the clamp on the extension tube during the last 0.2 cc of the injection.) Heparinization of the port is per the institution's policy. Usually the heparin dose is 5 cc of 100 units heparin per ml.
- Press down on the port with two fingers and remove the needle.
- Apply a Band-Aid to the site if bleeding occurs.

Preparing the Implanted Port for a Continuous Infusion

- Wash hands to maintain asepsis.
- Gather all equipment: IV tubing, IV pump, extension tubing attached to a noncoring needle, povidone-iodine swabs, alcohol swabs, sterile 2″ × 2″ gauze pad, tape, a 4″ × 4″ sterile gauze pad or an air-occlusive dressing, IV fluids.

- Prepare the infusion setup, prepriming all tubing. Set IV pump.
- Attach the extension tubing to a noncoring needle. Use a bent noncoring needle to stabilize the needle during the infusion. Choose the appropriate size needle gauge for the infusion.
- Attach the 10-cc syringe filled with normal saline to the extension tubing. Prime the tubing with the saline. Clamp the tubing to prevent air emboli.
- Access the port, using the procedure explained above for accessing the implanted port.
- Open the clamp and flush the port with 5 cc of normal saline to ensure the patency of the port and to clear heparin from the system.
- Clamp the extension tubing and remove the syringe. Attach the extension tubing to the IV tubing. All IV tubing should be connected with Luer-Lok connectors to ensure that the tubing will not become disconnected.
- Turn on the IV pump.
- Monitor the system for any infusion complications.
- Pad beneath the noncoring 90-degree bent needle with a sterile 2′ × 2′ gauze pad. Apply tape across the needle. The gauze pad and tape help stabilize the needle to prevent it from being dislodged.
- Cover the needle with an air-occlusive dressing or sterile 4′ × 4′ gauze pad. The proximal tubing should also be covered by the dressing to help stabilize the needle and tubing.

PATIENT TEACHING

- Prior to the implantation of the port, instruct the patient regarding the procedure used to place the implanted port, about the uses of the implanted port, and the care involved with the port. Include information regarding potential complications associated with the placement of the port and with usage of the port.
- Preoperative teaching includes instructing the patient to remain NPO the night before the surgery, and that the insertion site may be painful and that narcotics will be available to alleviate the pain. Instruct the patient to examine the insertion site for signs of excessive swelling or development of a hematoma.
- Instruct the patient to examine the area around the port for swelling, redness, tenderness, or warmth, especially while receiving an infusion. Instruct the patient to notify the physician if he or she develops a fever of 38.° C or greater. While receiving an infusion, the patient should check the placement of the needle in the port. Instruct the patient to notify a nurse if the needle appears to be dislodged, and instruct him or her in how to remove the needle.

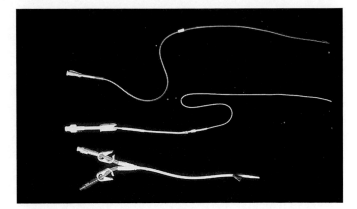

FIGURE 15-3
Long-term central venous catheters: dual-lumen Hickman, Broviac, and Groshong.

LONG-TERM CENTRAL VENOUS CATHETERS

Long-term central venous catheters are surgically placed by a physician under either local or general anesthesia. An incision is made between the nipple and clavicle, and the catheter is tunneled through subcutaneous tissue to a large vein such as the cephalic or internal or external jugular vein. The catheter is then threaded to a point where the tip of the catheter is in the right atrium. The end of the catheter is tunneled through subcutaneous tissue and exits the body at the lower anterior chest wall. The tunneling of the catheter assists in stabilizing the catheter, allowing the catheter to be used for long periods of time. One unique feature of the long-term central venous catheter is that there is a Dacron cuff. This serves three functions. It allows embedding of the catheter into the subcutaneous tissue; it allows stabilization of the catheter; and it minimizes the risk of an ascending infection. Long-term central venous catheters come with single, double, and triple lumens.

Long-term central venous catheters are referred to by many different names, including right atrial catheters, permanent catheters, and indwelling catheters. They are also referred to by their brand names, such as Hickman catheters, Groshong catheters, or Broviac catheters. These catheters can all be used immediately after their placement is verified by chest radiograph.

The Groshong catheter is designed differently from other long-term venous catheters. The end of the catheter is closed. At the end of the catheter is a slit valve that opens with positive and negative pressure. This valve keeps the catheter a closed system. Because of this closed system, the catheter is flushed weekly with 10 cc of normal saline.

INDICATIONS

Long-term central venous catheters are indicated when the patient has poor peripheral access or when the duration of therapy is long, defined as greater than 1 month. The catheter is recommended for those patients requiring continuous short- or long-term infusions of vesicant chemotherapeutic agents. Patients requiring cyclic hyperalimentation benefit from this type of catheter.

CONTRAINDICATIONS

Long-term central venous catheters are contraindicated in those patients who are unable to care for their catheters themselves, who do not have family or friends who can provide the assistance necessary to care for a catheter, who do not have the financial resources to care for a catheter, or who need infrequent venous access. For the patient with these considerations, the implanted port may be a better vascular access device.

COMPLICATIONS

Catheter infections are a common complication of this type of vascular access device. The infection could be localized to the catheter exit site only, or involve the lumen of the catheter. Antibiotic therapy is started after blood cultures are drawn from the catheter. If the cultures are positive from the catheter only, then antibiotic therapy is continued for 14 days. If the patient becomes afebrile and repeat cultures from the catheter are negative, then the catheter is maintained. Otherwise, the catheter is removed when the infection is not controlled effectively with antibiotics.

Occlusions are another common complication with long-term central venous catheters. They are caused by the formation of blood clots or by medication precipitants. Urokinase is used to dissolve blood clots and restore patency of the catheter. The catheter itself can tear or develop punctures. There are kits to repair catheters if this occurs. The last major complication seen with atrial catheters is when the IV tubing becomes disconnected from the hub of the catheter. This can result in blood loss if not corrected immediately.

NURSING CARE

Accessing the Long-Term Central Venous Catheter

- Wash hands well to maintain asepsis and to prevent the transmission of microorganisms.
- Gather all equipment needed for the procedure: sterile gloves, alcohol pads, povidone-iodine swab, syringe with or without a needle, IV tubing.
- Follow one of two procedures to access the catheter: (1) Cleanse the injection cap with an alcohol pad and allow to dry. (The alcohol prevents the transmission

of microorganisms.) Insert a needle attached to a syringe or IV tubing into the injection cap. Use a needle that is 1 inch or less because a needle longer than 1 inch could puncture the catheter. (2) If the catheter is to be accessed directly, cleanse the catheter hub and injection cap with povidone-iodine and allow to dry for approximately 30 seconds. Remove the povidone-iodine with an alcohol pad. Remove the injection cap and attach the IV tubing or syringe directly to the catheter. (Povidone-iodine prevents transmission of microorganisms; the alcohol also prevents transmission of microorganisms, and prevents povidone-iodine from entering the catheter.)

Accessing the Catheter for Blood Sampling

- Access the catheter using one of the two procedures described above.
- After accessing the catheter, draw and discard 5 cc of blood/solution from the catheter. The first 5 cc is discarded because it contains a mixture of blood and solution that can alter laboratory results. However, if the blood is being drawn for blood cultures, the first 5 cc is used and not discarded.
- Clamp the catheter to prevent an air embolus.
- Attach another syringe, unclamp the catheter, and aspirate the desired amount of blood. If several syringes are required to obtain the desired amount of blood, clamp the catheter before removing each syringe.
- Clamp the catheter to prevent an air embolus.
- Unclamp the catheter and flush the catheter with 10 cc of normal saline. Remove blood from the lumen of the catheter to prevent the catheter from becoming clotted.
- Clamp the catheter.
- While the catheter remains clamped, wipe the hub of the catheter with an alcohol pad to prevent the growth and transmission of microorganisms.
- The catheter is then heparinized or an IV tubing is attached. If the catheter is heparinized, an injection cap can be placed before or after the catheter is flushed. The catheter is flushed with heparin according to the institution's policy. Generally, 100 units per ml of heparin is used.
- Document the procedure, including what laboratory tests were drawn.

Changing the Injection Cap

- Wash hands to maintain asepsis.
- Gather all equipment needed: sterile gloves, injection cap, povidone-iodine swabs, and alcohol pads.
- Don sterile gloves to maintain asepsis.
- Cleanse the old injection cap with a povidone-iodine swab and allow to dry for 30 seconds to maintain asepsis.

- Wipe the povidone-iodine off with an alcohol pad to prevent povidone-iodine from entering the catheter.
- Clamp the catheter to prevent an air embolus.
- Remove the old injection cap and attach the new injection cap. It is recommended that injection caps be changed twice a week or when needed.

Changing the Dressing to the Exit Site

- Wash hands to maintain asepsis.
- Gather all appropriate equipment: sterile gloves, three povidone-iodine swabs, three alcohol swabs, sterile 4″ × 4″ gauze and tape, or a sterile, air-occlusive dressing, povidone-iodine ointment (optional).
- Remove old dressing and discard in the appropriate waste receptacle.
- Wash hands again.
- Inspect the exit site for redness, pain, drainage, and swelling. Inspect the tunnel tract for redness and tenderness.
- Apply sterile gloves to maintain asepsis.
- Cleanse the exit site of the catheter with an alcohol swab. Applying friction, start at the center of the exit site and move in a spiral motion about 2 inches from the center of the catheter. Always move from a clean area to a dirty area.
- Repeat the procedure above two more times, waiting 30 seconds before each application of the alcohol swabs.
- Cleanse the exit site of the catheter with a povidone-iodine swab. Applying friction, start at the center of the exit site and move in a spiral motion about 2 inches from the center of the catheter. Always move from a clean area to a dirty area.
- Repeat this procedure two more times, waiting 30 seconds before each application of the povidone-iodine.
- Apply povidone-iodine ointment to the exit site. This is an optional step and is to be performed according to the institution's policy. Some infection control nurses believe that ointment promotes the growth of microorganisms.
- Apply the dressing. It is recommended in the hospital that the patient keep an air-occlusive dressing over the catheter exit site. This dressing is changed every 3 days while the patient is in the hospital. When the exit site has healed after the insertion procedure, the patient can keep a bandage over the exit site when at home.
- Document the procedure. Document the assessment of the catheter site and the time and date of the dressing change. The nurse should note on the dressing the time and date and the initials of the nurse who changed the dressing.

EXTERNAL CATHETERS

External catheters are those catheters that provide short-term vascular access. These catheters, unlike the long-term central venous catheters, are not tunneled subcutaneously. They are placed percutaneously through either the subclavian or jugular veins. These catheters may also be placed peripherally through the basilic vein in the antecubital fossa. The external catheter may be placed at the patient's bedside, and the nurse may be asked to assist with the procedure. The multiple uses of the external catheter are the same as those of the long-term central venous catheter. The care of the external catheter is also the same as that for the long-term catheter.

PATIENT TEACHING

- Instruct the patient preoperatively about the procedure involved in the placement of the catheter, the purpose of the catheter, the care the catheter requires, and potential complications associated with placement and use of the catheter.
- Care of the catheter includes principles of good hand washing and maintaining aseptic technique when caring for the catheter.
- Teach the patient how to draw up heparin into a syringe, how to flush the catheter, how to care for the exit site, and how to change the injection cap.
- Teach assessment of the catheter exit site and the tunnel. This assessment includes evaluating the site for redness, swelling, tenderness, warmth, or drainage. If the patient develops a fever, the physician needs to be notified.
- Teach the patient to keep the catheter looped and taped to the dressing to prevent pulling on the catheter and accidental dislodgement.
- Instruct the patient that sharp objects such as scissors should not be used around the catheter. To prevent tears or pinhole leaks in the catheter, instruct the patient to use needles no longer than ¾ inch.
- Teach the patient the proper clamping procedures to avoid cuts and leaks in the catheter. This includes telling the patient that if he or she needs to use a clamp not attached to the catheter, then the clamp should have smooth edges or be covered in latex or plastic. Serrated clamps should never be used on the catheter, because they can damage the catheter. The clamp is not to be closed directly behind the hub, because this could crack the catheter. The clamp on the catheter should remain open unless the catheter is being accessed. The clamp can cause damage to the integrity of the catheter if left closed for long periods of time.

PUMPS

A vascular access device should be used in conjunction with a pump to ensure a positive pressure to prevent the catheter from becoming occluded. Pumps serve one or more purposes. Pumps provide a more accurate flow rate control than is available with a roller clamp administration set. Pumps can signal problems with the infusion, through a series of alarms. Positive pressure can be maintained for infusions requiring high pressure. Arterial infusions require high pressures that pumps can provide. Pumps allow the initiation and maintenance of very high or extremely low rates of flow. The pump allows safer administration of potent drugs by providing a specific and reliable infusion rate.

There are two classifications of pumps, based on their function: the external and the internal infusion system. The internal infusion system is an implanted pump used primarily to administer drugs such as chemotherapeutic agents or narcotics for pain control. The external infusion system comprises the pumps used most commonly by patients. This system is further divided into three groups: the large-volume infusion system, the small-volume infusion system, and the patient-controlled infusion system.

The large-volume system is an external system designed to deliver larger-volume infusions at rates as high as 2000 cc/hr. These pumps can deliver an infusion as a bolus, intermittent, and/or continuous infusion. There are three types of large-volume infusion systems. One, the controller, is an enhancement to the normal gravity-run system. The controller is essentially an electronic roller clamp capable of restricting the rate of flow of an infusion to a certain degree. If the resistance becomes too great for gravity to maintain the desired flow rate, the alarm will sound and the controller will stop infusing. Volumetric pumps, the second type, are pressure driven. They operate through a series of repetitive cycles where a known volume of fluid is forced into a reservoir, then expressed from the reservoir through the IV tubing into the vein. A variable flow system is a pressure-driven device that can be programmed to deliver an infusion at different rates. An example of the application of this type of pump is in the administration of cyclic TPN, where the rate of infusion is slower during the first and last 2 hours of administration.

INDICATIONS AND CONTRAINDICATIONS

Controllers are indicated for patients receiving intravenous fluids or medications at a constant rate. They are also used with infusions via peripheral lines where positive pressure is contraindicated. The controller is contraindicated when a patient is receiving infusions that

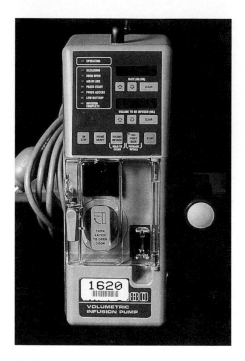

FIGURE 15-4
Volumetric pump.

are frequently interrupted to administer multiple medications on an intermittent basis. It is not utilized when a patient requires a pump that delivers positive pressure to maintain a prescribed rate of infusion. The controller is contraindicated for the administration of potent drugs, very low or very high flow rates, and any other but intravenous and fluid replacement infusions.

Volumetric pumps are indicated with infusions where it is important to have positive pressure to maintain the prescribed infusion rate. They are also used with infusions where positive pressure is needed to avoid clotting. The volumetric pump is not utilized when positive pressure is contraindicated for an infusion.

Variable flow systems are used in situations where the patient receives multiple fluids and medications and where both pumping and variable infusion rates are prescribed. The system is also used where the patient receives an intermittent administration of medications or fluids at predetermined times through the catheter. It is usually not utilized in patients who have an inadequate vascular access, who are receiving a single infusion of IV fluid or medications, or whose IV fluids are at a constant rate for all infusions.

Small-volume infusion systems are external devices designed to deliver small-volume infusions, from 2 to 250 cc/hour, as a bolus, intermittent, and/or continuous infusion. There are several types of small-volume infusion systems, including the intermittent syringe device, continuous and intermittent peristaltic devices, elastomeric device, and programmable portable infusion devices. The elastomeric pump is a nonelectric infusion

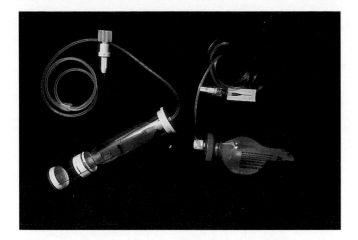

FIGURE 15-5
Elastomeric pump.

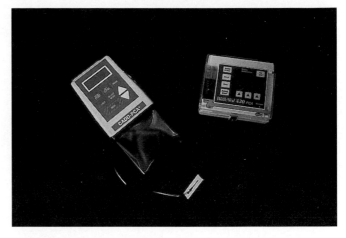

FIGURE 15-6
Ambulatory pumps by CADD for PCA (patient-controlled anesthesia).

system that consists of a solution container with a balloon that expands within a polycarbonate protective outer shell. It slowly, at a constant rate, deflates and ejects the medication. A syringe pump is a mechanical bed in which a typical hypodermic syringe is mounted after it has been filled. The syringe barrel is driven forward by a steady pressure from the driver device. A peristaltic pump operates in a manner similar to the way intestinal contents are propelled forward through the gastrointestinal tract. The pump has several fingers that are placed adjacently and are driven back and forth so that a wave motion is created, propelling the intravenous fluid forward.

The small-volume infusion system pump is indicated in patients who will receive small-volume infusions that require close monitoring or titration. It is a useful pump when delivering such medications as chemotherapeutic agents, antibiotics, and narcotics. It is also indicated for those patients who will receive their medications as outpatients. This pump is not utilized in patients who will receive infusions at rapid infusion rates or with large volumes.

Patient-controlled infusion devices are designed with the capacity to preset intermittent prescribed doses of medications. They permit the patient or caregiver to manage undesirable symptoms with self-control and independence. There are several different types of patient-controlled infusion systems: the continuous infusion, and the variable, intermittent, and basal rate pumps. These pumps are utilized for patients who do not get a response from medications administered via an oral, intramuscular, or rectal route. They are used for patients who require continuous dosing and/or intermittent bolus infusions for symptom control. They are not used for patients who have extreme variation in the amount of medication required to achieve symptom control.

COMPLICATIONS

Major complications associated with the use of pumps include occlusions, system malfunctions, and severed or leaking IV tubing.

Occlusions can be prevented by priming all IV tubing and regulating the infusion rate. The nurse ensures that all clamps are open on the IV tubing and the catheter and avoids simultaneously administering drugs that can precipitate. Occasionally, the occlusion is in the catheter or peripheral IV itself. To clear an occlusion, access the line from the catheter to the pump and correct any identified problems, such as closed clamps. An occlusion may be corrected by resetting or reprograming the pump itself.

System malfunctions can be prevented by ensuring that the pump system is plugged in or the batteries are charged. The nurse needs to ensure that the pump rate has been correctly entered and set into the system. There always has to be adequate fluid volume to prevent a system malfunction. In addition, all clamps must be open, or the pump will malfunction. If a pump malfunction occurs, assess the line from the catheter to the pump to look for the cause of the malfunction. Resetting and reprogramming the pump may correct the malfunction.

The last complication with the use of pumps is leaking IV tubing. This can be avoided by preventing undue tension on the IV tubing. No sharp objects, such as scissors, should be used around the catheter or tubing. IV connector sites should be secured using Luer-Loks. If leaking occurs, clamp the catheter and tubing between the patient and the leak. Once the catheter is clamped, the IV tubing needs to be replaced. If the catheter is damaged, then it needs to be repaired by a health care worker.

• • •

For additional readings on procedures covered in this chapter, see the bibliography for Chapter 15 at the end of this book.

CHAPTER 16

Pharmacology

Antibiotics, strictly defined, are substances produced by one living organism that may kill another living organism. **Antimicrobial** is a more generic term that applies to any substance—either natural or synthetic—that suppresses the growth of other microorganisms and may eventually destroy them. Many of the "antibiotics" are actually synthetic; however, they retain the classification of antibiotic because of their effect. Antimicrobial drugs may be described as either **bacteriostatic,** that is, they inhibit the growth of an organism, or **bactericidal** (or **fungicidal, amebicidal,** etc.), meaning that they destroy (or kill) the organism. The terms are often used interchangeably, since a drug that is bacteriostatic to one microorganism at a specific concentration may be bactericidal in higher concentrations or to other organisms. Infections that are treated with antimicrobial drugs often recur unless the body's own defense mechanisms are capable of eradicating the infection.

The treatment of infectious disease is based on the type of infecting organism, the location and severity of the infection, and the sensitivity (or susceptibility) of the organism to specific drugs. The goal of drug treatment is to eradicate the infecting organism by directly destroying it or suppressing growth so the body's own defenses are able to control the disease.

The number or range of organisms against which a drug is effective is referred to as its **spectrum** of activity. Often drugs are referred to as **broad-spectrum** antibiotics or **narrow-spectrum** antibiotics, referring to their effectiveness against a broad or narrow range of organisms.

A side effect common to most antimicrobials following prolonged or repeated administration is inhibition of normal flora, leading to overgrowth of nonsusceptible organisms. Secondary infection as a result of this overgrowth of bacteria or fungi is called a **superinfection.**

Dosing of antimicrobials is extremely varied. The infecting organism and the severity and location of the infection all influence the dose and route of administration. The age, size, and health of the host also are important considerations when determining antimicrobial doses.

In addition, in immunocompromised persons, antimicrobial drugs are often used in higher doses and in unusual combinations. These drugs may be given in prophylactic doses to prevent infection or in suppressive doses to prevent recurrence of diseases caused by organisms that have not been totally eradicated from the body. Also, because the phenomenon of HIV-related immunosuppression is so new, a great deal of empiric therapy is employed in treating HIV infection and opportunistic infections. Patients may have multiple pathologies, more frequent drug reactions, and poorly functioning renal and hepatic systems, which ordinarily work to clear drugs from the circulation. All of these conditions will necessitate use of lower than normal drug dosages. Conversely, the failure of the immune system to function properly may mean that high drug levels are necessary to eliminate opportunistic infections. Even more challenging for planning treatment, HIV-infected patients sometimes can do as well or better on moderate doses of drugs as compared to high doses.

As a result, antimicrobial therapy is often prescribed on a "best guess for dosage" basis, which is contingent on the patient's physical condition, the body site affected, the route of administration, the efficacy of the current dose of drug, how well the patient is tolerating the drug, the potential danger of side effects, and the potential interaction with other drugs. Therefore, no dosages will be given in this chapter. The reader should refer to previous chapters for recommended drug dosages according to body system affected and disease process, always recognizing that dosages may be adjusted according to the needs of individual patients.

This chapter lists each drug's potential side effects as well as its potential interactions with other drugs. In both cases the listed reactions are those that have been recognized and published at the time of this writing. Drug therapy in HIV infection, however, is a rapidly evolving arena and some of the information in this chapter is expected to become obsolete and/or incomplete in the future. Therefore, readers are encouraged to refer to recent publications on drug therapy, to read the package inserts for new drugs, and to consult with pharmacists regarding new and evolving therapies for HIV-infected patients.

GENERAL NURSING CONSIDERATIONS FOR ALL ANTIMICROBIAL DRUGS

When it is possible, assist with the identification of the infecting organism by obtaining cultures **before** antimicrobial therapy is instituted. Cultures should be sent to the laboratory and processed as soon as possible. Administer antimicrobials at the prescribed times, even when it means waking a patient or disturbing routines. Around-the-clock administration at regular intervals is often necessary to maintain antimicrobial therapeutic plasma or tissue levels. Many drugs have side effects; some are minor, whereas others are life threatening. The nurse must monitor and evaluate the patient for side effects that may develop. Serum levels should be drawn at appropriate times (see box below) and moni-

tored. Observe for development of superinfections. Reinforce the importance of completing the full course of therapy, even though the patient may be symptomless, and instruct the patient to not take "leftover" drugs for new illness. This is particularly important for the HIV-infected person who may receive multiple courses of treatment with the same drug over the years. Incompletely treated latent infections may recur with drug-resistant strains. Clients with drug allergies should be instructed in how to protect themselves from receiving the drug, by alerting health care providers and by carrying identification of the allergy, such as wallet cards or bracelets.

ANTIBACTERIALS

Antibacterial agents are commonly classified or grouped together based on their mechanism of action. Four primary mechanisms of antibacterial action are commonly recognized:

1. Inhibition of cell wall synthesis
2. Alteration of cell membrane permeability or active transport across the cell membrane
3. Inhibition of protein synthesis
4. Inhibition of nucleic acid synthesis

Dosages and routes of administration are based on the sensitivity of the infecting organism to the antibiotic and the location and severity of infection. Because different organisms require different concentrations of antibiotic for effectiveness, general guidelines for administration of many antibiotics cannot be given. In general, therapy should continue for at least 48 hours after the patient becomes symptomless. With all antibiotics, therapy should continue for the prescribed length of time even after symptoms have subsided.

SERUM DRUG LEVELS

The effects of some antibiotics are difficult to measure. Other antibiotics may have a narrow therapeutic index with either toxicity or lack of efficacy possible. To establish efficacy within safe ranges, a therapeutic range has been established for some antibiotics. The therapeutic range is the "safe range" in which serum levels are sufficient for desired drug effect but remain below the toxic level. Serum drug concentrations are used for adjustments of either dosage or dosing interval. Blood samples are often drawn to measure maximal drug concentration (peak level) and minimal drug concentration (trough level). Peak drug levels are drawn shortly following administration when serum levels are expected to be the highest. Exact timing is related to the route of administration. Peak levels are achieved immediately following IV administration and generally 30 to 60 minutes after IM or oral administration, but peak levels may vary significantly between drugs. Trough levels are drawn at the end of the dosing interval, immediately before the next dose is administered. The organism and site of infection also influence the desired concentration.

Penicillins

Penicillins are the most widely effective and widely used antibiotics. Penicillins and cephalosporins are two large groups of antibiotic drugs that share similar properties. These drugs are referred to as **beta-lactam drugs** because of their chemical structure, which includes a "beta-lactam" ring. Antibiotics in this class exert their antibacterial effect by inhibiting cell wall synthesis. Penicillin G, the prototype penicillin, was discovered in 1929 by Fleming. There are significant differences within the penicillins in degree of inactivation by gastric acids, protein binding, inactivation by penicillinase, and spectrum of antimicrobial activity.

Resistance to many of the penicillins may occur by organisms producing an enzyme, beta-lactase (also called penicillinase), which inactivates some penicillins by breaking the beta-lactam ring in their structure. Penicillins that are resistant to these enzymes are called **penicillinase resistant.** Combinations of a penicillin with a beta-lactamase inhibitor are now available. The combination is thought to increase the effectiveness of penicillin by inhibiting the beta-lactamase enzyme.

The amidinopenicillins are a new group of penicillins, of which amdinocillin is the prototype. Because this drug binds with different receptors rather than other penicillins, it may be synergistic with penicillins.

Indications: Penicillins are used to treat infections caused by penicillin-sensitive bacteria. They are commonly used in the treatment of infections attributable to gonococci, spirochetes, *Actinomyces. Haemophilius, Pseudomonas, Staphylococcus aureus. Streptococcus pneumoniae,* group A streptococci, and *Serratia.* Penicillins have been used prophylactically in treating persons exposed to S. *pyogenes,* gonorrhea, or syphilis; in preventing recurrences of rheumatic fever; and in preventing subacute bacterial endocarditis (in patients with valvular heart disease who are undergoing surgical or dental procedures). Various routes of administration of the penicillins are presented in Table 16-1.

Precautions/contraindications: All penicillins are cross-sensitizing and cross-reacting.

Side effects/adverse reactions: The incidence of allergic reactions to the penicillins has been estimated to be as high as 5% to 10% in adults. Original sensitizing exposure may come from exposure to environmental mold and dermatophytes living on the skin, which are capable of producing penicillin-like molecules. Another source of exposure is from penicillin in the milk of cows being treated for mastitis. Allergic reactions may be immediate (e.g., pruritus, urticaria, asthma, rhinitis, laryngeal edema, and anaphylaxis), intermediate (e.g., rashes and fever), or delayed even after the antibiotic is stopped (e.g., serum sickness, rash, thrombocytopenia, and anemia). Anaphylactic reactions, although rare,

most commonly occur following parenteral therapy. All penicillins are **cross-sensitizing,** which means that a patient allergic to any one penicillin may be allergic to other penicillins.

Penicillins are generally well tolerated by most patients. Penicillins may produce gastrointestinal (GI) upset, local pain may accompany intramuscular (IM) injections, and sclerosing phlebitis may follow intravenous (IV) administration. High doses of ticarcillin, carbenicillin, mezlocillin, piperacillin, azlocillin, or nafcillin have been reported to cause bleeding abnormalities.

Many penicillins have a high sodium content, which may lead to electrolyte imbalances when high doses are administered. Hypokalemia has been reported in patients receiving azlocillin, mezlocillin, ticarcillin, piperacillin, and carbenicillin.

Ampicillin frequently causes skin rashes, some of which are not related to allergy.

Bone marrow depression with granulocytopenia, or interstitial nephritis may occur with the penicillinase-resistant penicillins.

Pharmacokinetics: Penicillins are primarily eliminated through the kidney. Nafcillin is least dependent on renal elimination, with about 80% of a dose excreted in the bile. Penicillin is also excreted in saliva and breast milk in roughly 3% to 15% of serum levels. Penicillin G and several other penicillin drugs may be either partially or totally inactivated by gastric acids with a pH of 2 or less. Absorption of most penicillins is affected by food.

Penicillins have been formulated to provide a prolonged action following IM administration. Procaine or benzathine salts are used for IM administration to maintain effective serum concentrations for up to 4 weeks as the result of slow, prolonged absorption from the injection site.

Interactions: Administration of probenecid blocks renal tubular excretion of penicillin and prolongs blood levels. Probenecid is sometimes administered with the penicillin for this effect. An increased incidence of breakthrough bleeding and pregnancy has been reported following the use of some penicillins in patients using oral contraceptives. Probenecid increases AZT, acyclovir, ganciclovir, and dapsone levels, and decreases renal clearance of ciprofloxacin.

Nursing considerations: Oral penicillins (except amoxicillin) should not be administered at meal time, but at least 1 hour before meals or 1 to 3 hours after meals to minimize inactivation by gastric acid. All patients should be monitored closely for signs of immediate or delayed allergic reaction. When administering parenteral penicillins, emergency drugs for treating anaphylaxis should be immediately available. Caution women using oral contraceptives to use an alternate method of

Table 16-1

PENICILLINS

Generic name	Trade names	Routes of administration
Penicillin G	Pentids	Oral
		IM, IV
Penicillin V	Compocillin-V	Oral
	Penicillin V	Oral
	Pen-Vee K	Oral
	V-Cillin	Oral
Penicillinase-resistant		
Methicillin	Staphcillin	IM, IV
Nafcillin	Unipen	Oral, IM, IV
	Nafcil	Oral, IM, IV
	Nallpen	Oral, IM, IV
Oxacillin	Prostaphlin	Oral, IM, IV
	Bactocill	Oral, IM, IV
Cloxacillin	Cloxapen	Oral
	Tegopen	Oral
Dicloxacillin	Dynapen	Oral
	Pathocil	Oral
Ampicillins		
Ampicillin	Amcill	Oral, IM, IV
	Omnipen	Oral, IM, IV
	Polycillin	Oral, IM, IV
	Totacillin	Oral, IM, IV
Bacampicillin	Spectrobid	Oral
Amoxicillin	Amoxil	Oral
	Larotid	Oral
	Polymox	Oral
	Trimox	Oral
Cyclacillin	Cyclapen	Oral
Extended spectrum		
Carbenicillin	Geopen	IM, IV
	Pyopen	IM, IV
Ticarcillin	Ticar	IM, IV
Mezlocillin	Mezlin	IM, IV
Piperacillin	Pipracil	IM, IV
Azlocillin	Azlin	IV
Amidinopenicillins		
Amdinocillin	Coactin	IM, IV
Combined penicillin/beta-lactamase inhibitors		
Amoxicillin/clavulanic acid	Augmentin	Oral
Ticarcillin/clavulanic acid	Timentin	IV
Ampicillin/sulbactam	Unasyn	IM, IV

Table 16-2

CEPHALOSPORINS

Generic name	Trade names	Routes of administration
First generation		
Cephalothin	Keflin	IM, IV
Cefazolin	Ancef	IM, IV
	Kefzol	IM, IV
Cephapirin	Cefadyl	IM, IV
Cephradine	Anspor	Oral, IM, IV
	Velosef	Oral, IM, IV
Cephalexin	Keflet	Oral
	Keflex	Oral
	Keftab	Oral
Cefadroxil	Duricef	Oral
	Ultracef	Oral
Second generation		
Cefamandole	Mandol	IM, IV
Cefuroxime	Ceftin	IM, IV
	Kefurox	IM, IV
	Zinacef	IM, IV
Cefonicid	Monocid	IM, IV
Cefoxitin	Mefoxin	IM, IV
Cefaclor	Ceclor	Oral
Cefotetan	Cefotan	IM, IV
Ceforanide	Precef	IM, IV
Cefmetazole	Zefazone	IV
Third generation		
Cefotaxime	Claforan	IM, IV
Ceftriaxone	Rocephin	IM, IV
Moxalactam	Moxam	IM, IV
Cefoperazone	Cefobid	IM, IV
Ceftizoxime	Cefizox	IM, IV
Ceftazidime	Fortax, Fortaz	IM, IV
	Tazidime	IM, IV
Cefixime	Suprax	Oral

birth control during penicillin therapy. Monitor patients at risk for electrolyte imbalance for signs of potassium imbalance, sodium imbalance, or water retention.

Cephalosporins

The cephalosporins are beta-lactam drugs with activity similar to penicillins. They are bactericidal by interfering with the cell wall synthesis of bacteria. Cephalosporin antibiotics are classified as first-, second-, or third-generation agents. This terminology, which was developed for marketing, does not necessarily follow the chronologic development of the drugs, but it does follow their spectrum of antibacterial activity. As a patient progresses through first-, second-, and third-generation cephalosporins, the effectiveness against gram-negative organisms generally increases, whereas the effectiveness against gram-positive organisms decreases. Several second-generation agents are also active against anaerobic organisms.

Indications: Cephalosporins are used to treat cephalosporin-sensitive bacterial infections and for surgical prophylaxis. Various routes of administration for the cephalosporins are presented in Table 16-2.

Precautions/contraindications: Cross-reactivity with the

Table 16-3

ERYTHROMYCINS

Generic name	Trade names	Routes of administration
Erythromycin	E-Mycin, Ery-Tab, ERYC	Oral
Erythromycin estolate	Ilosone	Oral
Erythromycin stearate	Eramycin, Ethril, Erypar	Oral
Erythromycin ethylsuccinate	E.E.S., Pediamycin, Wayamycin, Eryped	Oral
Erythromycin lactobionate	Erythrocin Lactobionate	IV
Erythromycin gluceptate	Ilotycin Gluceptate	IV

penicillins has been reported rarely but is potentially serious when it occurs.

Side effects/adverse reactions: Allergic reactions and tissue irritation are similar in nature and incidence to penicillins. Renal toxicity has been reported with some of the early cephalosporins, especially when used concomitantly with an aminoglycoside antibiotic.

Pharmacokinetics: Many of the cephalosporins are poorly absorbed from the GI tract and therefore are administered parenterally. Cephalosporins are eliminated primarily by the kidney. Food may increase or decrease absorption, depending on which oral cephalosporin is used.

Interactions: Nephrotoxicity attributable to aminoglycosides may be potentiated. Oral anticoagulants may have an increased effect. Nausea and vomiting may occur if alcohol is consumed while the drug is in the body (the "Antabuse" reaction).

Nursing considerations: See Penicillins.

Erythromycin

Erythromycin exerts its antibacterial effect by interfering with protein synthesis. The base form of erythromycin is destroyed in stomach acid and therefore must be administered with an enteric coating.

Indications: Erythromycin is used to treat infections caused by erythromycin-sensitive bacteria, including pneumococcal pneumonia, bacillary angiomatosis, *Mycoplasma pneumoniae*, and *Legionella* infections. Erythromycin is also used as a substitute for penicillin in patients allergic to penicillin. Various routes of administration for the erythromycins are presented in Table 16-3.

Precautions/contraindications: Erythromycin should be used with caution in patients with impaired hepatic function. Erythromycin estolate and ethylsuccinate are contraindicated in the presence of liver disease.

Side effects/adverse reactions: Impaired liver function

and jaundice have been reported following use of erythromycin estolate and ethylsuccinate, but the effects appear to be reversible upon discontinuation. GI disturbances, including nausea, cramping, anorexia, and diarrhea, are common with oral administration. Discomfort at the site of infusion and phlebitis are commonly associated with parenteral administration. Reversible hearing loss can occur with high doses.

Pharmacokinetics: Erythromycin is concentrated in the liver and eliminated in the bile, with a small amount eliminated by the kidneys.

Interactions: Increased effects of digoxin, carbamazepine (Tegretol), xanthines, and oral anticoagulants may occur, most commonly from altered metabolism. Erythromycins may antagonize the effects of chloramphenicol or lincomycin.

Nursing considerations: Do not administer concurrently with chloramphenicol or lincomycin. Monitor for jaundice or other signs of liver dysfunction with erythromycin estolate and ethylsuccinate. When oral forms are used, instruct the patient to take the drug on an empty stomach (i.e., 1 hour before or 2 hours after meals). Erythromycin estolate, ethylsuccinate, and enteric-coated tablets may be taken without regard to meals. Oral doses should be taken with a full glass of water. Monitor for symptoms of GI intolerance.

Clindamycin

The lincosamides, which include clindamycin, exert their effect by inhibiting bacterial protein synthesis. Clindamycin resembles erythromycin in its spectrum of activity. The drug is administered by oral, IV, or IM routes.

Indications: Clindamycin is used to treat infections caused by erythromycin-sensitive bacteria; it is sometimes used to treat PCP and for prophylaxis for toxoplasmosis.

Precautions/contraindications: Clindamycin must be

Table 16-4 _____

TETRACYCLINES

Generic name	Trade names	Routes of administration
Short duration		
Tetracycline	Achromycin, Panmycin	Oral, IM, IV
	Sumycin, Tetralan	Oral, IM, IV
		IV
Chlortetracycline	Achromycin	Topical
		Ophthalmic
Oxytetracycline	Terramycin, Uri-Tet	IM, oral
Intermediate duration		
Demeclocycline	Declomycin	Oral
Methacycline	Rondomycin	Oral
Longer duration		
Doxycycline	Vibramycin, Doxychel,	Oral, IV
	Doxy Caps, Doryx	IV, Oral
Minocycline	Minocin	IV, oral

used cautiously in patients with impaired renal or hepatic function.

Side effects/adverse reactions: A rash occurs in about 10% of patients, and mild GI effects are common. Pseudomembranous colitis may occur. Hepatic and renal dysfunction has been reported, usually associated with prolonged therapy may cause neutropenia and/or eosinophilia.

Pharmacokinetics: Administration with food does not impair absorption of clindamycin. The drug is greater than 60% protein bound and is eliminated primarily via hepatic metabolism. A significant amount of the drug can be found in breast milk.

Interactions: Clindamycin has a neuromuscular blocking effect that may enhance the effect of other neuromuscular blocking drugs.

Nursing considerations: Administer with a full glass of water to prevent esophagitis.

Tetracyclines

The tetracyclines exert their antibacterial effect by inhibiting bacterial protein synthesis.

Indications: Tetracyclines are used to treat infections caused by a variety of gram-positive bacteria, gram-negative bacteria, spirochetes, *Leptospira* organisms, chlamydiae, mycoplasmata, amebae, and some rickettsiae. Tetracyclines are also used to treat shigellosis and campylobacteriosis. Various routes of administration for the tetracyclines are presented in Table 16-4.

Precautions/contraindications: Tetracyclines should not be administered to pregnant women or children under the age of 6 years to avoid bone and tooth discoloration and dysplasia.

Side effects/adverse reactions: GI upset and diarrhea may occur from direct irritation or altered gut flora. IV administration can cause severe hepatic and pancreatic injury. Tetracyclines are readily bound to newly formed bones and teeth, leading to brownish discoloration and possibly dysplasia. Systemic administration may lead to photosensitivity. Enterocolitis and pseudomembranous colitis may occur.

Pharmacokinetics: Absorption following oral administration is variable. Calcium and aluminum salts tend to impair absorption. Elimination is primarily through the kidney.

Interactions: A nonabsorbable complex is formed, leading to reduced absorption if given in combination with calcium, magnesium, or aluminum-containing antacid preparations and also iron-containing products. A buffer in ddI prevents absorption of tetracyclines.

Nursing considerations: Oral preparations should be taken on an empty stomach with a full glass of water to avoid esophageal or gastric irritation. Avoid dairy products or laxatives containing aluminum, calcium, or magnesium for 1 hour after or 2 hours before taking tetracyclines. Inform patients that the drug may cause photosensitivity and instruct them to avoid direct sunlight as much as possible and to use sunscreen.

Table 16-5

AMINOGLYCOSIDES

Generic name	Trade names	Routes of administration
Amikacin	Amikin	IM, IV
Gentamycin*	Garamycin	IM, IV
Kanamycin	Kantrex, Klebcil	IM, oral, IV
Neomycin	Mycifradin	IM, oral
	Neobiotic	Oral, IM
Netilmicin	Neo-IM, Netromycin	IM, IV
Paromomycin	Humatin	Oral
Streptomycin	None	IM
Tobramycin*	Nebcin	IM, IV

*Also available in cream, ointment, and solution forms for ophthalmic and topical use.

Aminoglycosides

The aminoglycoside antibiotics are effective against a wide range of bacteria, but their use is limited primarily to the treatment of serious gram-negative infections because of the toxicity of these drugs. The aminoglycosides exert their bactericidal effects by interfering with protein synthesis.

Indications: Parenteral administration of aminoglycosides is used to treat gram-negative infections caused by *E. coli*, *Proteus*, *Pseudomonas*, *Klebsiella*, *Enterobacter*, and *Serratia* organisms. Streptomycin is used as an antitubercular drug. Amikacin is a second-line antitubercular drug. Oral forms (Neomycin) are used to suppress GI flora in preparation for abdominal surgery and for reducing ammonia-forming bacteria in the treatment of hepatic coma. Paromomycin is used in the treatment of intestinal amebiasis and cryptosporidiosis. Various routes of administration for the aminoglycosides are presented in Table 16-5.

Precautions/contraindications: Aminoglycosides are not used for long-term therapy because of the high incidence of ototoxicity and nephrotoxicity. Dehydration and advanced age increase the risk of toxicity. These drugs may aggravate muscle weakness, especially in patients with neuromuscular disorders such as myasthenia gravis.

Side effects/adverse reactions: Aminoglycosides are associated with nephrotoxicity and ototoxicity even at conventional doses. Renal damage may be evidenced by decreased creatinine clearance levels, cells or casts in urine, oliguria, proteinuria, or increased serum BUN or creatinine levels. The renal damage may be reversible. The drugs are toxic to the eighth cranial nerve, causing both auditory and vestibular damage. The damage may appear as high-frequency hearing loss, tinnitus, or vertigo. Onset of deafness may occur several weeks after administration has been stopped and may be irreversible. High doses may be neurotoxic and exhibit a neuromuscular blocking effect.

Pharmacokinetics: Oral forms are not significantly absorbed, whereas absorption is rapid and complete following IM administration. Excretion of the unchanged drug is through the kidney and is markedly reduced in the presence of decreased renal function.

Interactions: The potential for ototoxicity or nephrotoxicity is enhanced when administered with other aminoglycosides or other nephrotoxic agents, such as amphotericin B, bumetanide, cephalosporins, cyclosporine, ethacrynic acid, furosemide, and vancomycin.

Nursing considerations: Doses should be reduced in patients with reduced renal function or in the elderly. Assessment of renal function and hearing and vestibular function should be done before and during high-dose or long-term therapy (>10 days). IV administration should proceed over a period of 30 to 60 minutes to reduce the possibility of toxic serum levels. Patients should be well hydrated and instructed to report any hearing loss, tinnitus, or dizziness. Peak and trough serum drug levels should be monitored.

Spectinomycin

Spectinomycin (Trobicin) is an aminocyclitol antibiotic related to the aminoglycosides. Its antibacterial action results from inhibition of protein synthesis. The drug is indicated only for treatment of gonorrheal infections using a single IM dose of 2 to 4 g. The dose should be administered deep in the gluteal muscle (2 g at each injection site). Pain at the injection site and occasionally fever, chills, urticaria, or nausea may occur.

Vancomycin

Vancomycin inhibits bacterial cell wall synthesis.

Indications: Parenteral forms of vancomycin are used to treat serious staphylococcal infection or endocarditis not responsive to other antibiotic treatment, as well as infections caused by *Streptococcus pneumoniae*. Oral therapy is used in the treatment of staphylococcal enterocolitis and antibiotic-associated pseudomembranous colitis caused by *Clostridium difficile*. Vancomycin is increasingly being used for the treatment of infections attributable to penicillinase strains of staphylococci.

Precautions/contraindications: IM administration is not used because pain and necrosis may result. Reduced doses are needed in the presence of renal impairment.

Side effects/adverse reactions: Thrombophlebitis and pain may occur following IV administration. If IV administration is too rapid, a sudden fall in blood pressure—with or without development of a rash over the face, neck, chest, and upper extremities—may occur. This is not an allergic reaction but is most likely the result of histamine release and resolves after administration is completed. Nephrotoxicity and ototoxicity may occur similar to the aminoglycoside antibiotics.

Pharmacokinetics: Oral doses are very poorly absorbed.

Interactions: There is an increased chance of nephrotoxicity if administered with other nephrotoxic antibiotics, such as aminoglycosides and amphotericin B.

Nursing considerations: The IV dose should be given over 1 to 2 hours in a dilute solution of at least 100 ml of fluid for each 500 mg. Renal and auditory function should be monitored, especially in patients over 60 years or in patients with already impaired renal function. Monitor blood pressure closely during IV infusion. Serum levels should be monitored and dosages adjusted accordingly.

Ciprofloxacin

Ciprofloxacin is a synthetic broad-spectrum antibacterial agent that works through inhibition of protein synthesis. It belongs to a class of drugs called fluoroquinolones. The drug is administered by oral and IV routes.

Indications: Ciprofloxacin is used to treat both urinary and systemic infections.

Precautions/contraindications: Ciprofloxacin must be used with caution in patients with known or suspected CNS disorders or with a predisposition to seizures. Reduced dosages may be needed in patients with diminished renal function.

Side effects/adverse reactions: CNS stimulation, including tremors, restlessness, light-headedness, seizures, nausea, vomiting, and diarrhea, may occur.

Pharmacokinetics: Ciprofloxacin is well absorbed and eliminated primarily through the kidney, with an increased half-life in the presence of decreased renal function. The rate of absorption of ciprofloxacin is delayed by the presence of food in the stomach, but the overall absorption is not altered.

Interactions: Antacids containing magnesium or aluminum hydroxide may interfere with ciprofloxacin absorption. Theophylline levels may be increased because of reduced theophylline clearance in patients taking fluoroquinolones. Absorption is decreased when the drug is taken with vincristine, doxorubicin, and ddI. Absorption is adequate if the drug is taken 2 hours after taking ddI.

Nursing considerations: Ciprofloxacin may be taken with or without meals. Patients should be well hydrated. Patients taking theophylline should be monitored for signs of toxic effects and have serum theophylline levels monitored.

Metronidazole

Metronidazole is effective against a variety of anaerobic bacteria and protozoa. It works by interfering with protein synthesis.

Indications: Metronidazole is used to treat anaerobic infections, antibiotic-associated pseudomembranous colitis, amebiasis, giardiasis, and trichomoniasis, and for prophylaxis during colorectal surgery.

Precautions/contraindications: Reduced doses may be needed in patients with liver disease.

Side effects/adverse reactions: Nausea, anorexia, vomiting, diarrhea, and other GI disturbances, as well as dry mouth and a "metallic" taste, are common side effects. Nausea and vomiting may occur if alcohol is consumed while the drug is in the body (Antabuse reaction). Darkened urine may occur, which is of no clinical significance. High cumulative doses have been associated with seizures or peripheral neuropathy. Pseudomembranous colitis may occur.

Pharmacokinetics: Food intake delays but does not alter total absorption. Elimination is primarily through the kidneys.

Interactions: Metronidazole may potentiate oral anticoagulants. Concurrent use with phenobarbital and phenytoin may increase metabolism of metronidazole and reduce its effectiveness unless the dosage is increased.

Nursing considerations: Administering the oral form with meals may reduce GI disturbances. Monitor for signs of nervous system toxicity, particularly dizziness, vertigo, incoordination, confusion, weakness, or numbness or paresthesia of an extremity. Warn patients not to consume alcohol.

Sulfonamides and Trimethoprim
Sulfonamides

The sulfonamides are bacteriostatic drugs. They competitively antagonize para-aminobenzoic acid (PABA),

Table 16-6

SULFONAMIDES AND TRIMETHOPRIM

Generic name	Trade names	Routes of administration
Sulfadiazine	Microsulfon	Oral
Sulfacytine	Renoquid	Oral
Sulfisoxazole	Gantrisin	Oral
		SC, IM, IV
Sulfamethoxazole	Gantanol	Oral
	Urobak	Oral
Sulfamethizole	Proklar	Oral
Multiple sulfonamides*		
Trisulfapyrimidines	Triple Sulfa	Oral
	Neotrizine	Oral
	Terfonyl	Oral
Trimethoprim	Proloprim	Oral
	Trimpex	
Trimethoprim (TMP)/	Bactrim	IV, oral
sulfamethoxazole	TMP-SMX	IV, oral
(SMX)	Comoxol	IV, oral
	Cotrim	IV, oral
	Sulfatrim	IV, oral
	Septra	IV, oral

*Multiple sulfonamides provide the same therapeutic effect as the total sulfonamide content but reduce the risk of precipitation in the kidneys.

which is essential for folic acid synthesis. Microorganisms that require endogenous folic acid are therefore susceptible to the sulfonamides.

Indications: The sulfonamides have a broad spectrum of activity; they are used in the treatment of urinary tract infections or in topical preparations. In HIV patients, they are used to treat *Pneumocystis carinii* infections, salmonellosis, shigellosis, toxoplasmosis, isosporiasis, and *H. influenzae* infections. Various routes of administration for the sulfonamides are presented in Table 16-6.

Precautions/contraindications: In patients with porphyria, these drugs may precipitate an attack. Photosensitivity can occur.

Side effects/adverse reactions: Nausea, vomiting, abdominal pain, photosensitivity, rashes, pruritus, and exfoliative dermatitis can occur. Cross-sensitivity can occur in patients sensitive to carbonic anhydrase inhibitors, thiazides, furosemide, bumetanide, and the sulfonylurea hypoglycemic agents. Sulfonamides can cause bone marrow depression and blood disorders, including anemia, granulocytopenia, and thrombocytopenia. The drugs can rarely precipitate in the urine, causing crystalluria, hematuria, or obstruction. They can also cause erythema multiforme in up to 50% of HIV-infected patients treated with these drugs.

Pharmacokinetics: Sulfonamides are readily absorbed from the GI tract and eliminated mainly through the kidneys.

Interactions: Sulfonamides may displace highly protein-bound drugs, such as oral anticoagulants, anticonvulsants, and oral antidiabetic agents, from protein binding sites, resulting in higher serum levels and increased therapeutic effects. There is increased potential for toxic effects when administered with hepatotoxic or bone marrow–suppressing drugs.

Nursing considerations: Instruct the patient to take each dose on an empty stomach with a large glass of water. If GI upset occurs, instruct the patient to take the drug with food. To minimize precipitation in urine, encourage patients to drink large amounts of liquids. Caution patients to avoid or minimize exposure to sunlight and to use sunscreens when outside.

Trimethoprim

Trimethoprim blocks the production of folic acid at a site different from that of the sulfonamides.

Indications: Trimethoprim is used to treat urinary tract infections.

Precautions/contraindications: Trimethoprim must be used with caution in patients with renal or hepatic impairment.

Side effects/adverse reactions: Rash, pruritus, exfoliative dermatitis, and GI disturbances can occur. Trimethoprim rarely causes bone marrow depression, which is usually associated with large doses or prolonged administration.

Pharmacokinetics: Trimethoprim is well absorbed after oral administration, with primary elimination through the kidneys.

Interactions: Trimethoprim may increase the effect of phenytoin through inhibition of metabolism.

Nursing considerations: The tablets should be protected from light.

Trimethoprim/sulfamethoxazole

The combination of trimethoprim and sulfamethoxazole results in a dual block of folate synthesis, which provides a synergistic effect with increased activity and antibacterial spectrum. The drug is used for prophylaxis, treatment, and suppression of *Pneumocystis carinii* infections. It also is used for treatment and suppression of *Isospora belli* infections. Drug profiles for trimethoprim and sulfonamides apply to the combined drug. In addition, the IV form should be administered over 60 to 90 minutes and must be diluted and used within 2 hours of mixing. The combined drug can result in bone marrow suppression and hepatotoxicity when administered with pyrimethamine.

ANTIFUNGAL DRUGS

Most fungi are resistant to the action of antibacterial drugs, whereas antifungal drugs generally have no effect on bacteria. Topical infections should be treated locally rather than with systemic therapy, which is associated with numerous adverse effects. The antifungal drugs available for systemic therapy are limited in both number and effectiveness. Therapy must continue for several weeks or months to prevent a recurrence of the infection. Table 16-7 presents various routes of administration for specific agents.

Amphotericin B

Amphotericin B, although highly toxic, is the most effective drug for treatment of systemic fungal infections and is widely used in treating HIV-infected patients. It is not absorbed following oral administration and must be given intravenously. Following IV administration, chills, fever, vomiting, and headache commonly occur. Aspirin, phenothiazines, antihistamines, antiemetics, and corticosteroids may be used to minimize or treat the adverse effects. The drug may impair renal and hepatic function and produce anemia. Hypotension, electrolyte imbalances (especially hypokalemia), and occasionally neurologic symptoms accompany therapy. The toxic effects are usually reversible following discontinuance of drug therapy. The drug is administered as an IV infusion over 2 to 6 hours. Rapid infusion is not recommended. The risk of nephrotoxicity is increased when the drug is administered with acyclovir, aminoglycosides, and foscarnet. The drug increases the hematotoxicity of AZT and increases all toxicities of flucytosine.

Fluconazole

Fluconazole is an antifungal drug widely used in the treatment of HIV-infected patients. It is used to treat local or systemic candidal infections, coccidioidomycosis, and cryptococcemia. The drug is used for both treatment and suppression in these conditions, al-

Table 16-7

SYSTEMIC ANTIFUNGAL DRUGS

Generic name	Trade names	Routes of administration
Amphotericin B	Fungizone	IV, intrabladder
Fluconazole	Diflucan	IV, oral
Flucytosine	Ancobon	Oral
Griseofulvin	Fulvicin	Oral
	Grifulvin	Oral
	Grisactin	Oral
Ketoconazole	Nizoral	Oral, topical
Miconazole	Monistat IV	IV, topical
		Intrathecal
		Intrabladder
Nystatin	Mycostatin	Oral, topical

though amphotericin B is the drug of first choice to treat meningitis due to coccidioidomycosis or cryptococcosis. Use of fluconazole has been associated with nausea, headache, skin rash, abdominal pain, diarrhea, elevated serum glutamic-oxaloacetic transaminase (SGOT) and, rarely, severe hepatotoxicity and severe skin disorders. Like most antimicrobials, fluconazole must be taken for the full course of treatment in order to prevent development of drug-resistant strains. It is important to emphasize this to the patient, because the effective length of treatment may be weeks. A nearly healed patient may no longer adhere to the treatment after the symptoms have subsided, thus precipitating a severe recurrence of the infection. The drug interacts with oral contraceptives and may reduce their effectiveness. Fluconazole increases prothrombin time in patients taking warfarin. Fluconazole blood levels are decreased when the drug is taken with rifampin.

Flucytosine

Flucytosine is effective against strains of *Candida* or *Cryptococcus*. The drug is well absorbed following oral administration and is excreted in the urine. Drug accumulation may occur in patients who have diminished renal function, and dosages should be reduced in these patients. Before initiation of therapy, renal and hematologic status should be evaluated. The possibility that bone marrow depression can occur necessitates monitoring of marrow function during therapy. Other adverse reactions include GI disturbances, rash, and elevation of serum liver enzymes, BUN, and creatinine levels. To avoid nausea or vomiting, advise the patient to take the capsules over 15 minutes rather than all at once. All side effects are increased when the drug is administered with amphotericin B. Hematotoxicity is increased with ganciclovir and AZT.

Griseofulvin

Griseofulvin is ineffective in *Candida* infections but is effective against *Microsporum, Epidermophyton,* and *Trichophyton* infections. The drug is most commonly used for treatment of ringworm infections of the skin, hair, and nails. Serum levels may be increased by giving the medication with a meal of high fat content. Side effects include headaches; rashes; GI disturbances; and, with long-term therapy, alterations in renal, hepatic, and hematopoietic function. The activity of oral anticoagulants and oral contraceptives is decreased. The drug may potentiate the effects of alcohol. Barbiturates may decrease the drug's effectiveness. Patients should be cautioned to minimize exposure to sunlight, because photosensitivity may occur.

Ketoconazole

Ketoconazole was the first antifungal drug found to be effective against systemic infections when administered orally. The drug is generally well tolerated. It is effective against a broad spectrum of fungi and is less toxic than amphotericin B. Side effects include GI disturbances and skin rashes. Ketoconazole blocks synthesis of adrenal steroids and androgens, which may lead to gynecomastia. High doses may cause liver dysfunction. An acid environment is needed for dissolution and absorption. Administration with food may minimize GI disturbances. Antacids and H_2 blockers should be given at least 2 hours after administration to avoid reduction in oral absorption. The patient should be instructed to notify the physician if signs of liver dysfunction (e.g., anorexia, jaundice, dark urine, and pale stools) occur. Nausea, vomiting, and skin reactions may occur if alcohol is consumed while the drug is in the body (Antabuse reaction). Ketoconazole's effectiveness is reduced by rifampin, isoniazid, and ddI.

Miconazole

A variety of fungi are susceptible to miconazole; however, frequent side effects are seen, including thrombophlebitis, rash, pruritus, nausea, vomiting, diarrhea, febrile reactions, anemia, thrombocytosis, hyponatremia, CNS toxicity, and hypersensitivity reactions. The effects of oral anticoagulants are enhanced when given concomitantly with miconazole. IV treatment should begin in a hospital with frequent monitoring of electrolyte, hematocrit, and lipid levels. The IV dose should be diluted with at least 200 ml of fluid and infused over 30 to 60 minutes. The effectiveness of both miconazole and amphotericin B is reduced if the drugs are used together.

Nystatin

Limited absorption, with no detectable blood levels following oral administration, makes nystatin useful in the treatment of oral, GI, or perineal infections. The drug is not useful for systemic infections. Nystatin is generally nontoxic and nonirritating, with few allergic reactions occurring.

ANTIVIRAL DRUGS

Because viruses are intracellular parasites, the drug treatment of viral infections is very difficult. The goal of drug therapy is to have the greatest effect on the virus-infected cells with minimal effect on other cells. The antiviral drugs discussed inhibit intracellular synthesis. Table 16-8 presents various routes of administration for specific agents.

Acyclovir

Acyclovir is a synthetic purine nucleoside analog that is active against herpes simplex viruses 1 and 2, the vari-

Table 16-8

ANTIVIRAL DRUGS

Generic name	Trade names	Routes of administration
Acyclovir	Zovirax	Oral, topical, IV
Didanosine (ddI)	Videx	Oral
Foscarnet	Foscavir	IV
Ganciclovir	Cytovene	IV
Vidarabine	Vira-A	IV
Zalcitabine (ddC)	HIVID	Oral
Zidovudine (azidothymidine [AZT])	Retrovir	Oral, IV

cella-zoster virus, and the Epstein-Barr virus. The drug interferes with viral polymerase and inhibits viral DNA replication. Recent reports of acyclovir-resistant strains of herpes viruses have led to caution in its use, particularly in mild cases of herpes simplex infections and in treatment of oral hairy leukoplakia, an essentially benign condition caused by the Epstein-Barr virus.

Indications: Treatment of severe herpes simplex and varicella-zoster infections.

Precautions/contraindications: When administered by rapid administration, acyclovir crystals can develop in the renal tubules.

Side effects/adverse reactions: Nausea, vomiting, diarrhea, headache, dizziness, fatigue, rash, anemia, and hypotension may occur.

Pharmacokinetics: Absorption of oral acyclovir is slow and incomplete but is not affected by food. Elimination is through the kidneys.

Interactions: Administering zidovudine and acyclovir together may cause severe drowsiness and lethargy. Probenecid decreases elimination of acyclovir. Use with foscarnet, aminoglycosides, and amphotericin B may result in nephrotoxicity.

Nursing considerations: Treatment may not reduce shedding of the virus. Caution patients to avoid sexual intercourse when visible herpes lesions are present because of the risk of infecting intimate partners. Avoid rapid bolus injections by infusing over at least 1 hour to reduce renal damage. Encourage fluids and ensure adequate hydration to prevent drug precipitation in the renal tubules following IV administration. Instruct the patient to wash hands after topical administration to avoid spreading the virus.

Didanosine (ddI)

Didanosine is a synthetic purine nucleoside analog that acts by converting itself intracellularly to didanosine tri-phosphate, which inhibits reverse transcriptase. Like other currently used antiretrovirals, ddI does not eliminate HIV but seems to slow the rate of replication of HIV, thereby reducing the rate of progression of the HIV infection. Viral resistance to ddI has been reported.

Indications: Didanosine is used in HIV infection as a single drug or in combination with zidovudine (AZT) after a decline in AZT's effectiveness or with development of intolerance to zidovudine. It is seldom used as a first-choice drug.

Precautions/contraindications: Didanosine should not be given to persons with impaired pancreatic function, elevated triglycerides, or a history of alcoholism. It must be used with caution in persons with neuropathy or a history of hepatic disease.

Side effects/adverse reactions: Peripheral neuropathy occurs in up to 12% of patients; acute pancreatitis, which occasionally is fatal, occurs in up to 5.9%; hepatitis occurs in fewer than 1%. Other side effects include diarrhea, leukopenia, confusion, rash, headache, and insomnia.

Pharmacokinetics: Because didanosine is rapidly degraded in low-pH environments, it must be taken with an antacid buffer. The drug is cleared primarily by the kidneys.

Interactions: Didanosine interacts with alcohol, asparaginase, azathioprine, estrogen, furosemide, methyldopa, nitrofurantoin, and thiazide diuretics to increase the risk of pancreatitis. Cisplatin, lithium, nitrofurantoin, nitrous oxide, and phenytoin may increase the risk of neuropathy. Because ddI must be taken with an antacid, dapsone, ketoconazole, fluoroquinolones, and tetracyclines must be taken 2 hours before ddI. Taking ddI with pentamidine increases the risk of pancreatitis. The risk of neuropathy increases with use of ethambutol, isoniazid, metronidazole, and vincristine.

Nursing considerations: Instruct the patient to chew or crush the tablets so that the buffer is immediately available in the stomach. Patients with oral lesions may need to use a buffered powder. Add powder to at least 1 ounce of water and stir or shake for 3 to 6 minutes to dissolve. Monitor serum amylase. Instruct the patient to report abdominal pain, nausea, or vomiting in order to evaluate for pancreatitis.

Foscarnet

Foscarnet is a nucleoside analog that is known to be effective in treating cytomegalovirus (CMV) infections. It also is used to suppress CMV and thereby prevent recurrence of CMV infections. A recent study suggests that foscarnet may work synergistically with zidovudine to inhibit replication of HIV.

Indications: Foscarnet is used to treat ganciclovir-resistant cytomegalovirus infections. It is seldom used as a first-line anti-CMV drug because of its high cost ($25,000 a year).

Precautions/contraindications: Foscarnet should not be used in patients with impaired renal function.

Side effects/adverse reactions: Almost all patients experience mild headaches, fatigue, and nausea. Fever and increased creatinine levels are common. Occasional seizures, increased liver enzymes, neuropathy, and penile ulcers have been reported.

Pharmacokinetics: Because foscarnet is not absorbed orally, it is administered only by the IV route; 43% of the drug is absorbed into CSF.

Interactions: The risk of nephrotoxicity is increased if foscarnet is taken with acyclovir, aminoglycosides, amphotericin B, and/or cyclosporine. The drug interacts with pentamidine to cause hypocalcemia.

Nursing considerations: Instruct patients that they are likely to experience headaches, fever, and nausea. Monitor creatinine levels. Most patients receive foscarnet for life once they start taking it, and most receive the drug through a central line.

Ganciclovir

Subclinical or latent cytomegalovirus (CMV) infection is common. When the patient is immunocompromised, as are chemotherapy or transplant patients or those who have AIDS, activation and dissemination of the infection are common. Ganciclovir enters cells infected with CMV and inhibits replication.

Indications: Ganciclovir is used to treat cytomegalovirus infection in immunocompromised patients.

Precautions/contraindications: Toxicity is increased in renal insufficiency.

Side effects/adverse reactions: Granulocytopenia, thrombocytopenia, anemia, headache, nausea, renal impairment, fever, rash, and abnormal liver function test results can occur.

Pharmacokinetics: Ganciclovir is eliminated through the kidneys and is not metabolized.

Interactions: Toxicity is increased when ganciclovir is administered with other cytotoxic drugs. Probenecid increases blood levels of ganciclovir. Dapsone, pentamidine, flucytosine, vincristine, vinblastine, doxorubicin, amphotericin B, and TMP/SMX may reduce renal clearance of ganciclovir. Increased hematotoxicity may occur when the drug is used with AZT, amphotericin B, antineoplastic drugs, and flucytosine.

Nursing considerations: The IV dose should be administered over 1 hour. Neutrophil and platelet counts should be monitored every 2 days initially and reduced to every week with continued therapy.

Vidarabine

The antiviral mechanism of vidarabine has not been established; however, it is one of the least toxic of the antiviral agents. As with most antiviral drugs, therapy is not curative but aims at reducing the duration and severity of symptoms.

Indications: Vidarabine is used to treat acyclovir-resistant herpes simplex infections and herpes zoster in immunosuppressed patients.

Precautions/contraindications: Patients with renal impairment may need reduced dosages. Because of the large amount of fluid required with IV administration, fluid overload is possible and may be life threatening in patients with cerebral edema or renal impairment.

Side effects/adverse reactions: GI disturbances occur but seldom are severe enough to stop therapy. Anemia, thrombocytopenia, neutropenia, and elevated liver enzymes have been reported. CNS symptoms, including tremor, headache, hallucinations, confusion, and ataxia, can occur.

Pharmacokinetics: Vidarabine is eliminated through the kidneys, mostly as active metabolites. The metabolite can accumulate in patients with reduced renal function.

Interactions: Allopurinol may interfere with vidarabine metabolism. Interactions are possible with any hemotoxic drugs or with drugs that are cleared by the kidney.

Nursing considerations: Monitor CBC during therapy. Infuse the total daily dose slowly over 12 to 24 hours. The drug has very low solubility. IV fluid for infusion may be prewarmed to aid in dissolving the drug, and an in-line membrane filter is necessary during infusion.

Zalcitabine (ddC)

Zalcitabine is a synthetic pyrimidine nucleoside that interferes with reverse transcriptase and thereby slows the rate of HIV replication. Like other antiretroviral drugs currently used, ddC does not eliminate HIV but may slow the rate of progression of HIV infection.

Indications: Zalcitabine has been approved for use in combination with zidovudine (AZT) for HIV-infected persons with CD4+ counts of less than 300/mm³. The drug is also added to AZT therapy when rapid immune deterioration is noted or when the person experiences opportunistic infections while taking AZT.

Precautions/contraindications: Caution must be used in administering ddC to patients with peripheral neuropathy or a history of pancreatitis.

Side effects/adverse reactions: The principal side effects of ddC are peripheral neuropathy (less likely at lower doses) and pancreatitis (more common in persons with a previous history of pancreatitis). Oral and esophageal ulcers, nausea, vomiting, diarrhea, rash, pruritus, fever, headache, and fatigue have been reported.

Pharmacokinetics: Zalcitabine is 70% to 80% absorbed and achieves 20% penetration into CSF.

Interactions: Use with cisplatin, lithium, nitrofurantoin, nitrous oxide, phenytoin, dapsone, ethambutol, isoniazid, metronidazole, and vincristine may increase the risk of peripheral neuropathy.

Nursing considerations: Monitor for signs of peripheral neuropathy. Instruct the patient to report signs of pancreatitis (abdominal pain, nausea, vomiting) to the treating clinician.

Zidovudine (AZT)

Zidovudine has been considered the first-choice drug for treatment of HIV infection. It is a nucleoside analog that interferes with replication of HIV by inhibiting reverse transcriptase. AZT does not eliminate the virus but seems to reduce CD4+ lymphocyte destruction and may slow the progression of HIV infection. Recent studies have suggested that AZT-resistant strains of HIV may develop rapidly (within 2 to 4 months) in some persons. AZT is currently used in combination with ddC for some patients.

Indications: Zidovudine is used in the management of patients with HIV infection who have some evidence of impaired immunity. It is also used for prophylaxis, after exposure to the HIV virus, although there is no evidence of efficacy for this use.

Precautions/contraindications: Zidovudine must be used cautiously in patients with impaired renal or hepatic function; patients may need dosage adjustments. It must also be used cautiously in patients with preexisting bone marrow suppression.

Side effects/adverse reactions: The drug may cause granulocytopenia and anemia, which may require transfusions or dosage modification. Headache, GI disturbances, insomnia, rash, myalgias, and CNS symptoms are among the many undesirable effects that may occur during therapy. Many minor side effects subside after the first weeks of therapy.

Pharmacokinetics: Zidovudine is well absorbed orally and is metabolized in the liver, with renal elimination of the drug and metabolites.

Interactions: Administration with other cytotoxic, nephrotoxic, hepatotoxic, or bone marrow–suppressing drugs may increase the toxicity of zidovudine. AZT hematotoxicity may be increased when the drug is used with dapsone, ganciclovir, pentamidine, TMP/SMX, vincristine, vinblastine, doxorubicin, interferon, flucytosine, or amphotericin B. Probenecid increases AZT levels. AZT may reduce the effectiveness of pyrimethamine.

Nursing considerations: Closely monitor the patient's blood count. Warn patients that the use of other medication may increase toxicity. Monitor patients closely for development of opportunistic infections or other complications that may develop during therapy.

ANTIPARASITIC DRUGS

Amebicidal drugs may affect amebae in the gut (intraintestinal or luminal) or amebae that have penetrated into the body tissue (systemic or extraintestinal), or both. When extraintestinal infections are being treated, an intraintestinal drug should also be used because of the nature of the disease. These amebicides are all administered orally, as shown in Table 16-9.

The other antiparisitic drugs described in this section are used for treatment of *Pneumocystis carinii* infections and are also shown in Table 16-9.

Atovaquone

Atovaquone is a recently discovered drug that has proved useful in treating *Pneumocystis carinii* pneumonia. Studies have shown it to be less effective than TMP/SMX; however, it has fewer side effects.

Indications: Atovaquone is used to treat mild to moderate *Pneumocystis carinii* pneumonia in HIV-infected patients.

Precautions/contraindications: Not yet established.

Side effects/adverse reactions: Rash, liver dysfunction, vomiting, fever, nausea, and pruritus may occur.

Pharmacokinetics: Not yet described.

Interactions: Not yet described.

Dapsone

Dapsone is a sulfone derivative that was originally used to treat leprosy. It is highly effective against *Pneumocystis carinii*.

Indications: Dapsone is used to treat pulmonary and extrapulmonary infection with *Pneumocystis carinii*. It

Table 16-9

ANTIPARISITIC DRUGS

Generic name	Trade names	Route of administration
Atovaquone	None	Oral
Dapsone	Anlosulfon	Oral
Paromomycin	Humatin	Oral
Iodoquinol	Yodoxin	Oral
Metronidazole	Flagyl	Oral, IV
	Protostat	Oral, IV
Pentamidine	Pentam 300	IM, IV
Pentamidine	NebuPent	Aerosol

is usually used in mild pneumonia caused by that organism and as prophylaxis against more severe episodes of *Pneumocystis carinii* pneumonia.

Precautions/contraindication: Dapsone should not be given to patients who are hypersensitive to sulfones. It should be used with caution in patients with renal or hepatic disease or in cases of refractory anemia.

Side effects/adverse reactions: Nausea, vomiting, rash, hemolysis, and anemia may develop if the patient has a G6PD deficiency. The drug is usually well tolerated even if the patient developed a rash when taking TMP/ SMX.

Pharmacokinetics: Dapsone is absorbed completely and rapidly from the GI tract. It is metabolized in the liver and is primarily excreted in urine.

Interactions: Together with AZT, dapsone increases bone marrow toxicity. Absorption of dapsone is reduced by ddI unless dapsone is taken 2 hours before ddI. Probenecid increases blood levels of dapsone. Rifampin decreases the half-life of dapsone. When dapsone is used with trimethoprim, blood levels of both drugs are increased, and there is an increased likelihood of methemoglobinemia.

Nursing considerations: Dapsone should be taken with food to minimize the possibility of gastric distress. Suspect methemoglobinemia if the patient becomes cyanotic with mucous membranes that develop a brownish hue.

Paromomycin

Paromomycin is an amebicidal and bacterial aminoglycoside. The drug is used to treat chronic intestinal amebiasis and as adjunct therapy in hepatic coma. The drug is very poorly absorbed from the GI tract, and large doses can cause GI disturbances. The drug profile and nursing considerations are similar to other aminoglycosides. Doses are administered with meals.

Iodoquinol

Iodoquinol is effective against the trophozoites and cysts of *Entamoeba histolytica* in the large intestine.

Indications: Iodoquinol is used to treat intraintestinal amebiasis.

Precautions/contraindications: Iodoquinol must be used cautiously in patients with thyroid disease. Optic neuritis, optic atrophy, and peripheral neuropathy have occurred during long-term therapy.

Side effects/adverse reactions: Pruritus, diarrhea, urticaria, skin eruptions, GI disturbances, fever, chills, vertigo, and thyroid enlargement can occur.

Pharmacokinetics: The drug is very poorly absorbed from the GI tract, increasing its effectiveness against intraintestinal amebiasis.

Interactions: Interference with thyroid function tests can occur and persist for up to 6 months after therapy is stopped.

Nursing considerations: Observe and monitor closely for adverse effects, especially optic changes. Administer the drug after meals.

Metronidazole

Metronidazole possesses both antibacterial and amebicidal activity. The mechanism of its amebicidal activity is not known. The drug has both extraintestinal and intraintestinal effectiveness and is indicated for treatment of acute amebiasis and amebicidal liver abscess. Because of a high failure rate when used alone, it is usually combined with an intraintestinal drug. The drug profile and nursing considerations are covered with antibiotics.

Pentamidine Isoethionate

Pentamidine, in its IV form, was the first drug used to treat *Pneumocystis carinii* pneumonia (PCP). It is still used to treat patients who are unable to tolerate TMP/

SMX or other oral drugs. The aerosolized form of pentamidine was also the first drug used for PCP prophylaxis. It is most effective in prophylaxis when used with either of two nebulizers, Respirgard II or System 22 Mizer Jet. However, orally administrated drugs, if tolerated, are considered more effective than IV or aerosolized pentamidine. IV, rather than aerosolized, pentamidine must be used for extrapulmonary infections.

Indications: Pentamidine is the second-choice drug for treatment of pulmonary and extrapulmonary *Pneumocystis carinii* infections and for use as an aerosol in prevention of PCP.

Precautions/contraindications: Caution must be used in administering pentamidine to patients with hypertension, hypotension, hypoglycemia, hypocalcemia, blood dyscrasias, diabetes, and hepatic or renal dysfunction.

Pharmacokinetics: Pentamidine leaves the blood circulation rapidly and binds extensively with body tissues. It is excreted primarily in the urine.

Side effects/adverse reactions: For IV use: Sudden hypotension may occur if the drug is infused too rapidly; rash, nausea, vomiting, nephrotoxicity, cardiac arrhythmia, neutropenia, thrombocytopenia, pancreatitis, hypocalcemia, and hypoglycemia followed by hyperglycemia also may occur. For aerosol administration: A cough may develop, which may respond to bronchodilators.

Interactions: Use with foscarnet may increase the risk of hypocalcemia; use with ddI, alcohol, asparaginase, azathioprine, estrogens, furosemide, methyldopa, nitrofurantoin, sulindac, and thiazide diuretics may increase the risk of pancreatitis; use with amphotericin B, cyclosporine, or vancomycin may increase the risk of nephrotoxicity.

Nursing considerations: Infuse pentamidine over 60 minutes (at least) to avoid sudden hypotension. The patient should be in a reclining position while receiving the IV. Monitor BP during IV administration and afterward until BP stabilizes. Upper lobe PCP has a higher likelihood of developing if aerosolized pentamidine is administered to a patient in a sitting position. Therefore, the patient should be in a reclining chair while receiving the aerosolized form. Administration of aerosolized drugs increases the risk of spread of TB to staff and other patients. Administer aerosolized pentamidine in a separate room that has negative air pressure vented to the outside. Staff must wear masks and should minimize their contact with the patient during administration and during the patient's subsequent coughing.

Pyrimethamine Combinations

Pyrimethamine is a folic acid antagonist that has long been used in prophylaxis for malaria. It also has been used in combination with a sulfonamide to treat toxoplasmosis. Recent reports have suggested that pyrimethamine in combination with either sulfadoxine or dapsone is effective as anti–*Pneumocystis carinii* prophylaxis. However, controlled studies have not been conducted to test these agents.

ANTIMYCOBACTERIAL AGENTS

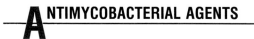

Drug treatment of tuberculosis is made difficult by two factors: relatively poor blood supply to the organism and rapid development of resistance by the organism. Because of the relatively poor blood supply to the organism, therapy must continue on a long-term basis to prevent recurrence. To prevent the development of resistance, three or four drugs are often given simultaneously. Isoniazid, rifampin, pyrazinamide, and ethambutol are the most widely used antitubercular drugs. Streptomycin is occasionally used, as are a variety of other secondary drugs. The primary antimycobacterial drugs are listed in Table 16-10.

Table 16-10

ANTIMYCOBACTERIAL DRUGS

Generic name	Trade names	Routes of administration
Isoniazid	Laniazid	IM, oral
Ethambutol	Myambutol	Oral
Rifampin	Rifadin	Oral, IV
	Rimactane	Oral, IV
Streptomycin	None	IM
Pyrazinamide	Tebrazid	Oral
Rifabutin	None	Oral

The secondary drugs are used in retreatment regimens in patients whose infection did not respond to the initial treatment. The secondary agents include aminosalicylate, ethionamide, cycloserine, and capreomycin, and are generally less effective and more toxic. If therapy lasts less than 6 months, the relapse rate is high. Patients must complete the entire course of treatment in order to prevent further development of drug-resistant strains of mycobacteria. Recommendations for initial treatment regimens are discussed with respiratory manifestations in Chapter 9. Patients who are taking antitubercular drugs for treatment of active TB pose the threat of transmitting the bacilli to health care workers and other patients. Anyone suspected of having, or known to have, active TB should be in AFB isolation (see Chapter 14 for CDC recommendations for preventing transmission of TB).

Isoniazid

Isoniazid (also called INH for isonicotinic acid hydrazide) is bactericidal by interfering with lipid and nucleic acid synthesis. The drug acts only on actively growing bacilli.

Indications: Isoniazid is used in the treatment and prophylaxis of tuberculosis caused by susceptible organisms. This drug is used in nearly all treatment regimens for tuberculosis.

Precautions/contraindications: Severe and occasionally fatal hepatitis has occurred in patients receiving INH. The incidence of hepatitis increases with age and in patients who consume alcohol daily.

Side effects/adverse reactions: CNS disorders (most commonly peripheral neuropathy with symmetrical numbness and tingling of extremities), rash, fever, and hepatotoxicity may occur. Children generally tolerate the drug with fewer side effects.

Pharmacokinetics: Absorption is complete following oral administration but may be delayed by food. Metabolism occurs in the liver, with elimination through the kidneys.

Interactions: Aluminum salts (in antacid preparations) may impair absorption. Enhanced effects of oral anticoagulants, some benzodiazepines, and hydantoins can occur. Daily ingestion of alcohol has been associated with an increased incidence of hepatitis.

Nursing considerations: Monitor liver enzymes during therapy, and assess the patient for signs of hepatotoxicity, including anorexia, nausea, malaise, and weakness. Pyridoxine (B_6) is often administered to reduce or treat peripheral neuropathies. Advise patients to limit intake of alcohol while taking the drug and to notify their physician if they develop weakness, fatigue, nausea and vomiting, yellowing of the skin, darkened urine, or numbness and tingling in the extremities.

Ethambutol

Ethambutol diffuses into the cells of tubercle bacilli and inhibits metabolism.

Indications: Ethambutol is used in conjunction with another drug to treat pulmonary tuberculosis.

Precautions/contraindications: Reduced doses are needed in patients with renal failure. Ethambutol is not recommended for children under the age of 13 years.

Side effects/adverse reactions: A reduction of visual acuity and color discrimination can occur with use of the drug. The visual changes may be unilateral or bilateral and are usually reversible if the drug is discontinued.

Pharmacokinetics: Absorption is not affected by food. About 20% of the dose is metabolized in the liver, whereas the rest is eliminated by the kidney and, to a lesser extent, in the feces.

Interactions: Aluminum salts (in antacid preparations) may reduce or delay absorption.

Nursing considerations: Administer with food to reduce GI disturbances. Monitor for visual changes during therapy. Because visual changes may be unilateral, both eyes should be checked for visual acuity and color discrimination.

Rifampin

Rifampin is always used in conjunction with other agents. The drug inhibits bacterial RNA polymerase activity in susceptible organisms.

Indications: Rifampin is used in conjunction with another drug to treat pulmonary tuberculosis.

Precautions/contraindications: Rifampin must be used with caution in patients with liver impairment or in patients who are taking other hepatotoxic drugs.

Side effects/adverse reactions: A "flulike" syndrome has occurred in 20% to 50% of patients taking high doses of the drug on an intermittent schedule, but it is not likely to occur at recommended doses. Elevations of liver enzymes and hepatitis can occur. Skin reactions, GI disturbances, and increases in BUN and serum uric acid levels can occur.

Pharmacokinetics: Rifampin is well absorbed orally; absorption is impaired by food. Metabolism occurs in the liver, with renal elimination of the metabolites. Dosage reduction may be needed in patients with severe liver disease but not in patients with renal failure.

Interactions: Rifampin induces hepatic enzymes, which increases the metabolism of many drugs and may decrease their therapeutic effect. The combination of rifampin with INH may lead to a higher incidence of hepatotoxicity. Rifampin decreases serum levels of methadone and may lead to withdrawal symptoms. Patients may stop taking rifampin to avoid withdrawal if the methadone dosage is not adjusted.

Nursing considerations: Monitor for signs of hepatotoxicity (see Nursing Considerations for INH). The medication should be administered 1 hour before or 2 hours after meals. Rifampin may cause a reddish-brown discoloration of the urine, stool, tears, saliva, and other body fluids; warn patients of this effect. Permanent discoloration of contact lenses can occur. The nurse may need to act as the patient's advocate in obtaining an increase in the methadone dosage.

Streptomycin

Streptomycin is an aminoglycoside drug that is effective against susceptible strains of tuberculosis. It is discussed with the other aminoglycoside drugs. When used in the treatment of tuberculosis, therapy is combined with additional medications.

Pyrazinamide

Pyrazinamide is a bacteriostatic agent used in combination with other drugs to treat active infections caused by *M. tuberculosis* and *M. kansasii*. Pyrazinamide should never be used as a single drug for treatment, because resistance develops in 6 to 7 weeks.

Indications: Pyrazinamide is used in conjunction with isoniazid (INH), rifampin, and ethambutol to treat active infections caused by *M. tuberculosis* and *M. kansasii*. It usually is given with these other drugs for up to 2 months and then is withdrawn from the treatment regimen. Treatment with the other drugs continues (see TB treatment, Chapter 9).

Precautions/contraindications: Pyrazinamide cannot be given to a patient with severe hepatic damage. It must be used with caution if the patient has gout or diabetes, or a family history of these diseases. It must also be used cautiously in patients with impaired renal function; peptic ulcer; or acute, intermittent porphyria.

Side effects/adverse reactions: Arthralgia, active gout, headache, difficulty in urination, photosensitivity, rash, sideroblastic or hemolytic anemia, hemoptysis (can be fatal), aggravation of peptic ulcer, hepatotoxicity, and a decrease in plasma prothrombin may occur.

Pharmacokinetics: Pyrazinamide is readily absorbed from the GI tract, and it crosses the blood-brain barrier. It is metabolized in the liver and excreted slowly in the urine.

Interactions: Use with ketoconazole, INH, rifampin, and other hepatotoxic drugs increases the risk of severe liver damage.

Nursing considerations: Observe for jaundice and gouty attacks; discontinue administration of the drug if these occur. Instruct the patient to complete the entire course of therapy to prevent development of resistant strains of bacilli.

Rifabutin

Rifabutin is a recently developed, semisynthetic rifamycin with demonstrated activity against *M. avium* complex. A recent large study demonstrated that the drug prevented development of *M. avium* bacteremia in HIV-infected patients.[123] This has led the U.S. Public Health Service to recommend lifelong use of the drug for *M. avium* complex prophylaxis for all HIV-infected individuals with CD4+ counts below 100/mm^3.

Indications: Rifabutin is used for anti-*Mycobacterium* prophylaxis in HIV-infected individuals with CD4+ lymphocyte counts of less than 100/mm^3.

Precautions/contraindications: Not yet established.

Side effects/adverse reactions: Neutropenia, thrombocytopenia, rash, nausea, flatulence, serum aminotransferase elevation, and myositis have been described.

Pharmacokinetics: Not yet described.

Interactions: Not yet described.

CHAPTER 17

Patient Teaching Guides

Patient education is important in all areas of nursing care, but nowhere is it more critical than in the area of HIV/AIDS. First, infection with HIV is preventable. Nurses, regardless of where they practice, must teach about prevention. This includes providing information about safer sexual practices and how to use condoms.

Second, once infected with HIV, the person begins a long course, which can range from 3 to 20 years, of coping with the chronic HIV infection and its multiple, eventually fatal consequences. During the course of these years an infected person may experience many acute, life-threatening diseases, hospitalizations, and complex treatments, for which information is needed. At the same time, infected persons need help and information on how to manage life with a chronic disease. They may have questions about the signs and symptoms of opportunistic diseases and how to manage the symptoms, such as nausea or pain. They need to know how to take their many medications, the side effects of their drugs, and how to manage the side effects. They may need to learn how to self-administer IV therapies at home and how to care for a central venous catheter or an implanted port.

Third, compliance with antiinfective therapy is critical in this day of expanding drug-resistant organisms. HIV-infected persons are prescribed multiple antiinfective drugs for multiple opportunistic infections during the course of HIV infection. Patients often stop therapy when their symptoms disappear, assuming they are cured before the therapy is completed. This can result in a superinfection with a more virulent form of the organism or recurrence of the initial infection that is more difficult to eradicate. For example, development of life-threatening, multidrug-resistant tuberculosis (MDRTB) has been attributed to failure of patients to complete the prescribed therapy. Every time an antiinfective drug is prescribed, the patient or caregiver should be taught about the drug,

dosage, length of treatment, mode of administration, side effects, and what to do if side effects appear. The nurse can emphasize in teaching that the patient must report to the health care provider if he or she stops taking the drug for any reason.

Fourth, HIV infection invades every aspect of a person's life and relationships. Infected individuals and their significant others require information on how to manage the many changes happening in their lives. Management may deal with simple changes, such as inability to climb stairs in one's home, to more complicated issues, such as whether to get pregnant, to participate in a clinical trial of a new drug, or to designate a power of attorney.

What is the implication of this for nurses caring for HIV-infected persons? Nurses need to be prepared to teach at all phases of the infection, to persons of both genders and of all age groups and risk groups, about a variety of topics, depending on where the person is in the course of the infection.

Chapter 11 provides guidance for patient teaching on many of these critical topics, and Chapter 2 contains the information that should be taught before and after a person receives an HIV test. In addition, this chapter provides written materials on a few selected topics to help reinforce patient teaching. These Patient Teaching Guides can be photocopied and used as handouts for patients or their caregivers. Although handouts do not replace direct teaching, they provide basic information that the patient or caregivers can refer to at a later time.

The handouts are designed to be used singly or in combination. For example, a person who is sexually active might be given "Facts About Sexually Transmitted Diseases," "About Condoms," and "Facts about HIV Infection and AIDS." All females would receive "The Female Condom."

Mosby's
**Clinical Nursing
Series**

About Condoms

Condoms ("rubbers") were once used mainly for birth control. Today, condoms are an important weapon in preventing the spread of HIV/AIDS and other sexually transmitted diseases (STDs). Total abstinence from sex is the only completely safe method of preventing AIDS and STDs. Condoms are the next best way to be safe—but only if they are used correctly. If you are sexually active, learn how to use condoms and **always use them from start to finish!**

Buying and storing condoms

There are many brands and styles of condoms on the market. Whether you choose plain or fancy condoms is up to you—as long as you **buy only condoms made of latex.** You should also use a contraceptive foam or jelly that contains non-oxynol-9. In addition to being a spermicide, non-oxynol-9 may kill the AIDS virus on contact, and it gives extra protection against other STDs. Applying a nonoxynol-9 spermicide foam or jelly on the outside of the condom will give you protection in case the condom breaks. (Some condoms are packaged with nonoxynol-9 jelly, but the amount is too small to protect against the AIDS virus, so you should use the foam or jelly even with these kinds of condoms.) Other instructions include:

- Store condoms in a cool, dry place away from sunlight and heat.
- If the package is damaged, don't use the condom because it may also be damaged.
- Do not use a condom that is brittle, discolored, or sticky because these are signs of age. An old condom can break easily.

Using condoms correctly

- Handle condoms carefully to prevent puncture.
- Always use a condom **from start to finish.** Even the briefest sexual contact can result in infection.
- If you use a lubricant, be sure it is water based, such as K-Y Jelly. Lubricants that contain petroleum (e.g., Vaseline) or oil weaken the latex and may cause the condom to break.
- Before sexual contact, apply the nonoxynol-9 contraceptive foam or jelly on the outside of the condom and intravaginally or rectally.
- If a condom breaks, replace it immediately. If ejaculation occurs with a broken condom, use ad-ditional nonoxynol-9 to reduce the risk of getting an infection.
- Never reuse a condom!
- The penis must be erect to put on a condom correctly.
- Hold the tip of the condom with one hand (see diagram below). With the other hand, slip the rolled-up portion over the head of the penis and unroll the condom down the shaft of the penis. A space should be left at the tip to collect semen, but be sure the tip is not filled with air, since this could cause the condom to break.
- After ejaculation, the penis should be withdrawn while still erect.
- Hold the base of the condom during withdrawal to prevent accidental slipping. Wrap the used condom in tissue and discard.

From Grimes, 1991.

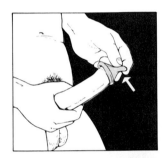

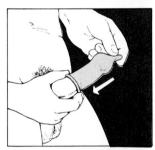

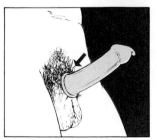

The Female Condom

The female condom is a polyurethane barrier device that is new on the market and is sold under the brand name "Reality." The condom is inserted into the vagina to protect against pregnancy and transmitting or acquiring a sexually transmitted disease. Like the male condom, the female condom does not eliminate the risk of pregnancy or disease, but it does lessen the chance. The only certain means of avoiding pregnancy or sexually transmitted diseases, such as HIV/AIDS, is to abstain from direct sexual contact.

In order for the female condom to be effective in preventing pregnancy or disease, it must be used properly. This means that it must be undamaged, be properly inserted, remain in place during sexual activity, be removed properly, and be used for every act of sexual intercourse.

Inserting the female condom

The Reality condom is a flexible sheath that is closed at one end and open at the other (like a long, narrow bag). In order to insert it, three steps are required. First, squeeze the closed end, compressing the flexible inner ring (Figure 1). Next, insert the squeezed end into the vagina like a tampon (Figure 2). Third, insert your finger in the center of the condom and push the inner ring up as far as it can go until it covers the cervical opening to the uterus (Figure 3). The action is similar to inserting a diaphragm for contraceptive purposes. Be careful to avoid puncturing the condom with a sharp fingernail or ring. Figure 4 shows a condom that is properly in place, with the large open ring extending out of the opening of the vagina. The Reality condom can be inserted while standing up (putting one foot on a chair or toilet seat helps) or while lying down. Either way, inserting it requires some skill that improves with practice. You may wish to practice several times before using it in an act of sexual intercourse.

The female condom during sex

During sex the penis is inserted into the center of the open ring at the opening of the vagina. Until both partners are familiar with the Reality condom, the penis should be guided by hand into the open ring. Otherwise there is the chance that the penis will be inserted outside the condom into the vagina, thus defeating the condom's purpose. Use of the male condom with the female condom is not recommended, because rubbing the latex male condom against the polyurethane female condom creates friction that may make intercourse difficult.

Removing the female condom

The female condom should be removed following intercourse and before standing up. To remove, squeeze and twist the outer ring to ensure that semen remains inside the condom. Gently pull the condom from the vagina. Discard in the trash. Do not attempt to flush the condom down the toilet, as it may clog the toilet or sewer lines. Do not reuse.

Important points to remember when using the female condom

1. The female condom works only if you use it every time you have sex.
2. Use a new condom each time you have sexual intercourse. **Do not reuse the female condom.**
3. You can still become pregnant and transmit or acquire a sexually transmitted disease while using the female condom. The risk is less than if you do not use the condom, but there still is a slight risk.
4. Although the Reality condom is prelubricated, it also comes with a tube of lubricant in the package. You may wish to add a few drops of lubricant to the opening of the condom or to the penis. Lubricant reduces friction and noise that results from friction.
5. Remove tampons before inserting the female condom.
6. Use caution to avoid tearing the female condom with a sharp fingernail, ring, or other jewelry when inserting and removing the condom.

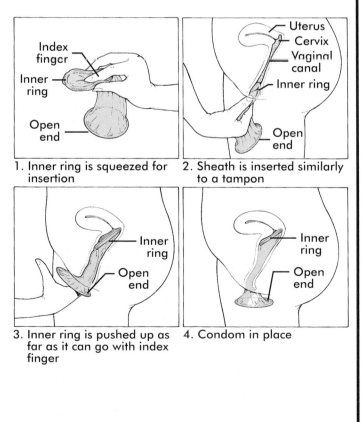

1. Inner ring is squeezed for insertion
2. Sheath is inserted similarly to a tampon
3. Inner ring is pushed up as far as it can go with index finger
4. Condom in place

Facts About Sexually Transmitted Diseases

Gonorrhea

Neisseria gonorrhoeae is the bacterium that causes gonorrhea, or "clap." It is often symptomless, especially in women. When symptoms do occur, they appear 2 to 14 days after exposure in men, and 7 to 12 days in women. Women may have painful urination and a vaginal discharge. Men have painful urination and a puslike discharge from the urinary opening. Rectal gonorrhea can cause anal discomfort and a rectal discharge, and the stool may be coated with pus. Infection of the throat (called **gonococcal pharyngitis**) is often symptomless, but some patients develop a sore throat. Babies born to mothers with gonorrhea may develop an eye infection (neonatal ophthalmitis), which can cause blindness if not treated.

Complications of untreated gonorrhea can be serious. In men, painful infection or abscesses involving the testicles and sperm duct can cause sterility. Pelvic inflammatory disease (PID), or salpingitis, in women usually requires hospitalization and can also cause sterility. Occasionally, the bacteria spread through the bloodstream, causing disease elsewhere in the body.

Gonorrhea can be completely cured with antibiotics. There are several different courses of treatment, some involving only one injection of an antibiotic, some consisting of oral antibiotics for 7 days, and some requiring a combination of injections and oral drugs. If an oral antibiotic is prescribed, take it exactly as ordered, for as long as you are supposed to. Do not have sexual contact until you have finished treatment and the infection is cured. If symptoms persist after completing the medication, return to your doctor. You may require treatment with a different antibiotic.

Chlamydia and nongonococcal urethritis

These diseases are caused by a bacterium called *Chlamydia trachomatis* and can cause symptoms similar to gonorrhea. Like gonorrhea, *Chlamydia* is often symptomless in women. Men usually have burning during urination and a clear or puslike discharge. Women may have a vaginal discharge, burning on urination, and pain similar to menstrual cramps. The symptoms usually appear 5 to 10 days after exposure. Untreated infection can

lead to the same serious complications as gonorrhea, including blindness in newborns.

Treatment consists of taking an oral antibiotic for 7 to 10 days. Be sure to take the antibiotic exactly as prescribed, for as long as prescribed. Do not have sexual contact until you have finished therapy and are completely cured.

Syphilis

Syphilis is caused by an organism called *Treponema pallidum.* The organism rapidly travels through the blood and invades the bones, brain, heart, and other organs. Untreated syphilis can cause serious disability. There are four stages that mark the progression of this disease: primary syphilis, secondary syphilis, latent syphilis, and tertiary (late) syphilis. Treatment at early stages will stop the progression to later stages.

A chancre, the sign of primary syphilis, usually appears within 4 weeks of exposure. The chancre starts as a small red pimple or blister that soon becomes an ulcer. It is not painful, but a clear fluid oozes from the ulcer. This fluid contains many organisms. One or more chancres can appear anywhere on the body exposed to the infection—on the penis, vulva, anus, rectum, inside the vagina, or on the lips or mouth. Even without treatment, the chancres disappear in about 4 to 6 weeks. Without treatment, however, many organisms continue their destructive path through the body.

In secondary syphilis, skin rashes appear 6 to 12 weeks after infection. The rashes may come and go on different parts of the body or they may be persistent. Swollen lymph nodes in the groin, armpit, and neck are common, as are fever and other flulike symptoms.

The latent stage begins about 1 year after exposure. Skin rashes sometimes erupt, but by the second year, all symptoms usually disappear. This stage can last a few years. In the tertiary stage (about 3 to 10 years after exposure—much sooner in patients with HIV infection), a type of ulceration called a **gumma** develops on the skin, bone, or internal organs. Heart, brain, and nervous system complications are common at this stage.

Untreated syphilis, even in the absence of chancres, can be transmitted sexually and to the fetus. Infections can cause serious malformations and even death of the fetus.

Often a single dose of penicillin injected into a muscle will cure early syphilis. For syphilis that has been present for over 1 year, several injections are necessary. Do not have sexual contact until you have finished treatment. See your doctor 3 months after finishing treatment to ensure that you are cured.

Genital herpes

Genital herpes is caused by the herpes simplex virus. About 4 to 7 days after exposure, a small cluster of blisters appears on the external genitals, around the anus, or inside the vagina. The blisters, which may be very painful and itchy, form ulcers. The tissue around the ulcers is very red and inflamed. After a few days, the ulcers crust over, and by about the tenth day, they heal. Some people have swollen lymph nodes, fever, and flulike symptoms.

If you are pregnant, tell your doctor if you have ever been infected with herpes. Babies born to mothers with active herpes can be infected during passage through the birth canal. This can cause serious, life-threatening infection in newborns. For this reason, cesarean delivery may be performed.

Unfortunately, the virus stays inside the body, and herpes nearly always recurs, although subsequent attacks are milder. Treatment with an antiviral drug (acyclovir) for 7 to 10 days helps lessen the symptoms and speeds healing of the ulcers. Do not have sexual contact while the herpes is active. Tell your sex partner(s) that you have herpes, because there is a chance you can transmit the virus even between attacks.

Genital warts

Genital warts (also called **venereal warts** or **condylomata acuminata**) are caused by papillomaviruses. The warts appear 1 to 20 months (within an average of 4 months) after exposure. They begin as small, soft, moist, red or pink swellings and quickly develop into the taglike pendulum-shape typical of warts. Often they grow in clusters and have a texture similar to cauliflower. Genital warts can appear on the outer genitals (penis or vulva) and around the anus or inside the urinary opening, vagina, or rectum.

Genital warts are removed by cauterization, freezing (cryosurgery), or surgery. In some cases drugs are applied directly to the warts. Genital warts are not easily cured, and repeated treatments are often necessary. No therapy kills the virus; the warts may reappear after treatment. Do not have unprotected sex while the warts are present.

Trichomoniasis

Trichomoniasis is caused by the protozoan *Trichomonas vaginalis.* In women this STD causes a heavy greenish-yellow, frothy discharge with a strong odor. Irritation and soreness in the genital area and pain on urination are common. Many women are symptomless carriers of *Trichomonas* for a long period, although symptoms can appear suddenly. Most men are symptomless but can carry and transmit the disease.

The drug metronidazole, which is taken orally in one large dose or in smaller doses for 7 days, cures the infection completely. Both the woman and her sexual partner(s) must be treated. Do not have sexual contact until treatment is completed.

Protecting yourself in the future

To protect yourself from getting an STD, you have three choices: (1) complete abstinence from sex, (2) having a totally monogamous relationship, and (3) using a condom correctly from start to finish. Abstinence is not acceptable to many people; for this reason, learn to use a condom and use one every time you have sex. There is no way to be certain whether your partner is sexually active with others.

If you get an STD during pregnancy, seek treatment immediately. If you are treated for an STD, make sure that your sexual partner is treated also to avoid being reinfected.

From Grimes, 1991.

Facts About HIV Infection and AIDS

HIV infection and AIDS: the difference

AIDS (which is an abbreviation for acquired immune deficiency syndrome) is caused by the human immunodeficiency virus, or HIV. HIV weakens the body's natural defenses, making the person more susceptible to infections.

HIV infection. Most people have absolutely no symptoms for several months or even years after they are infected with HIV. Some people have a mild, temporary illness early in the infection, consisting of fatigue, fever, and swollen glands—much like mononucleosis. Later, the person has repeated bouts of viral and fungal infections, such as herpes and *Candida* (thrush or yeast infections).

AIDS. AIDS occurs when an HIV-infected person becomes ill with an AIDS-defining condition such as Kaposi's sarcoma (a rare form of cancer), *Pneumocystis carinii* pneumonia, widespread severe bacterial or fungal infections, or brain disease.

How is HIV infection diagnosed?

A positive result on both of two blood tests (ELISA and Western blot) confirms infection with HIV.

Who gets the AIDS virus?

Anyone—women, men, and children—can get the AIDS virus. It is not a "gay disease" or a "drug addict's disease." All it takes is being exposed one time!

People are at greatest risk of getting the AIDS virus if (1) they or their sexual partner have sex with homosexual males, bisexual males, intravenous (IV) drug users, male or female prostitutes, or many different people; (2) they inject IV drugs and share "works" (e.g., needles, syringes, and cookers); (3) they have gotten other sexually transmitted diseases; or (4) they had a blood transfusion or were given blood products between 1978 and March 1985. Babies born to infected mothers can also have the AIDS virus.

How the AIDS virus is transmitted

There are only two ways of getting the AIDS virus: (1) by having direct sexual contact with someone who is already infected or (2) by getting infected blood into your bloodstream.

How can the AIDS virus get in your bloodstream? This can occur by injecting IV drugs and sharing "works" (e.g., needles, syringes, and cookers) with someone who is infected, by getting a blood transfusion or blood products that are infected with the AIDS virus, by having body fluids from an infected person enter your body through a wound, and through the mother's blood to the fetus during pregnancy.

You **cannot** get the AIDS virus through casual contact with an infected person. The virus is **not** spread through the air, so you can't get it if an infected person coughs or sneezes. You **can't** get the virus by shaking hands, hugging, or kissing. And you **can't** get AIDS from a toilet seat or swimming pool, or by sharing food with an infected person.

Protecting yourself from sexual exposure

Next to total abstinence, the only protection against the AIDS virus is using condoms plus contraceptive foam or jelly containing nonoxynol-9. Learn to use a condom correctly, and use a condom every time. The AIDS virus can also be transmitted during oral sex, so you must use a condom for all activity that involves penetration of any part of the body. Ask for information about correct use of condoms.

If someone close to you has HIV infection

Your friend or family member needs your help now more than any other time. Be supportive and try to keep a positive attitude. Encourage the person to seek professional counseling to help him or her cope. A good diet, plenty of sleep, and avoiding stress are important. If the person has a drug or alcohol problem, encourage him or her to get help to quit.

You can be physically affectionate with an HIV-infected person without worrying about getting the virus yourself. Hugging, stroking each other, and dry kissing (avoid deep, wet, or "French" kissing) are safe. Do not share personal items that might carry small amounts of blood—things like toothbrushes and razors.

From Grimes, 1991.

HIV Testing

What are the HIV tests?

HIV antibody tests can tell if you have HIV antibodies in your blood. HIV tests are performed on a small amount of blood drawn from a vein in the arm. Two laboratory tests are used. The blood is tested first with the ELISA test. If the results are negative, no further testing is done. If the results of the ELISA are positive, the ELISA is repeated. If the second ELISA is positive, then the Western blot test is performed. If this test is positive, the person is considered infected with HIV.

Who should be tested?

Anyone who believes they have been exposed to HIV or whose life-style puts them at risk of exposure should be tested. HIV is passed from one person to another through sexual contact and through the blood. People are considered to be "high risk," meaning they are more likely to be infected, if (1) they have sex with homosexual males, bisexual males, injection (IV) drug users, male or female prostitutes, or many different partners; (2) their sexual partner has had sex with someone in this group; (3) they inject drugs and share "works" (e.g., needles, syringes, and cookers); (4) they have gotten other diseases from having sex; or (5) they had a blood transfusion or were given blood products between 1978 and March 1985. An unborn child whose mother has the AIDS virus can also be infected.

Will anyone find out about my test?

There are two procedures for HIV testing: confidential testing and anonymous testing. **Confidential testing** is like any other medical test—the results become part of your medical record. Insurance companies and employers may obtain a copy of your medical record with the results of your HIV antibody test, if you give a release to see the records. Some states allow **anonymous testing,** in which the person does not give a name. Each person is assigned a code number, and you must give the code to find out the test results. With anonymous tests, the decision to tell anyone—even a doctor—is up to the individual.

What does a negative test mean?

If your test results are negative, it means no HIV antibodies were found in your blood. However, it takes about 1 to 6 months after a person is infected for HIV antibodies to form. This means that a person recently infected can have a negative HIV test. If you are in a "high risk" category or suspect you may have been exposed to the AIDS virus, you may want to be tested again 6 months after your last exposure. Even if your test is negative, you and your partner(s) should protect yourself during sex by always using condoms **from start to finish.** You should not inject drugs, but if you do, you should never share works with anyone.

What if the test is positive?

A positive HIV test does not mean that you necessarily have AIDS now, but you could have it in the future. We do not know whether everyone infected with HIV eventually develop AIDS. We know that some people have had HIV infection for several years and have not developed AIDS. It seems that by taking very good care of themselves—both physically and emotionally—many of these people are leading normal, productive lives for many years with the HIV infection.

The main thing is not to panic. HIV infection is only part of your total life picture. Take care of your health, see your doctor regularly, seek emotional support from a trained counselor, protect yourself and others from further exposure to the AIDS virus, and continue with productive, satisfying activities.

Whom should you tell?

Tell your doctor and dentist, so they will be able to give you the best possible care. You should also tell your current and past sex partner(s) and encourage them to get tested. Discuss with them how you can protect each other. And if you have injected drugs, you should tell anyone with whom you have shared "works."

It is important to have people to help you cope—friends, relatives, or other people who are HIV positive. But you should choose with care the people you tell. In spite of the tremendous efforts made in recent years to educate the public, there are still many people with misconceptions about HIV infection and AIDS.

From Grimes, 1991.

Use of Antiretroviral Drugs

No drug cures infection with the human immunodeficiency virus (HIV). However, a number of drugs have been shown to reduce the rate at which HIV multiplies within the body. Each of these drugs seems to be reasonably effective for certain time periods. However, after some time passes, the drug seems to lose some or all of its ability to prevent multiplication of the virus. When this occurs, you may be switched to another antiretroviral drug or you may be given a second drug to take with the first drug. The length of time it takes for a drug to lose its potency varies with each person. For some this takes only a few months, whereas others obtain benefit from the same antiretroviral drug for years.

Because it is not clear why some people do well for only a short time and others do well for a long time, your response to the drugs will be watched closely. Your doctor will schedule you to return for examination and blood testing on a regular basis. It is important that you keep your medical appointments so that your doctor can determine if your drug therapy is working. If it is not, your physician will want to change drugs or add another drug to the one you are taking.

Antiretroviral drugs are very powerful and may cause physical reactions, called side effects, even while they are doing their job of preventing HIV from multiplying. Some of the side effects are temporary and go away after a few weeks. Other side effects will continue as long as you take the drugs. Most of these side effects can be described as being uncomfortable or inconvenient but not harmful. Other side effects, however, may be permanently damaging or even life threatening. Therefore, it is important that you learn what to expect when you take these drugs. You are the best judge of how you feel and what is happening to your body. The physicians and nurses caring for you need your assistance in watching for potentially harmful side effects. Therefore, the following guide has been prepared to help you understand and report your symptoms.

If you are taking AZT (zidovudine)
Possible side effects: What you should do

Nausea and/or vomiting: Usually disappear within 4 to 6 weeks of starting the drug. Report these symptoms to your health care provider if they last longer than this, cause you to lose weight, or return after being absent.

Headache: Usually disappears within 4 to 6 weeks of starting the drug. Report this symptom to your health care provider if it persists past 6 weeks, does not respond to usual pain-relieving remedies, or returns after being absent.

Fatigue: Usually disappears within 4 to 6 weeks. You can cope with it by reducing the amount you expect to accomplish and by getting plenty of rest. Report this symptom to your health care provider if fatigue persists past 6 weeks, returns after being absent, or interferes with your ability to live your life.

Muscle pain, severe upper abdominal pain, shortness of breath, unusual bleeding or bruising, sore throat, fever, injury that will not heal: These may indicate more serious reactions; report any of these symptoms to your health care provider.

If you are taking ddI (didanosine)
Possible side effects: What you should do

Diarrhea: A fairly common side effect; discuss remedies with your health care provider at the next visit. Report this symptom sooner if the diarrhea is severe, lasts for several days, or causes you to lose weight.

Upper abdominal pain, persistent nausea and vomiting; pain, tingling, or numbness in your hands or feet; convulsions, shortness of breath, mental confusion, unusual bleeding or bruising: Report these symptoms to your health care provider as soon as possible.

If you are taking ddC (zalcitabine)
Possible side effects: What you should do

Canker sores in mouth; rashes and itching skin: See your dentist; avoid using soaps or powders that may further dry or irritate the skin; use lotions to moisturize the skin. Report these symptoms to your health care provider if they persist.

Upper abdominal pain, persistent nausea and vomiting; pain, tingling, or numbness in your hands or feet; convulsions, shortness of breath, mental confusion, unusual bleeding or bruising: Report these symptoms to your health care provider as soon as possible.

Other reactions while taking antiretrovirals

All three of these drugs may cause side effects that are not listed here in some people, because individuals respond differently to different drugs. In addition, unusual symptoms may be related to other infections and not to the drugs that you are taking. Symptoms that are disabling or that interfere with your ability to live a reasonably normal life should be reported to your health care provider as soon as possible. Also, symptoms that involve pain, weakness, unusual weight loss, or bleeding should be reported soon. Problems that are merely annoying can usually wait until the next scheduled visit.

When Your HIV Test Is Positive

A positive HIV test does not mean that you have AIDS. It means that you are infected with the HIV virus and must take steps to protect your health and prevent transmission.

Your medical care

Your positive test is only part of the picture—your overall health counts for a great deal. Your doctor may suggest drugs or other treatment that can help you stay healthy and avoid other infections. Drugs such as AZT are proving beneficial in slowing the progression of HIV infection. And a great deal of research is under way to find other treatments and, hopefully, a cure. You should be alert for changes in your body because HIV-positive people are more susceptible to other infections. See your doctor if a sudden acute illness occurs or if you notice a change (e.g., fever, pain, cough, shortness of breath, bleeding, or an unusual skin condition).

The importance of a healthy life-style

The better you care for your body, the better your body can fight the HIV infection. A nutritious diet and adequate rest are essential. Exercise is important because it strengthens your body, increases your energy and stamina, and makes you feel better mentally. Do not abuse alcohol or inject drugs because they can make the HIV infection worse and you will be more likely to develop AIDS. Alcohol and drugs can also impair your judgment, and you might take risks you ordinarily would not. If you have a problem with drugs or alcohol, get help to quit.

Coping

Coping with a diagnosis of HIV can be difficult. Many people feel they are all alone, that no one can understand what they are going through. **But help is out there—you don't have to face this alone.** Seek professional help from a trained counselor, psychologist, or psychiatrist. These professionals can provide emotional support and guidance in helping you cope with the variety of social problems that HIV-positive people may face. Friends and family members can be valuable in helping you cope. Share information about HIV infection and AIDS with these people so they can better help you.

How can you protect others?

Most people would not deliberately place their friends, sex partner(s), or even total strangers in jeopardy by exposing them to the AIDS virus.

Sex. The only sure way to protect your sexual partner(s) is to not have sex. It is safe to hug, cuddle, masturbate each other (as long as the skin isn't broken), rub, or "dry kiss." If you have sex, here are ways to minimize the chance of spreading the infection: (1) Use a latex condom **from start to finish,** with a birth control foam or jelly that contains nonoxynol-9. (2) Do not do anything that might cause a tear, abrasion, or bleeding (such as anal intercourse). (3) Use only a water-based lubricant, such as K-Y Jelly. Do not use saliva or oily lubricants, such as petroleum jelly or vegetable oil. (4) Avoid oral sex. (5) Avoid deep, wet, or French kissing.

Drug use. If you inject drugs, please get help to quit because drugs can make your HIV infection worse. Until you quit: (1) do not share "works" with anyone else, (2) never use works that someone else has used, and (3) if you reuse your own works, clean them with bleach and water between uses.

Women. If you don't want to pass the virus to your child, do not get pregnant, because there is a strong chance you could pass the virus to your unborn baby. Babies with the AIDS virus usually die before age 2 years. If you already have a baby, do not breast-feed, because you could pass the virus to your baby in your milk.

Personal items. Even during normal use, some personal items may carry small amounts of blood that can be passed on to other people if you share them. Items such as toothbrushes, razors, and sex toys should not be shared.

Donations. Do not donate blood, sperm, or body organs.

From Grimes.[82]

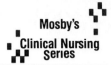
Managing Pain Without Drugs

There are several techniques you can use to relieve pain without taking drugs or to enhance the effect of your pain medication—**relaxation, imagery, distraction,** and **skin stimulation.**

Relaxation

Relaxation relieves pain by easing muscle tension. Easing muscle tension can also help you feel less tired and anxious and help other pain-relieving methods work better.

How to relax. Sit or lie down, preferably in a quiet place. Be sure you are comfortable. Do not cross your legs or arms.

Take a deep breath, and tense your muscles (you may tense up your whole body or concentrate on one set of muscles at a time, such as your facial muscles or those in your arms and hands).

Hold your breath, and keep your muscles tense.

Release your breath and your muscles at the same time. Let your body go limp (repeat for other muscle areas if you are concentrating on one set at a time).

You can add imagery (see below) or music to help you relax. Relaxation tapes are also available.

Don't be discouraged if relaxation doesn't help immediately. Practice the relaxation technique for 2 weeks before you give it up. If you find that it aggravates your pain, try another method.

Imagery

Imagery involves using your imagination to create mental scenes that use all your senses: sight, sound, touch, smell, and taste. You can imagine exotic locations or revisit one of your favorite places. You can create stories and characters to add to your scenes. Imagery can take your mind off your anxiety, boredom, and pain.

How to use imagery. Close your eyes. A few moments of the relaxation technique (see above) will help your body and mind prepare for imagery.

Let your mind begin forming its image. The following is an example of imagery:

Imagine that you are at the seashore. You are sitting in the wet sand; the afternoon sun is warm on your shoulders. The ocean rolls into the shore in gentle waves, and the water laps teasingly at your toes. A hungry pair of seagulls cry overhead and take swift, darting dives at a dog that is scavenging along the shore. Your tension lessens with each wave that touches your toes and retreats. You close your eyes and take a deep, slow breath of salt-filled air. You are completely relaxed. Stay on the beach as long as you like.

To end the image, count to three and open your eyes. Resume your regular activities slowly.

Distraction

A distraction is any activity that takes your mind off your pain and focuses your attention elsewhere. Doing crafts, reading a book, watching television, or listening to music through headphones can all help distract your mind. Distraction works well when you are waiting for drugs to take effect or if you have brief bouts of pain. Sometimes people can take their minds off their pain for long periods, especially if the pain is mild.

Skin stimulation

Skin stimulation is used to block pain sensation in the nerves. Pressure, massage, hot and cold applications, rubbing, and mild electrical current are all ways to stimulate the skin. However, if you are undergoing radiation treatment, consult your doctor before applying any skin stimulation.

You can do skin stimulation at the site of the pain, near it, or on the opposite side of pain. For example, stimulating the left wrist when the right wrist is in pain can actually ease the pain in the right wrist.

Pressure. Using your entire hand, the heel of your hand, your thumb, your knuckles, or both hands, apply at least 15 seconds of pressure at the point where you feel pain. Keep trying spots around the painful area if you find no relief the first time. You may extend the time you apply pressure to 1 minute.

Massage. You or someone else can perform the slow, circular motions of massage. The feet, back, neck, and scalp can be massaged to relieve tension and pain anywhere in the body. Some people prefer to use oils or lotions during the massage. If deep massage is too uncomfortable, try light stroking. Do not massage red, raw, or broken skin.

Heat and cold. Some people prefer cold; others prefer heat. Use whichever works best for you. A convenient way to use cold is to freeze gel-filled packs and wrap them in towels. Ice cubes can also be used. Heat can be applied with a heating pad; hot, moist towels; or a hot water bottle or by taking a hot bath. Be careful not to burn your skin with water that is too hot or to go to sleep with a heating pad on. Don't expose your skin to intense cold for very long.

Transcutaneous electrical nerve stimulation. TENS can be used to eliminate or ease pain. A TENS unit is a pocket-sized, battery-operated device that provides a mild, continuous electrical current through the skin by the use of two to four electrodes, which are taped onto the skin. Lead wires connect the electrodes to the device. It is this mild electrical current that blocks or modifies the pain messages and replaces them with a buzzing, tingling sensation. It is also thought that TENS may stimulate the body's production of endorphin, a natural pain reliever.

From Belcher, 1992.

Fever

Fever—a temperature of 100.4° F (38° C) or above—is usually a sign of infection. A person with a fever may be flushed, irritable, and tired and may complain of aching. Fever may start with chills, which are caused by the body temperature rising. Sweating often occurs with high temperatures and when the fever "breaks"—a sign that the temperature is decreasing. Some infections produce little or no fever, so a normal temperature by itself does not necessarily mean that no infection is present.

Fever should always be watched carefully. Although most of the time fever is an expected reaction to infection, a very high fever is dangerous because it can cause convulsions, especially in children. Therefore it is important to know how to take a temperature correctly, what you can do to help reduce the fever, and when to call the doctor.

The most accurate reading is done with an oral temperature. However, taking an oral temperature requires cooperation, so do not attempt this method with young children or anyone who is not conscious and cooperative. A regular thermometer can also be used under the arm. Authorities advise against taking temperatures rectally, even in children.

Although 98.6° F is considered the "normal" oral temperature, a healthy person's temperature actually ranges from about 97° F to 99.5° F during a 24-hour period. Underarm temperature is 1° or 2° lower than oral readings.

Mercury thermometers

A mercury thermometer is a glass tube with a bulb at one end that contains mercury. A scale on the tube shows degrees of temperature, with an arrow marking the normal point of 98.6° F. The bulb is placed under the tongue or in the armpit. As the mercury is heated, it rises up the tube to a point that shows the person's temperature. To read a thermometer, hold it at eye level in good light and rotate it slowly until you see the thin silver line of mercury.

Never leave a child alone, even for a minute, with a mercury thermometer! Injury can occur from broken glass, and mercury is a poison.

- First, clean the thermometer with soap and then rinse it with cool tap water. Hot water will cause the thermometer to break. Hold the thermometer at the end opposite the mercury bulb and shake it a few times to make the mercury go below the arrow.
- To take an oral temperature, place the bulb of the thermometer under the tongue as far toward the back as possible. Have the person close his or her mouth and hold the thermometer in place for 4 to 5 minutes.
- To take an underarm temperature, place the bulb of the thermometer snuggly in an armpit and have the person keep the upper arm clasped tightly to the side, with the elbow bent and the lower arm folded across the chest. Leave the thermometer in place for 10 minutes.
- After you're done, wash the thermometer again with soap and cool water and shake it to return the mercury to the bulb.

Managing a fever

Rest and plenty of liquids are needed when someone is running a fever. Encourage the person to drink water and juice to prevent dehydration. Try to make the person as comfortable as possible—extra covers during the chill stage, and sponging with a cool wet cloth when the person feels hot. Keep the room air cool or use a fan.

A moderate amount of fever is actually beneficial, so unless the fever is high (above 100.4° F) or headache or other pain is present, it is not necessary to take aspirin or an aspirin substitute to bring down fever. However, you should call the doctor if the temperature exceeds 102° F or lasts longer than 24 hours.

From Grimes, 1991.

Dealing with Loss of Appetite, Nausea, and Vomiting

Loss of appetite and nausea and vomiting are common symptoms of HIV infection opportunistic infections, and treatment. There are a variety of ways to relieve nausea and vomiting and help increase appetite.

Loss of appetite

Loss of appetite can be a serious problem; it can lead to malnutrition and severe weight loss. When your body is trying to fight infection, it needs nutrition. It needs enough protein and calories to function at its best, to give you energy, and to help reduce the effects of the disease and its treatment.

Eating enough of the right kinds of foods can be difficult when you don't feel like eating at all. Here are some tips to help you increase your appetite:

Take a walk before mealtime. Mild exercise can stimulate your appetite.

Avoid drinking liquids before a meal, because they can fill you up. If you want to drink, then drink juices or milk—something nutritious.

Eat with family or friends if possible. If eating is a social event, it will seem less of a chore.

Eat a variety of foods. Spice up your food with herbs, spices, and sauces. Use butter, bacon bits, croutons, wine sauces, and marinades to provide taste-pleasing meals.

Don't fill up on salads or "diet" foods. Eat vegetables and fruits along with meats, poultry, and fish to make sure you get enough calories and nutrition.

Eat smaller meals more often, especially if you fill up before you've eaten all your meal.

If you still are not getting enough calories or protein, your health care provider may recommend dietary supplements that can be added to milk, soup, or pudding.

Nausea and vomiting

Nausea and vomiting are common side effects of many treatments and infections. Doctors frequently prescribe an *antiemetic* to combat this. The antiemetic usually is given a few hours before the treatment and then every 3 or 4 hours after the treatment for a day or two. It may take some ex-perimenting with dosage and timing to come up with the best schedule for you.

The following are other remedies and preventive measures you can try to help prevent or alleviate nausea and vomiting:

Eat soda crackers and suck on sour candy balls throughout the day to relieve queasiness.

Choose cold or room-temperature foods instead of hot ones; hot and warm foods seem to cause nausea.

Avoid salty, fatty, and sweet foods or any food with strong odors—opt instead for bland, creamy foods such as cottage cheese, toast, and mashed potatoes.

Stay away from nauseating odors, sights, and sounds. Get as much fresh air as possible. A leisurely walk can help alleviate nausea.

Don't eat right before your treatment. Eat lightly for a few hours after your treatment.

Try relaxation therapy, self-hypnosis, or imagery to alleviate nausea-inducing tension.

Distract yourself with a book, TV, or activity.

Sleep during episodes of nausea if possible.

If vomiting does occur, eat or drink nothing until your stomach has settled, usually a few hours after the last vomiting episode. Then begin sipping clear liquids or sucking on ice cubes. If you tolerate the liquids, you may begin eating bland foods a few hours after you started the liquids.

Adapted from Belcher, 1992.

Clinical Trials—What Are They?

Research studies that use patients are called clinical trials. As a person with HIV infection, you may be asked to help evaluate a new treatment.

What are clinical trials?

When a new treatment becomes available, it must first go through rigorous testing in a laboratory and then in a clinical setting. The testing is carefully monitored, and the results are evaluated and published in medical journals, where other researchers and clinicians further evaluate the data.

There are three types of clinical trials: phase I trials, phase II trials, and phase III trials. Each of these trials is a carefully controlled, highly ethical human experiment designed to test a new drug or procedure that could cure or halt the spread of a disease. The drug or procedure usually is tested in all three phases before it can be accepted as a treatment.

Phase I trials determine the best way to provide a new treatment and how much can be given safely. These trials involve patients with advanced disease who have tried every possible treatment with no long-term success. These patients are willing to undergo treatments that probably will not cure their disease but that give them some hope and that might help similar patients in the future. Any treatment given these patients has first undergone testing on animals and has been approved for human trials.

Phase II trials study the effect of a new treatment on patients whose disease has not been cured by standard treatments. There is some possibility that the treatment may benefit these patients. A treatment reaching phase II trials has gone through phase I trials.

Phase III trials compare a new treatment to current treatments. These trials require large numbers of patients to control the effects that age, race, gender, and other factors may have on the experimental treatment.

One group of patients receives the experimental treatment, and another is given a standard treatment. Randomization (selection by chance to be in one group or the other) is used to keep bias out of the trial.

Informed consent

Informed consent means that you have been given the information you need to decide whether to participate in a clinical trial. This information includes what is involved, possible benefits and risks, the length of the study, the cost (if any), and how your anonymity and the confidentiality of your participation will be protected. Ask any questions you have. Then, if you wish to be a part of the study, you can sign the form. You can refuse to participate or withdraw from the study at any time without penalty.

Should you participate in a trial?

Those who participate in clinical trials have the opportunity to receive the latest in treatments or a new, experimental treatment that could be even more effective. In fact, according to published studies, patients who participate in trials often have a better survival rate.

You and your doctor should discuss the possibility of your participating in a clinical trial. If you are interested, your doctor should be aware of the different trials being conducted so he or she can recommend the best one for you. Many patients benefit both physically and mentally from participating in clinical trials.

For more information, call 1-800-TRIALS A.

Adapted from Belcher, 1992.

Mosby's
Clinical Nursing
Series

Safety Tips for the Caregivers of Persons with Confusion or Impaired Judgment

The mental status of a person with HIV infection may change suddenly, leading the person to exhibit symptoms ranging from confusion and forgetfulness to severe dementia and psychosis.

The person who has confusion or impaired judgment may be unable to remember where dangers lie, or to judge what is dangerous (steps, stoves, medications). Fatigue and inability to make the body do what one wants also can lead to injury. Therefore it is very important that this person live in an environment that has been made as safe as possible. The following are some safety guidelines to use in your home:

- Keep clutter out of the hallway and off stairs or anywhere the person is likely to walk. Remove small rugs that could cause tripping.
- Remove breakables and dangerous objects (matches, knives, guns).
- Keep medications in a locked cabinet or drawer.
- Limit access to potentially dangerous areas (bathrooms, basement) by locking doors if the person tends to wander. Have the person wear an identification bracelet in case he or she wanders outside.
- Dress appropriately for the season.
- Put name labels in clothing. Make sure clothing is not too baggy and that shoes fit well and have nonskid soles.
- Keep the person's bed low. If he or she falls out, you may want to place the mattress on the floor or install siderails.
- Make sure rooms are well lit, especially in the evening. Night-lights can help prevent falls.
- Have someone stay with the person who is severely confused or agitated or place the person in a day care center.
- Encourage rest periods if the person tires easily.
- Keep exit doors locked. Consider some type of exit alarm, such as a bell attached to the door.
- Consider a mat alarm under a bedside rug to alert others of the person getting up during the night.

Encourage the person to do the following:
- Rest frequently. Don't let the person get fatigued.
- Avoid crowded places such as shopping malls and stadiums.
- Have someone with the person when he or she goes outdoors.
- Keep meal times quiet and calm.
- Limit the number of visitors.
- Have the person do one activity at a time.
- Keep activities simple—this will minimize fatigue.
- Plan activities ahead of time.
- Ensure that medications are taken as prescribed.
- Keep a calendar of activities visible on the wall. Cross off days as they pass.
- Maintain a photo album with labeled pictures of family members, friends, home, and so on.
- Include the person in family activities and conversations.
- Remember to treat the person with respect and maintain his or her privacy.
- Discuss all medication use with the health care provider.

Some things to avoid during periods of confusion

- Alcohol
- Contact sports
- Horseback riding
- Swimming
- Hunting
- Power tools or sharp implements
- Driving
- Riding recreational vehicles such as bicycles, skateboards, motorcycles, or snowmobiles
- Cooking without supervision

Adapted from Chipps, Clanin, and Campbell, 1992.

Tuberculosis

Tuberculosis (TB) is caused by *Mycobacterium tuberculosis,* a bacterium that is transmitted by inhaling moist secretions coughed into the air by an infected person. Although TB is an infection in the lungs, the bacteria do enter the bloodstream and infect other parts of the body. TB infection progresses in stages, the primary stage and a secondary stage, with a latency stage sometimes intervening between the two.

During the primary stage, the bacteria reside in tissue in the lungs and elsewhere in the body. During this stage, most people have no symptoms. The body's natural defenses are activated to produce antibodies to fight the infection. If the body's defenses are successful, the bacteria are walled off within a capsule, and the infection doesn't progress. The person is now in latency stage. However, the bacteria are still alive and can escape and become active later. This can happen if the body's immune system becomes impaired by illness, poor nutrition, certain drugs, or infection with AIDS.

The secondary stage (active stage) begins several months after the primary stage if the body's defenses were not successful. Bacteria begin destroying body tissue, particularly lung tissue. Symptoms include a slight fever, weight loss, fatigue, and night sweats. TB in the lungs causes a chronic cough that is initially dry but eventually produces sputum that contains blood and pus. Symptoms will also appear in other areas of the body where the bacteria have spread.

Diagnosing TB

A skin test is given when a person is suspected of having TB or has been exposed to people with TB. A positive test detects antibodies against the mycobacterium. Antibodies are detectable 4 to 12 weeks after exposure and will produce a positive test for the remainder of a person's life. A positive test does not indicate active disease—only the presence of antibodies.

The most widely used test, the **Mantoux test,** involves injecting a solution containing a small amount of harmless bacteria just under the skin on the inside of the forearm. A skin reaction consists of a rash, blisters, or swelling around the injection site. An early reaction is not significant. Swelling in 48 to 72 hours may indicate a positive reaction, de-

pending on the size of the swelling. If a skin test is positive, further procedures are necessary to determine whether the TB is active. The only way to diagnose active TB is by laboratory examination of a sputum specimen to detect live mycobacteria. Chest x-rays may show an area of lung disease. To diagnose TB of other organs, a small sample from the infected area is examined.

Treatment

Treatment of TB consists of taking a combination of drugs for 9 to 12 months (or longer), depending on the extent of the TB. Isoniazid and rifampin are nearly always prescribed, and other drugs may also be added. **It is important that you take the drug exactly as your doctor orders, and for as long as necessary.** If you do not finish the treatment, the TB can reappear and may be even harder to treat.

Avoid alcohol while taking isoniazid and rifampin because this can cause serious liver problems. Take both drugs on an empty stomach with a full glass of water. If stomach upset is a problem, take them with a small amount of food. Avoid taking antacids that contain magnesium or aluminum within 1 hour of taking isoniazid, since this can interfere with drug absorption. Rifampin can make oral contraceptives less effective, so if you are on the pill, use another method of birth control. Rifampin gives a reddish or brownish color to urine, saliva, sputum, stools, sweat, and tears and will discolor soft contact lenses. Other possible side effects are dizziness, stomach upset, diarrhea, or rash.

Report to the doctor blurred vision, eye pain, chills, joint pain and swelling, breathing difficulty, fever, weakness, vomiting, or yellowing of the skin or eyes.

Preventing the spread of TB

TB is not extremely contagious, but you need to protect close contacts. TB bacteria are spread by coughing, so cover your nose and mouth and dispose of soiled tissues properly and wash hands thoroughly. Good room ventilation helps to reduce the amount of bacteria in the air. Sometimes household members are required to take antituberculosis drugs for 6 to 9 months (as a precaution).

From Grimes.[82]

Food Safety

Food contaminated with bacteria, viruses, or parasites can cause illness. The following tips are designed to help you guard against contaminated food. **Wash hands with soap before and after handling food.** Most food contamination happens at home.

Commercially packaged food

The U.S. government has strict standards aimed at protecting the consumer from improperly canned and packaged foods. Even so, contaminated foods occasionally find their way to the grocery shelves. Observe the following guidelines and remember: **If in doubt, throw it out! Do not even taste a small amount.**

- Do not buy containers that appear to have been opened or have broken seals on jar lids.
- Do not buy or use cans that have bulging ends, leaks, or rust.
- Do not use food that shows spoilage, such as mold, an off-color, or an off-odor. A can that spurts liquid when opened is unsafe.
- Be sure to refrigerate after opening a jar if the label so instructs.

Home canned foods

Home canning requires following very precise methods of preparing the food, using the proper kind of jars, and sealing the jars carefully. Nonacid foods are especially susceptible to the bacteria responsible for botulism. (Note: Nonacid foods include all vegetables, tomatoes, meat, poultry, and fish.) Pressure canning using 10 pounds of pressure at 240° F is the only method recommended for nonacid foods. The botulism bacteria does not cause an odor, a change in color or texture, or the formation of gas. **Never taste home canned nonacid food before first cooking!** To cook nonacid home canned foods, vigorously boil in an uncovered pot (vegetables for 3 to 5 minutes, meat, poultry, and fish for 10 minutes).

Meat and poultry

Salmonella and other bacteria may be present in raw meat and poultry. Any kitchen equipment that comes in contact with raw meat or poultry should be washed thoroughly before it is used with other foods.

- Use hot water and detergent to wash utensils that have touched raw meat or poultry before using the equipment with other food.
- When cutting raw meat or poultry, use a nonporous cutting board (plastic, marble, or glass) and wash it immediately.
- Keep meat refrigerated at 35° to 40° F. Ground meats are very perishable and should be cooked (or frozen) within 24 hours after purchase. Roasts will keep for 3 or 4 days without freezing. Poultry should be eaten within 2 days. Before cooking, check the odor of meats and poultry. Do not risk it if there is an unpleasant smell. Wash hands between handling raw meat and other foods and **cook** all meat.

Pork

Pork may contain a parasite that causes trichinosis. The only way to destroy the parasite is to cook pork thoroughly until the meat is white or grayish all the way through or registers 137° F on a meat thermometer.

Eggs

Eggs may be infected with *Salmonella* or other bacteria. Never use an egg that has an unpleasant odor or that has a cracked shell. Only eat eggs that have been cooked. Refrigerate eggs and prepared food that contains eggs (mayonnaise and other salad dressings) until ready to serve.

Milk and dairy products

Milk and other dairy products made from raw (unpasteurized) milk have caused TB. Buy only pasteurized dairy products.

Fish and shellfish

Because of environmental pollution, hepatitis has been caused by eating raw oysters, and several types of bacterial food poisoning can occur from eating raw shellfish or fish. Avoid eating any uncooked fish and shellfish.

Travel outside the U.S.

Travelers to developing countries should not drink local water or eat uncooked vegetables. Fruits that require peeling are safe, but peel them yourself. Do not eat food from street vendors.

From Grimes.[82]

PATIENT TEACHING GUIDE

Facts About Your Prescription

Your doctor has prescribed one or more drugs to treat an infection. It is important that you take the drugs exactly as prescribed, for as long as needed. Even if you feel better, **don't stop taking the drug before you are supposed to!** This could cause the infection to reappear, and it is sometimes harder to get rid of the second time.

From Grimes, 1991.

MEDICATION INFORMATION FORM

Here is some information about the medication your doctor prescribed:

Name of drug:_____
       (generic and brand)

Dose:_____

When to take:_____

Special instructions for taking:_____
_____

Cautions:
Do not take on an empty stomach_____
Do not take with milk or antacids_____
Avoid alcohol_____
Avoid sun exposure while taking_____
Take with food_____
Drink plenty of fluids_____
May cause drowsiness_____
Do not take while pregnant_____
Do not take while breast-feeding_____
Do not take with these other drugs:_____
                       _____
                       _____

Side effects:_____
_____

Cease taking medicine and call your doctor if any of the following occur:
_____
_____

Doctor's phone number_____

Mosby's
Clinical Nursing
Series

Dealing with the Effects of Immune and Bone Marrow Suppression

HIV infection impairs a person's immune system and leaves the person susceptible to infection. Zidovudine (AZT) and several drugs used to treat opportunistic infections can cause suppression of the bone marrow's ability to produce cells to control bleeding.

Preventing infection

Infection is a serious problem, and you should do everything possible to prevent it by following the guidelines below:

Eat nutritious meals, drink plenty of fluids, get enough rest, and avoid stress as much as possible.

Keep your mouth, teeth, and gums clean. Use a soft toothbrush and salt-water rinse.

Wash your hands frequently with soap and water, especially before eating and after using the toilet.

Cleanse your perianal area after each bowel movement. Women should avoid bubble baths, douches, and feminine hygiene products such as tampons. Sanitary napkins should be changed frequently. Use a commercial lubricant and a condom during sexual intercourse. Urinate before and after intercourse.

Avoid the following:

People who are ill.

People vaccinated recently with a live virus (e.g., polio virus).

Crowded places (waiting rooms, malls).

Raw fruits and vegetables, raw eggs, and raw milk; eat only cooked food and pasteurized milk and milk products.

All sources of stagnant water (water in flower vases, pitchers, denture cups, humidifiers, and respiratory equipment). Water in these containers should be changed daily.

Dog, cat, and bird feces. Let someone else change bird cages or litter boxes.

Even if you follow these guidelines carefully, an infection may occur. Call your doctor immediately if you develop any sign of infection:

Fever over 100.4° F

Redness, swelling, or pain around any wound

Coughing, sore throat, and stuffy or runny nose

Nausea, vomiting, or diarrhea

Chest pain or shortness of breath

Burning or frequency of urination, or a change in the color or odor of urine

Sores or white patches in the mouth

Even if your symptoms seem mild, they may indicate a life-threatening infection.

Preventing bleeding

Patients receiving certain drugs run a greater risk of bleeding from the skin and mucous membranes or inter-nally. The bleeding results because the bone marrow is producing few or no platelets (special blood cells that cause the blood to clot), or because platelets already in the blood are being destroyed. Allergic reactions to medication, radiation therapy, or chemotherapy can cause this reduction in the number of platelets; the condition is called **thrombocytopenia**.

Because the lack of platelets makes bleeding hard to stop once it has begun, it is *very* important that patients with thrombocytopenia take great care to prevent bleeding. Check your skin each day for bruises, and call the doctor if any get larger after you first notice them.

To prevent bleeding from the skin mucous membranes, or internally:

Avoid physical activities that could cause injury.

Shave with an electric razor.

Keep your nails short. File rough edges.

Brush with a soft toothbrush. If you still have trouble with bleeding gums, use sponge-tipped applicators or a Water-Pik. Do not floss. Keep your lips moist with petroleum jelly. Check with your health care provider before having dental work.

Avoid hot foods that might burn your mouth.

Blow your nose gently. Humidify your house if the air is too dry, because dry air can cause nosebleeds. If your nose does bleed, pinch your nostrils shut for a few minutes. If the bleeding persists, put an ice bag on the back of your neck.

Use stool softeners and drink plenty of water if you are constipated. Do not use enemas or suppositories.

Take acetaminophen (e.g., Tylenol) or ibuprofen instead of aspirin. Aspirin can increase the risk of bleeding.

Avoid douches and vaginal suppositories. Use a lubricating jelly before sexual intercourse.

Try to arrange furniture so you won't bruise yourself on it. Keep clutter off floors.

Avoid tight-fitting clothing and any buttons or ornaments that could bruise or chafe your skin.

Do not lift heavy objects.

If bleeding does occur, apply pressure to the site for 5 to 10 minutes and elevate.

Any bleeding that does not stop after 5 minutes should be reported to your health care provider.

Preventing anemia

In anemia there are not enough red blood cells to carry oxygen to the cells and take away carbon dioxide. (With bone marrow suppression the marrow is producing fewer red blood cells.) You may tire easily and need to rest more often.

To lessen the effects of anemia:

Schedule activities with frequent rest periods.

Eat a diet high in protein. Take a multivitamin supplement with minerals.

Be alert for any of these signs: pallor, dizziness, ringing in the ears, chest pain, or shortness of breath. Report these problems to your health care provider.

Adapted from Belcher, 1992.

Care of the Hickman-Broviac Central Venous Catheter

A central venous catheter is a convenient way to deliver medications, including drugs for chemotherapy, and to take the many blood samples needed without having to insert a needle into your vein. The catheter is a soft, plastic tube that is implanted in your chest. One end of the tube is placed in a large vein close to your heart; the other end stays outside your body. The catheter has a cap that can be removed when blood samples are needed or drugs for chemotherapy must be given.

You will need to follow three procedures to care for your central venous catheter: changing the dressing, changing the cap, and flushing the catheter. Follow the procedures carefully to prevent infection and clotting of the tube.

Changing the dressing

You must change the dressing on your catheter frequently (at least 3 times a week) until the wound site has healed. (After the site has healed, your health care provider may allow you to clean around the wound site with soap and water while you shower; then dry the area and apply a small gauze pad or adhesive bandage to the exit site.) Assemble the following equipment:

- Povidone-iodine swabs
- Alcohol swabs
- Povidone-iodine ointment (optional)
- Air-occlusive dressing or sterile 4″ × 4″ gauze with tape
1. Wash your hands.
2. Remove the old dressing and wash your hands again.
3. Starting at the wound site and using a circular motion, clean the skin with an alcohol swab, working your way out approximately 2 inches.
4. Repeat the process 2 more times, allowing the alcohol to dry for 30 seconds.
5. Repeat steps 3 and 4 with the povidone-iodine swabs.
6. Apply povidone ointment to the exit site (optional).
7. Apply either an air-occlusive dressing or a sterile 4″ × 4″ gauze pad.
8. Loop the catheter and tape over dressing.

Changing the catheter cap

Catheter caps should be changed twice a week.
Assemble the following equipment:
- Catheter cap
- Catheter clamp
- Alcohol wipes
- Povidone-iodine swabs
1. Wash your hands.
2. Clamp the catheter.
3. Wipe the injection cap with a povidone-iodine swab. Allow to dry for 30 seconds.
4. Wipe the injection cap with an alcohol pad.
5. Remove the old injection cap. Screw on a new cap. Unclamp the catheter.

Flushing the catheter

You need to flush your catheter as directed by your health care provider (as often as once a day) to prevent blood clots from forming inside it.
Assemble the following equipment:
- Vial of heparin-saline solution
- Disposable syringe and needle
- Alcohol wipes
1. Wash your hands.
2. Open the bottle of heparin-saline solution; wipe the vial opening with an alcohol wipe.
3. Remove the needle guard from the syringe, and pull back the plunger. Insert the needle into the vial, turn the vial upside down, and pull back on the syringe to fill it (tap on the side of the syringe to remove air bubbles).
4. Clean the catheter cap with an alcohol wipe. Insert the needle into the cap, and push down on the plunger to inject the solution into the catheter.
5. Remove the needle and carefully discard it and the syringe.

Catheter maintenance

Be sure to buy a catheter repair kit to use when a leak occurs.

Call your health care provider if:

Pain, redness, or puffiness develops around the catheter site.

You notice drainage from the catheter site.

Your temperature is above 100.4° F.

The catheter slips.

There is blood in the catheter.

You are unable to flush the catheter.

Vein

Exit site

Adapted from Belcher, 1992.

Care of the Implanted Port

An implanted port is a convenient way to deliver medications, including drugs for chemotherapy, and to take the many blood samples needed without damaging your veins. The implanted port consists of a soft, plastic catheter that is placed in a large vein close to your heart and a port with a metal base and rubber top through which medications will be administered and blood will be drawn. The implanted port is surgically placed in your chest or abdomen, and there are no external parts.

Because an implanted port is completely under the skin, it doesn't require a lot of care. You must watch for signs of infection, protect the needle during ambulatory infusion pump treatments, and prevent the skin over the port from becoming irritated.

Watching for signs of infection

Call your health care provider if:
Redness, pain, or puffiness develops around the port.
You notice drainage from the incision site.
Your temperature is above 100.4° F.
You become short of breath.
You have chest pain.

Protecting the needle during infusion

Sometimes you may need to receive treatments over an extended period. For these occasions, a bent needle (Huber needle) is inserted into the port and connected to an ambulatory infusion pump. The needle is left in the port until the treatment is finished, sometimes for several days. The pump is attached to your body by a belt or pouch and is worn for the duration of the treatment.

During this time you will need to prevent the needle from becoming dislodged. A dressing will be taped over the needle, and you must check it to make sure the tape is holding the dressing and the needle hasn't slipped. You may need to change this dressing periodically.

Protecting the skin over the port

It is important that you prevent irritation of the skin over and around the port. Do not wear any bra straps or clothing that may rub the port site. Adjust your seat belt if it rubs the port site.

Unless you are receiving an infusion, you may shower, bathe, and swim without worry. When re-ceiving an infusion, you need to keep the site dry and protected.

Changing the drug reservoir bag

If you are receiving treatment over several days, you may be taught to change the drug reservoir bag. Directions for changing the bag vary with the type of pump. Your health care provider will provide you with a diagram and complete instructions.

Adapted from Belcher, 1992.

Portal   Lock   Catheter

Huber needle
Skin
"Pocket"
Catheter
Large vein

References

1. Allen MH, Marte C: HIV infection in women: presentations and protocols, *Hosp Pract* 27(3):155-162, March 15, 1992.
2. Amantea M, Drutz D, Rosenthal J: Antifungals: a primary care primer, *Patient Care* 24(11):58, 1990.
3. American College of Obstetricians and Gynecologists: *Prevention of HIV infection and AIDS*, Washington, DC, 1987, The College.
4. American Dental Association: *Facts about AIDS for the dental team*, ed 3, Chicago, 1991, American Dental Association.
5. Anastos K, Marte C: Women—the missing persons in the AIDS epidemic, *Health/PAC Bull* 19(4):6-13, Winter, 1989.
6. Andiman W et al.: Rate of transmission of human immunodeficiency virus type I infection from mother to child and short-term outcome of neonatal infection: results of a prospective cohort study, *Am J Dis Child* 144:758-766, July 1990.
7. Araneta MR, Lemp GF, Cohen JB, Derisk PA, Carmona I, Clevenger AC: Survival trends among women with AIDS in San Francisco. In Abstracts of the VII International Conference on AIDS, Vol 1, p 328, abstract M.C. 3122, Florence, Italy, 1991.
8. Bartlett JG: *1992-93 Recommendations for the medical care of persons with HIV infection*, ed 2, Baltimore, 1992, The Johns Hopkins School of Medicine.
9. Bartlett JG: *1991-92 Pocketbook of infectious dis-*
ease therapy, Baltimore, 1991, Williams & Wilkins.
10. Belcher A: *Cancer nursing*, St Louis 1992, Mosby.
11. Benenson AS, editor: *Control of communicable diseases in man*, ed 15, Washington, DC, 1990, American Public Health Association.
12. Beral V, Peterman TA, Berkelman RL, Jaffe HW: Kaposi's sarcoma among persons with AIDS: a sexually transmitted infection? *Lancet* 335:123-8, 1990.
13. Berger J: Neurological complication of HIV disease, *PAAC Notes*, September, 1992, pp 236-240.
14. Berger TG: Dermatologic care in the AIDS patient: a 1990 Update. In Sande MA, Volberding PA, editors: *The medical management of AIDS*, Philadelphia, 1990, WB Saunders.
15. Berger TG, Obuch ML, Goldschmidt RH: Dermatologic manifestations of HIV infection. *Am Fam Physician* 41(6):1729-1742, 1990.
16. Berkow R, Fletcher AJ, editors: *Merck manual of diagnosis and therapy*, vol 1, ed 16, Rahway, NJ, 1992, Merck Research Laboratories.
17. Bhasker S, Lilly G, Pratt L: A practical high yield mouth exam, *Patient Care* 24(1):53, 1990.
18. Bird AG: Monitoring of disease progression of HIV infection. In Bird AG, editor: *Immunology of HIV infection*, Boston, 1992, Kluwer Academic Publishers.
19. Braun J, Solvetti A, Xakellis G: Decubitus ulcers:

what really works? *Patient Care*, Oct 15, 1988, pp. 22-34.

20. Brenner ZR: *Diagnostic tests and procedures: applying the nursing process*, Norwalk, Conn, 1987, Appleton & Lange.

21. Brettle R: Clinical issues of injecting drug users related to HIV, International Seminar Series: Aspects of HIV Management in Injecting Drug Users. Highlights of a seminar meeting, October 14, 1989, Madrid, Spain. Colwood House Medical Publications, 1990.

22. Broadhead RS: Social constructions of bleach in combating AIDS among injection drug users, *J Drug Issues*, 21:713-737, 1991.

23. Brown LS, Siddiqui N: Relationship between cocaine use and HIV disease progression in injecting drug users (IDUs). Program and abstracts of the VII International Conference on AIDS, abstract MC 3156, Florence, Italy, June 16-21, 1991.

24. Carpenter C, Mayer K, Stein M, Leibman B, Fisher A, Fiore T: Human immunodeficiency virus infection in North American women: experience with 200 cases and a review of the literature, *Medicine* 70:307-25, 1991.

25. Centers for Disease Control: Impact of new legislation on needle and syringe purchase and possession—Connecticut, 1992, *MMWR* 5; 42(8):145-148, March 1993.

26. Centers for Disease Control: Initial therapy for tuberculosis in the era of multidrug resistance, *MMWR*, 42(RR-7), 1993.

27. Centers for Disease Control: *HIV/AIDS surveillance*, Atlanta, January, 1993, The Centers.

28. Centers for Disease Control: Childbearing and Contraceptive-use plans among women at high risk for HIV infection—selected U.S. sites, 1989-1991, *MMWR* 28;41(8):135, 141-144, Feb 1992.

29. Centers for Disease Control: 1993 Revised classification system for HIV infection and expanded surveillance case definition for AIDS among adolescents and adults, *MMWR* 41(RR-17), December, 1992.

30. Centers for Disease Control: *HIV-related tuberculosis*, Washington, DC, 1992, U.S. Government Printing Office.

31. Centers for Disease Control: Update: investigations of patients who have been treated by HIV-infected health care workers, *MMWR* 41(19):344-346, May, 1992.

32. Centers for Disease Control: Publicly funded HIV counseling and testing—United States, 1991, *MMWR* 41(34):613-617, Aug 1992.

33. Centers for Disease Control: *HIV/AIDS surveillance*, Atlanta, January, 1992, The Centers.

34. Centers for Disease Control: Update: acquired immunodeficiency syndrome—United States, *MMWR* 42(28):547-57, 1992.

35. Centers for Disease Control: Update: transmission of HIV infection during invasive dental procedures—Florida, *MMWR* 40(23):377-381, June 1991.

36. Centers for Disease Control: Guidelines for preventing the transmission of tuberculosis in health-care settings, with special focus on HIV-related issues, *MMWR* 39(RR-17): Dec 17, 1990.

37. Centers for Disease Control: Guidelines for prevention of transmission of human immunodeficiency virus and hepatitis B virus to health-care and public-safety workers, *MMWR* 38(S-6), 1989.

38. Centers for Disease Control: Recommendations for prevention of HIV transmission in health-care settings, *MMWR* 36(2S), Aug 21, 1987.

39. Centers for Disease Control: Recommendations for assisting in the prevention of perinatal transmission of human T-lymphotrophic virus type III/lymphadenopathy associated virus and acquired immune deficiency syndrome, *MMWR* 34:721-732, Dec 6, 1985.

40. Centers for Disease Control: CDC guidelines for isolation precautions in hospitals, HHS pub no (CDC) 83-8314, Atlanta, 1983, The Centers.

41. Chevret S, Roquin H, Ganne P, Lefrere J: Prognostic value of an elevated CD8 lymphocyte count in HIV infection: results of a prospective study of 152 asymptomatic HIV-positive individuals, *AIDS* 6:1349-1352, 1992.

42. Chipps E, Clanin N, Campbell B: *Neurologic disorders*, St Louis, 1992, Mosby.

43. Chu SY, Buehler JW, Fleming PL, Berkelman RL: Epidemiology of reported cases of AIDS in lesbians, United States 1980-89, *Am J Public Health* 80:1380-1381, 1990.

44. Clinical Insight: Drug Interactions. *Clinical Insight: Guidelines for Management of HIV Infection* 2(2):6, March 1992.

45. Cockerell CJ: Off-label treatment of HIV-associated skin conditions, *PAACNotes* 5(4):155-157, 1993.

46. Cockerell CJ, Conant MA, Sadick NS: When the skin is a harbinger of AIDS, *Patient Care* 53-76, May 1992.

47. Cohen FL, Durham JD, editors: *Women, Children and AIDS*, 1993, Springer.

48. Contoreggi C, Jones SW, Simpson PM, Lange WR, Meyer WA: A model of syringe disinfection as measured by polymerase chain reaction for human leukocyte antigen and HIV genome. VIII International Conference on AIDS/III STD World

Congress, vol 2, p C291, abstract PoC 4280, Amsterdam, The Netherlands, July 19-24, 1992.

49. Cooney T: Clinical management of the complications of HIV infection, *J Gen Intern Med* 6(S12): 1991.

50. Corbett JV: *Laboratory tests and diagnostic procedures with nursing diagnoses*, ed 2, Norwalk, Conn, 1987, Appleton & Lange.

51. Crocchiolo P, Lizioli A, Goisis F, Giorgi C, Buratti E, Bedarida G, et al.: Cervical dysplasia and HIV infection, *Lancet* 1:238-239, 1988.

52. Cumming PD et al: Exposure of patients to human immunodeficiency virus through the transfusion of blood components that tested antibody negative, *N Engl J Med* 321:941-946, 1989.

53. Curran JW, Scheckel LW, Millstein RA: HIV/AIDS Prevention Bulletin: provisional recommendations for bleach disinfection of injection equipment. Jointly issued by Centers for Disease Control and Prevention, Center for Substance Abuse Treatment, and National Institute on Drug Abuse, 1993.

54. Denenberg R: *Gynecological care manual for HIV positive women*, Essential Medical Information Systems, Inc, 1993.

55. Denenberg R: Women, immunity, and sex hormones, *Treatment Issues*, 6(7):6-10, 1992 (special edition).

56. Department of Health and Human Services: *National HIV serosurveillance summary*, vol 2, HIV/NCID/11-91/011, Washington, DC, 1991, US-DHHS, USPHS.

57. Dieterich D: CMV infection, *PAAC Notes*, Oct 92, pp 277-280.

58. Dieterich DT, Kotler DP, Busch DF, Crumpacker C, DuMond C, Dearmand B, Buhles W: Ganciclovir treatment of cytomegalovirus colitis in AIDS: a randomized, double-blind, placebo-controlled multicenter study, *J Infect Dis* 167:278-282, 1993.

59. Doughty DB, Jackson DB: *Gastrointestinal disorders*, St Louis, 1993, Mosby.

60. Easterbrock PJ, Keruly JC, Creagh-Kirk T, et al: Racial and ethnic differences in outcome in zidovudine-treated patients with advanced HIV disease, *JAMA* 266(19):2713-2718, 1991.

61. Ekstrand M, Stall R, Kegeles S, Hays R, DeMayo M, Coates T: Editorial Comment: Safer sex among gay men: what is the ultimate goal? *AIDS* 7:281-282, 1993.

62. Ellerbrock T, Bush T, Chamberland M, et al: Epidemiology of women with AIDS in the United States, 1981 through 1990: a comparison with heterosexual men with AIDS, *JAMA* 265:2971-2975, 1991.

63. European Collaborative Study: Children born to women with HIV-1 infection: natural history and risk of transmission, *Lancet* 337:253-258, Feb 2, 1991.

64. Faltz BG, Rinaldi J: *AIDS and substance abuse: a training manual for health care professionals*, The AIDS Health Project, University of California—San Francisco, 1987.

65. Farizo KM, Buehler JW, Chamberland ME, et al: Spectrum of disease in persons with human immunodeficiency virus infection in the United States, *JAMA*, 267(13):1798-1805, 1992.

66. Fegan C: Cryptosporidial disease in the adult HIV infected patient, *J Assoc Nurses AIDS Care* 3(4):11-20, 1992.

67. Fernandez F, Holmes V, Levy JK, Ruiz P: Consultation-liaison psychiatry and HIV related disorders, *Hosp Community Psychiatry* 40(2):146-153, 1989.

68. Flegg PJ, Brettle RP, Robertson JR, Clarkson RC, Bird GA: Beta 2-microglobulin levels in drug users: the influence of risk behavior, *AIDS* 5:1021-1024, 1991.

69. Fleming P, Cleslelski CA, Berkelman RL: Sex-specific differences in the prevalence of reported AIDS-indicative diagnosis, United States, 1988-1989. In Abstracts of the VII International Conference on AIDS, vol 1, p 350, abstract M.C. 3210, Florence, Italy, 1991.

70. Folstein MJ, Folstein FE, McHugh PR: Mini Mental State, *J Psychol Res* 12:189-198, 1975.

71. Friedman SL: Gastrointestinal symptoms in AIDS, *AIDS Clin Care* 1(3):17-20, 1989.

72. Gabuzda DH, Hirsch MS: Neurologic manifestations of infection with human immunodeficiency virus, *Ann Intern Med* 107:383, 1987.

73. Galgiani J et al: Fungal infections in AIDS, *Patient Care* 23(10):118, 1989.

74. George R: Pulmonary mycoses: new concepts and new therapy, *Postgrad Med* 84(1):185, 1988.

75. Godofsky EW, Zinreich J, Armstrong M, Leslie JM, Weikel CS: Sinusitis in HIV-infected patients: a clinical and radiographic review, *Am J Med* 93:163-170, 1992.

76. Goldschmidt RH, Dong BJ: Treatment of AIDS and HIV-related conditions, *J Am Board Fam Pract* 5(3):335-350, 1992.

77. Gottlieb M, Polsky B, Safrin S: Opportunistic viruses in AIDS, *Patient Care* 23(10):139, 1989.

78. Grant IH, Anastos K, Ernst J: Gender differences in AIDS-deficiency illnesses. In Abstracts of the VII International Conference on AIDS, vol 1, p 356, abstract M.C. 3192, Florence, Italy, 1991.

79. Greenspan D: Oral manifestations of AIDS, *AIDS Clin Care* 1(6):45-48, 1989.

80. Greenspan JS, Greenspan D, Winkler JR: Diagnosis and management of the oral manifestations of HIV infection and AIDS. In Sande MA, Volberding PA, editors: *The medical management of AIDS*, Philadelphia, 1990, WB Saunders.

81. Greenspan D, Greenspan JS: Oral lesions of HIV infection: features and therapy. In Volberding P, Jacobson MA, editors: *AIDS clinical review 1992*, New York, 1992, Marcel Dekker.

82. Grimes DE: *Infectious diseases*, St Louis, 1991, Mosby.

83. Grimes RM: *Managing the HIV infected/AIDS patient*, Austin, 1990, Texas Medical Association.

84. Gubuzda DH, Hirsch MS: Neurologic manifestations of infection with human immunodeficiency virus, *Ann Intern Med* 107:383-391, 1987.

85. Guidry HM, Grimes RM: Management of HIV infection: a summary of summaries, part 1, *Hosp Pract*, Nov 15, 1992.

86. Hamilton JD, Hartigan PM, Simberkoff MS, the VA Cooperative Group: Early versus later zidovudine treatment of symptomatic HIV infection, *Clin Res* 39-216A, 1991.

87. Hankins C, Handley M: HIV disease and AIDS in women: current knowledge and a research agenda, *J Acquir Immune Defic Syndr* 5:957-976, Oct 1992.

88. Handsfield HH: Recent developments in STDs. I. Bacterial diseases, *Hosp Pract* 26(7):47, 1991.

89. Haverkos HW, Lange WR: Serious infections other than human immunodeficiency virus among intravenous drug abusers, *J Infect Dis* 161:894-902, 1990.

90. Herbert JR, Barone J: On the possible relationship between AIDS and nutrition, *Med Hypothesis* 27:51-4, 1988.

91. Hoegsberg B, Abulafia O, Sedlis A, Feldman J, DesJalais D, Landesman S, Minkoff H: Sexually transmitted diseases and human immunodeficiency virus infection among women with pelvic inflamatory diseases, *Am J Obstet Gynecol* 163 (4pt 1):1135-1139, Oct 1990.

92. Hollander H: Care of the individual with early HIV infection. In Sande MA, Volberding PA, editors: *The medical management of AIDS*, ed 7, Philadelphia, 1990, WB Saunders.

93. Hughes W, Leoung G, Kramer F, et al: Comparison of atovaquone (566c80) with trimethoprim-sulfamethoxazole to treat *Pneumocystis carinii* pneumonia in patients with AIDS, *N Engl J Med* 328(21):1521-1527, 1993.

94. Hutchinson M, Kurth A: "I need to know that I have a choice": a study of women, HIV, and reproductive decision-making, *AIDS Patient Care*, Feb 1991, pp 17-25.

95. Imam N, Carpenter C, Mayer K, Fisher A, Steiun M, Danforth S: Hierarchical pattern of mucosal *Candida* infections in HIV-seropositive women, *Am J Med* 89:142-146, 1990.

96. Janssen RS, St Louis ME, Satten GA, et al: HIV infection among patients in U.S. acute care hospitals, *N Engl J Med* 327(7):445-452, 1992.

97. Johnson MA, Webster A: Human immunodeficiency virus infection in women, *Br J Obstet Gynaecol* 96:129-134, 1989.

98. Karan L, Hoegerman G: Chemical dependency, HIV infection, and motherhood: a case presentation and discussion, *Pediatric AIDS and HIV Infection: Fetus to Adolescent* 2(5):284-9, 1991.

99. Kelly P: Fertility, menstruation, and birth control in HIV, *Treatment Issues* 6(7):10-14, 1992 (special edition).

100. Kelly P, Holman S: The new face of AIDS, *Am J Nursing*, March 1993, pp 26-36.

101. Kim MJ, McFarland GK, McLane AM: Pocket guide to nursing diagnoses, ed 5, St Louis, 1993, Mosby.

102. Kline MW, Shearer WT; Impact of human immunodeficiency virus infection on women and infants, *Infect Dis Clin North Am* 6(1):1-17, March 1992.

103. Kravis NM, Weiss C: Working with the IVDU: an approach to management in the inpatient medical setting, Cornell University Medical College, The New York Hospital, Memorial Sloan-Kettering Cancer Center, Training for Health Care Providers to Address AIDS, Module no. 1.

104. Lagakos S, Fischl MA, Stein DS, Lim L, Volberding P: Effects of zidovudine therapy in minority and other subpopulations with early HIV infection, *JAMA* 266(19):2709-2712, 1991.

105. Lassoued K, Clauvel J-P, Fegueux S, Matheron S, Gorin I, Oksenhendler E: AIDS-associated Kaposi's sarcoma in female patients, *AIDS* 5:877-880, 1991.

106. Leedom JM, Yu VL: Pneumonia in compromised patients, *Patient Care* 22(2):153, 1988.

107. Levy JA: Transmission of HIV and factors influencing progression to AIDS, *Am J Med* 95:86-100, 1993.

108. Levy RM, Bredsen DE, Rosenblum ML: Neurologic complications of HIV infection, *Am Fam Phys* 41(2):517-535, 1990.

109. Lynn LA: Primary care for HIV infection, *Hospital Pract* 48-64, Feb 1992.

110. Maiman M, Fruchter RG, Serur E, Remy JC, Feuer G, Boyce J: Human immunodeficiency virus infection and cervical neoplasia, *Gynecol Oncol* 38:377-382, Sept 1990.

111. Markowitz R-B, Thompson HC, Mueller JF, Co-

hen JA, Dynan WS: Incidence of BK virus and JC virus viruria in human immunodeficiency virus–infected and –uninfected subjects, *J Infect Dis* 167:13-20, 1993.

112. Marmor M, Weiss L, Lynden M, et al: Possible female-to-female transmission of human immunodeficiency virus, *Ann Intern Med* 105:969, 1986.

113. Matorras R, Ariceta J, Rementeria A, Corral J, Gutierrez de Teran G, Diez J, et al: Human immunodeficiency virus–induced immunosuppression: a risk factor for human papillomavirus infection, *Am J Obstet Gynecol*, 164:42-44, 1991.

114. McKusick L: Center for AIDS Prevention Studies, University of California: Issues of specific groups in the hospital, *HIV Frontline*, no 5, p 5, San Francisco, November 1991.

115. Mehta JB, Morris F: Impact of HIV infection on mycobacterial disease, *Am Fam Phys* 45(5):2203-2211, 1992.

116. Millstein RA: NIDA Community Alert Bulletin: U.S. Department of Human Services, Public Health Service, National Institutes of Health, National Institute on Drug Abuse: Using bleach to decontaminate drug injection equipment, March 25, 1993.

117. Minkoff H, DeHovitz J: Care of women infected with the human immunodeficiency virus, *JAMA* 266:2253-2258, Oct 23-30, 1991.

118. Monforte A et al.: Maternal predictors of HIV vertical transmission, *Eur J Obstet Gynecol Reprod Biol* 42:131-136, Nov 1991.

119. Monzon OT, Capellan JMB: Female-to-female transmission of HIV, *Laucet* 2:40-41, 1987 (letter).

120. Nanda D, Minkoff HL: Pregnancy and women at risk for HIV infection; *AIDS and HIV Infection in Office Practice* 19(1):157-168, 1992.

121. Nichols S: Psychosocial reactions of persons with the acquired immunodeficiency syndrome, *Ann Intern Med* 103:765-767, 1985.

122. Nightingale SD, Cal SX: Medical management of HIV-positive patients, *Dallas Med J*, Jan 1993.

123. Nightingale SD, Cameron DW, Gordin FM, et al: Two controlled trials of rifabutin prophylaxis against *Mycobacterium avium* complex infection in AIDS, *N Engl J Med* 329(12):828-33, 1993.

124. Novack DH: Therapeutic aspects of the clinical encounter, *J Gen Intern Med* 2:346-55, 1987.

125. Obstetrics and Gynecology Clinics of North America; Minkoff HL, guest editor: *HIV disease in pregnancy* 17(3), Philadelphia, September 1990, WB Saunders, Ordering information 1-800-654-2452.

126. Peiperl L: *Manual of HIV/AIDS therapy: current clinical strategies*, Newport Beach, Calif, 1992, Publishing International.

127. Peterson HB, Galaid EI, Zenilman JM: Pelvic inflammatory disease: guidelines for prevention and management, *Rev Infect Dis* 12:S656-664.

128. Petersen L, Doll L, White C, Chu S, the HIV Blood Donor Study Group: *J Acquir Immune Defic Syndr* 5:853-855, 1992.

129. Plummer FA, Simonsen JN, Cameron DW, Ndinya-Achola JO, Kriess JK, Gakinya MN, Waiyaki P, Cheang M, Piot P, Ronald AR, Ngugi EN: Cofactors in male-female sexual transmission of human immunodeficiency virus type 1, *Infect Dis* 163:233-239, 1991.

130. Poulton TB: Chest manifestations of AIDS, *Am Fam Phys* 45(1):163-168, 1992.

131. Price R, Brew B: The AIDS dementia complex, *J Infect Dis* 156:1079, 1988.

132. Quinn TJ, Strober W, Janoff EN, Masur H: Gastrointestinal infections. In Smith PD, moderator: *Ann Intern Med* 116:63-77, 1992.

133. Reese RE, Douglas RG: *A practical approach to infectious diseases*, ed 2, Boston, 1986, Little Brown & Co.

134. Regan-Kubinski MJ, Sharts-Engel N: The HIV-infected woman: illness cognition assessment, *J Psychosocial Nurs Mental Health Serv* 30:(2):11-15, 1992.

135. Rhoads J, Wright D, Redfield R, Burke D: Chronic vaginal candidiasis in women with human immunodeficiency virus infection, *JAMA* 257:3105-3107, 1987.

136. Rosenstein DI, Reviere GR, Scott KS: HIV associated periodontal disease: a new spirochete found, *J Am Dent Ass* 124:76-80, 1993.

137. Rossitch E, Carrazana EJ, Samuels MA: Cerebral toxoplasmosis in patients with AIDS, *Am Fam Physician* 867-873, Mar 1990.

138. Royce RA, Tu X, Pagans M: Gender differences in survival after AIDS diagnosis: U.S. surveillance data. In Abstracts of the VII International Conference on AIDS, vol 1, p 331, Abstract M.C. 3135, Florence, Italy, 1991.

139. Safrin S, Dattel BJ, Hauer L, Sweet RL: Seroprevalence and epidemiologic correlates of human immunodeficiency virus infection in women with acute pelvic inflammatory disease, *Obstet Gynecol* 75:666-670, 1990.

140. Sande MA, Volberding PA: *The medical management of AIDS*, ed 3, Philadelphia, 1992, WB Saunders.

141. Sande MA, Volberding PA: *The medical management of AIDS*, Philadelphia, 1990, WB Saunders.

142. Sanford JP, Sande MA, Gilbert DN, Gerberding JL: *Guide to HIV/AIDS therapy*, Dallas, Texas, 1992, Antimicrobial Therapy, Inc.

143. Santa Cruz Women's Health Collective: *Lesbian health matters!*, 1979. Order from: the Santa Cruz Women's Health Center, 250 Locust Street, Santa Cruz, Calif. 95060.

144. Schram NR: Refining safer sex, *Focus* 5(7):3-4, 1990.

145. Schwartz EL, Brechbuhl AB, Kahl P, Miller MA, Selwyn PA, Friedland GH: Pharmacokinetic interactions of zidovudine and methadone in intravenous drug-using patients with HIV infection, *J Acquir Immune Defic Syndr* 5:619-626, 1992.

146. Selwyn PA, Alcabes P, Hartel D, Buono D, Schoenbaum EE, Klein RS, Davenny K, Friedland GH: Clinical manifestations and predictors of disease progression in drug users with human immunodeficiency virus infection, *N Engl J Med* 327:1697-1703, Dec 10, 1992.

147. Selwyn P, Schoenbaum E, Davenny K, Robertson V, Feingold A, Shulman J, et al: Prospective study of human immunodeficiency virus infection and pregnancy outcomes in intravenous drug users, *JAMA* 261:1289-1294, 1989.

148. Shernoff M: *Counseling chemically dependent people with HIV illness*, New York, 1991, Harrington Park Press.

149. Sperling RS, Friedman F Jr, Joyner M, Brodman M, Dottino P: Seroprevalence of human immunodeficiency virus in women admitted to the hospital with pelvic inflammatory desease, *J Reprod Med* 36:122-124, 1991.

150. Sperling RS, Stratton P, O'Sullivan MG, Boyer P, Watts DH, Lambert JS, Hammill H, Livingston EG, Gloeb DJ, Minkoff H, Fox HE: A survey of zidovudine use in pregnant women with human immunodeficiency virus infection, *N Engl J Med* 326(13):857-861, 1992.

151. Springer E: Effective AIDS prevention with active drug users: the harm reduction model. In Shernoff M, editor: *Counseling chemically dependent people with HIV illness*, New York, 1991, The Hayworth Press.

152. Stowe A, Ross MEW, Wodak A, Thomas GV, Larson SA: Significant relationships and social supports of injecting drug users and their implications for HIV/AIDS services, *AIDS Care* 5(1):23-33, 1993.

153. Tanowitz HB, Simon D, Wittner M: Gastrointestinal manifestation, *Med Clin North Am* 76(1):45-62, 1992.

154. Thompson M, Whyte B, Morris A, Rimland D, Thompson S: Gender differences in the spectrum of HIV disease in Atlanta. In Abstracts of the VII International Conference on AIDS, vol 1, p 326, Abstract M.C. 3115, Florence, Italy, 1991.

155. *Treatment team workshop handbook update*, New York, 1991, World Health Communications, Inc.

156. U.S. Department of Health and Human Services, National Institute of Allergy and Infectious Diseases and the National Cancer Institute: Understanding the immune system, NIH Publication No. 92-529, Washington, DC, October, 1991.

157. Valenti WM: *Early intervention in the management of HIV*, Rochester, NY, 1992, Community Health Network Inc.

158. Vermund SH, Galbraith MA, Ebner SC, Sheon AR, Kaslow RA: Human immunodeficiency virus/ acquired immunodeficiency syndrome in pregnant women, *AEP* 2(6):773-803, 1992.

159. Volberding P, Jacobson MA, editors: *AIDS Clinical Review 1992*, New York, 1992, Marcel Decker.

160. Walker CM, Moody DJ, Stites DP, Levy JA: CD8+ lymphocytes can control HIV infection in vitro by suppressing virus replication, *Science* 234:1563-1566, 1986.

161. Wartenberg A: HIV disease in the intravenous drug user: role of the primary physician, *J Gen Intern Med* 6(Jan/Feb suppl):S35-S40, 1991.

162. Weber R, Ledergerber B, Opravil M, Luthy R: Cessation of intravenous drug use reduces progression of HIV-infection in HIV+ drug users. Program and Abstracts of the VI International Conference on AIDS, Abstract ThC36, San Francisco, June 19-23, 1990.

163. Weber R, Ledergerber B, Opravil M, Siegenthaler W, Luthy R: Progression of HIV infection in mis-users of injected drugs who stop injecting or follow a program of maintenance treatment with methadone, *Br Med J* 301:1362-1365, 1990.

164. Wehrle PF, Top FH, editors: *Communicable and infectious diseases*, St Louis, 1981, Mosby.

165. Weisberg L, Ross W: Aids dementia complex: characteristics of a unique aspect of HIV infection, *Postgrad Med* 86:213, 1989.

166. Weller IVD, editor: International Seminar Series. Aspects of HIV management in injecting drug users: highlights of a seminar meeting 14 October 1989, Madrid, Spain. Colwood House Medical Publications (UK) Limited, 1990.

167. Wheat J: Diagnosis of histoplasmosis, Histoplasmosis Reference Laboratory, 1001 West 10th Street, WOP 430, Indianapolis, Ind 46202.

168. Wilson B, Shannon M: Govoni and Hayes Nurses' drug guide 1993, Norwalk, Conn, 1993, Appleton & Lange.

169. Wilson S, Thompson J: *Respiratory disorders*, St Louis, 1990, Mosby.

170. Winkler JR, Robertson PB: Periodontal disease

associated with HIV infection, *Oral Surg Oral Med Oral Path* 73:145-150, 1992.

171. Wofsy CB, Padian NS, Cohen JB, Greenblatt R, Coleman R, Korvick J: Management of HIV Disease in Women. Chapter 13 in Volberding P and Jacobson MA, editors: *AIDS Clinical Review 1992*, New York, 1992, Marcel Dekker, Inc.

172. World Health Organization: *Current and future dimensions of the HIV/AIDS pandemic*, Geneva, 1992, WHO.

173. Worth D, Drucker E, Erik K, Pivnick A: Sexual and physical abuse as factors in continued risk behavior of women IV drug users in a South Bronx methadone clinic. The VII International Conference on AIDS: Final Programs and Abstracts, Abstract Th.D. 786, 1990.

174. Zurlo JJ: Sinusitis in HIV-1 infection, *Am J Med* 93:157-162, 1992.

BIBLIOGRAPHY FOR CHAPTER 15

Ausman RK: *Intravascular infusion systems*, Lancaster, 1984, MTP Press Limited.

Barton-Burke M, Wilkes GM, Berg D, Bean CK, Ingwersen K: *Cancer chemotherapy*, Boston, 1991, Jones & Bartlett Publishers.

Brager BL, Yasko J: *Care of the client receiving chemotherapy*, Reston, Va, 1984, Reston Publishing Co.

Camp DL: Care of the Groshong catheter, *Oncology Nursing Forum* 15(6):745-749, 1988.

Coco CD: *Intravenous therapy: a handbook for practice*, St Louis, 1980, Mosby.

Crocker KS: Parenteral nutritional delivery systems. In Grant J, Kennedy-Caldwell C, editors: *Nutritional support in nursing*. Philadelphia, 1988, Grune & Stratton, pp. 133-190.

Englert DM, Lawson M: Ambulatory home nutrition support. In Grant J, Kennedy-Caldwell C, editors: *Nutritional support in nursing*. Philadelphia, 1988, Grune & Stratton, pp. 281-306.

Hennessy KA: Now TPN therapy begins at home, *RN* 51(6):81-84, 1988.

Hutman S: How to treat AIDS-related lymphoma, *AIDS Patient Care* 6(5):214-219, 1992.

Kovacs JA: Diagnosis, treatment, and prevention of *Pneumocystis carinii* pneumonia in HIV-infected patients, *AIDS Update* 2(2):1-12, 1989.

Kovacs JA, Masur H: AIDS commentary: *Pneumocystis carinii* pneumonia: therapy and prophylaxis, *J Infect Dis* 158(1):254-259, 1988.

MMWR: Recommendations for prophylaxis against Pneumocystis carinii pneumonia for adults and adolescents infected with human immunodeficiency virus, vol 41 (RR-4), pp. 1-11, 1992.

Nentwich PF: *Intravenous therapy: a comprehensive application of intravenous therapy and medication administration*, Boston, 1990, Jones & Bartlett Publishers.

Oncology Nursing Society: Module I-1: Catheters, 1989.

Oncology Nursing Society: Module II-1: Implanted ports and reservoirs, 1989.

Oncology Nursing Society. Module III-Pumps (infusion systems), 1990.

Oncology Nursing Society: Safe handling of cystotoxic drugs, 1989.

Plumer AL, Cosentino F: *Principles and practice of intravenous therapy*, Boston, 1987, Little, Brown & Co.

Raiten DJ: *Nutrition and HIV infection: a review and evaluation of the extant knowledge of the relationship between nutrition and HIV infection*. November. Prepared for Center for Food Safety and Applied Nutrition, FDA, Dept of Health and Human Services. FDA contact no 223-88-2124, task order no 7. Rockville, Md, 1990.

Tenenbaum L: *Cancer chemotherapy a reference guide, Philadelphia, 1989, WB Saunders Co.*

Ungvarski PJ: Administration of pentamidine aerosol therapy, *Journal of the Association of Nurses in AIDS Care* 2(1):12-14, 1991.

Your guide to total parenteral nutrition, *Nursing '92*. March, 1992.

Index

RESOURCES

INFORMATION RESOURCES

AIDS Clinical Trials Information Service
P.O. Box 6003
Rockville, MD 20849-6003
800-874-2572 (800-TRIALS-A)
800-243-7012 (TTY/TDD)
301-738-6616 (FAX)

Provides information on federally and privately funded clinical trials for people with HIV/AIDS.

American Foundation for AIDS Research
733 Third Avenue
12th Floor
New York, NY 10017
212-682-7440
212-682-9812 (FAX)

Funds HIV/AIDS related research in biomedicine, the social sciences, education for prevention, and public policy development. Publishes a quarterly newsletter which provides updates on HIV/AIDS clinical trial results, ongoing studies, and their locations and eligibility criteria.

CDC National AIDS Clearinghouse
P.O. Box 6003
Rockville, MD 20849-6003
800-458-5231
800-243-7012 (TTY/TDD)
301-738-6616 (FAX)

Maintains databases which contain information on 20,000 organizations providing HIV/AIDS services, 12,000 educational materials on HIV/AIDS, and HIV/AIDS funding sources. Also has an on-line database of AIDS/HIV news from the newswires.

CDC National AIDS Hotline
P.O. Box 13827
Research Triangle Park, NC 27709
800-342-AIDS
800-344-7432 (Spanish)
800-243-7889 (TTY/TDD)

Provides current and accurate information about HIV/AIDS to the general public. Good phone number to give to clients who may wish general information about HIV infection.

Hemophilia and AIDS/HIV Network for the Dissemination of Information
The National Hemophilia Foundation
110 Greene Street
Suite 303
New York, New York 10012
212-431-8541
800-42-HANDI
212-431-0906 (FAX)

Provides information, resources, and referrals on hemophilia and HIV/AIDS to people with hemophilia, their families, and the professionals who care for them.

HIV Telephone Consultation Service from San Francisco General Hospital
800-933-3413

Provides patient specific consultation to health care professionals on HIV/AIDS related problems. Phone is answered by an HIV experienced nurse practitioner, clinical pharmacist, or physician. Written materials supplementing the telephone discussions may also be sent. Phone is staffed from 7:30 AM to 5:00 PM Pacific time, Monday through Friday. Phone recorder is used at other times.

National Association of People with AIDS
1413 K Street NW
Eighth Floor
Washington, DC 20005
202-898-0414
202-898-0435 (FAX)
703-998-3144 (BBS)

Assists in conducting education programs, provides speakers for HIV/AIDS programs, assists local groups in establishing PWA groups. French and Spanish speaking staff are available.

National Library of Medicine
8600 Rockville Pike
Bethesda, MD 20894
301-496-6308 (public information)

This is the largest medical library in the world; it has a variety of computerized databases which can be accessed by modem. It can arrange inter-library loans through 8 regional medical libraries, 131 resource libraries, and over 3000 hospital libraries. Maintains AIDS-LINE, a computer file with over 70,000 AIDS/HIV references published since 1980.

Project Inform
1965 Market Street
Suite 220
San Francisco, CA 94103
415-558-8669
800-822-7422
415-558-0684 (FAX)

Provides information on AIDS/HIV funding, access to care, and research. An excellent source of information on treatment trials (including nonconventional treatments), standards of care, and drugs in development. Very useful for both professionals and patients.

AIDS EDUCATION AND TRAINING CENTERS (ETCs)

The ETCs are a national network of centers, each of which is responsible for a designated geographic area in which it conducts targeted, multidisciplinary education and training for health care providers. Nurses and nurse practitioners are among the targeted groups. ETCs also serve as centers for current, accurate information about HIV resources, drug trials, and referrals.

Central Office:

AIDS ETC Program
5600 Fishers Lane
Room 4C-03
Rockville, MD 20857
301-443-6364
301-443-8890 (FAX)

The Regional ETCs are:

Serving Texas and Oklahoma

AIDS ETC for Texas and Oklahoma
The University of Texas
1200 Herman Pressler Street
P.O. Box 20186
Houston, Texas 77225
Richard Grimes, Ph.D.
(713) 794-4075, Fax (713) 794-4877

Serving Pennsylvania

Pennsylvania AIDS ETC
University of Pittsburgh
Graduate School of Public Health
130 DeSoto Street, Room A425
Pittsburgh, Pennsylvania 15261
Linda Frank, Ph.D., M.S.N., R.N.
(412) 624-1895, Fax (412) 624-4767

Serving New Jersey

New Jersey AIDS ETC
University of Medicine and Dentistry of N.J.
Office of Continuing Education
30 Bergen Street, ADMC #710
Newark, New Jersey 07107-3000
Charles McKinney, Ed.D.
(201) 982-3690, Fax (201) 982-7128

Serving Florida

Florida AIDS ETC
University of Miami
P.O. Box 016960 (D-90)
Miami, Florida 33101
Howard Anapol, M.D.
(305) 585-7836, Fax (305) 324-4931

Serving Puerto Rico

Puerto Rico AIDS ETC
University of Puerto Rico
Medical Sciences Campus

S
S

Digital SLR Video
& Filmmaking
FOR
DUMMIES®

3/1/13